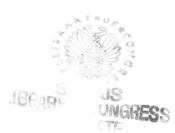
MICRONUTRIENTS AND HEALTH RESEARCH

MICRONUTRIENTS AND HEALTH RESEARCH

TAKUMI YOSHIDA
EDITOR

Nova Biomedical Books
New York

Copyright © 2008 by Nova Science Publishers, Inc.

For permission to use material from this book please contact us:
Telephone 631-231-7269; Fax 631-231-8175
Web Site: http://www.novapublishers.com

NOTICE TO THE READER

The Publisher has taken reasonable care in the preparation of this book, but makes no expressed or implied warranty of any kind and assumes no responsibility for any errors or omissions. No liability is assumed for incidental or consequential damages in connection with or arising out of information contained in this book. The Publisher shall not be liable for any special, consequential, or exemplary damages resulting, in whole or in part, from the readers' use of, or reliance upon, this material.

Independent verification should be sought for any data, advice or recommendations contained in this book. In addition, no responsibility is assumed by the publisher for any injury and/or damage to persons or property arising from any methods, products, instructions, ideas or otherwise contained in this publication.

This publication is designed to provide accurate and authoritative information with regard to the subject matter covered herein. It is sold with the clear understanding that the Publisher is not engaged in rendering legal or any other professional services. If legal or any other expert assistance is required, the services of a competent person should be sought. FROM A DECLARATION OF PARTICIPANTS JOINTLY ADOPTED BY A COMMITTEE OF THE AMERICAN BAR ASSOCIATION AND A COMMITTEE OF PUBLISHERS.

LIBRARY OF CONGRESS CATALOGING-IN-PUBLICATION DATA

Micronutrients and health research / Takumi Yoshida (editor)
        p.; cm.
 Includes bibliographical references and index.
 ISBN: 978-1-60456-056-5 (hardcover)
 1. Trace elements in nutrition. I.Yoshida, Takumi.
 [DNLM: 1. Micronutrients—pharmacology. 2. Micronutrients—therapeutic use. 3. Dietary Supplements. QU 130.5 M6265 2007]
 QP534.M517 2007
 612.3'924—dc22

                              2007039047

Published by Nova Science Publishers, Inc. ✦ New York

CONTENTS

0173469787

PREFACE

Called micronutrients because they are needed only in minuscule amounts, these substances are the "magic wands" that enable the body to produce enzymes, hormones and other substances essential for proper growth and development. As tiny as the amounts are, however, the consequences of their absence are severe. Iodine, vitamin A and iron are most important in global public health terms; their lack represents a major threat to the health and development of populations the world over, particularly children and pregnant women in low-income countries. This new book presents the latest research from around the world.

Expert Commentary - In this work were reported analytical procedures applying X-ray spectrometry and its variants in the characterization of trace elements present in biological, environmental and food samples in an effort to better understand the participation of trace elements in bioinorganic and in the biologic processes.

Short Communication - Interactions between drugs and micronutrients have received only little or no attention in the medical and pharmaceutical world in the past. Since more and more pharmaceutics are used for the treatment of patients, this topic is increasingly relevant. As such interactions – depending on the duration of treatment and the status of micronutrients – impact the health of the patient and the action of the drugs, physicians and pharmacists should pay more attention to such interactions in the future. The following article intends to point out the relevance of mutual interactions between micronutrients and drugs, without claiming to be exhaustive.

Chapter I - The main focus of this chapter is to provide an overview of the significance of zinc in human health research. The following issues are discussed: (1) the history of our understanding of human zinc deficiency; (2) the biochemistry and biology of zinc with an emphasis on the relevance of zinc in human nutrition and the importance of human zinc deficiency; (3) the clinical spectrum of zinc deficiency; (4) the lack of biomarkers for milder zinc deficiency states to ascertain their prevalence and clinical outcomes, including growth retardation, diarrhoea, pneumonia, other infections and abnormalities in neuropsychological performance; (5) human zinc requirements with special focus on estimation of average dietary zinc requirements and zinc toxicity; (6) the causes of zinc deficiency, particularly in the developing world; and (7) potential strategies for the prevention and management of human zinc deficiency. The chapter concludes with an emphasis on the immediate need for expanded research on human zinc metabolism and homeostasis at a molecular, cellular, organ and whole body level.

Chapter II - *Background:* Vitamin A is fundamentally required in physiological processes and growth and low folate level is implicated with neural tube defects.

Aim: To evaluate retinol and folate serum levels in mothers and their newborns of two ethnic group.

Methods: Data concerned 710 Greeks and 686 Albanian mothers along with their newborns. Immediately after delivery blood from the umbilical cord and from the mothers were collected into light-protected tubes. Retinol serum level was measured with a reversed-phase HPLC method and serum folate with Bayer Advia-Centaur System. A 60d dietetic diary was kept by each woman during the last two months of pregnancy.

Results: Retinol values (0.9 ± 0.1 and 18.5 ± 3.47 µmol/L) were considered to be normal in Greek mothers and most of their newborns, respectively, whereas in Albanian mothers the lipid soluble vitamin was found low (0.6 ± 0.1 µmol/L) $p<0.001$ and in 1/3 significantly low (< 0.45 µmol/L). Consequently retinol was found to be very low in their newborns (0.4 ± 0.1 µmol/L) and in half cases extremely low. However, in 12% of the Albanian cord blood samples, retinol levels were dectected higher, than those of their mothers. Folate serum concentration in mothers and newborns were similar (18.7 ± 9.1 and 26.5 ± 15.2 nmol vs 18.1 ± 8.6 and 24.6 ± 14.7 nmol) in the two ethnic groups. Vitamin A intake was found extremely low in the group of immigrants.

Conclusions: The decreased vitamin A intake and their low blood status in the immigrant mothers may be due to their low socio-economic and nutritional status. In contrast, normal folate levels in the mothers of the two ethnic groups could be due to their normal intake of this vitamin. Immigrant programs for the elevation of the socio-economic status, along with a close follow up of the immigrant-pregnant women should be planned in Greece.

Chapter III - Well-balanced and adequate maternal nutrition prior conception and during pregnancy affects the course and outcome of pregnancy, and enables achievement of a: 1) healthy pregnancy, 2) uncomplicated delivery of a full-term and well-developed baby, 3) lower risk of maternal postpartum complications, and 4) sufficient source for lactation. Adequate maternal nutrition also improves future maternal health in general and reproductive health in particular. As it is now widely recognized that the risk of various chronic diseases in adulthood might have their origins in intrauterine life, the new goal of the contemporary approach in pregnancy nutrition is to establish the nutritional foundations for a healthy adults during intrauterine life.

Pregnancy represents a special maternal demand for high-quality nutrients, as it is regarded as a metabolic stress that is increasing according to the course of the gestation. Although it is not completely clear how nutritional status of the mother influences her own health as well as fetal growth/development, nutrition imbalance could be harmful to the pregnant woman, influencing both the outcome of pregnancy and the composition of breast milk.

In well-nourished women these increased needs are best met by biological and metabolic adaptation to pregnancy. Increasing demands should be achieved by appropriate dietary intake, which contains all nutrition requirements. In cases of imbalanced dietary intake, preexisting deficiencies of micronutrients, previous adverse pregnancy outcomes, and in all cases of high-risk pregnancies micronutrient supplementation is especially important. However, until now there is insufficient evidence to define whether there is a need for routine antepartum supplementation or should nutritional intervention be restrained to deficient populations and high-risk pregnancies. As the data on the effectiveness of supplementation in preventing or treating pregnancy-related disorders and perinatal complications are contradictory, future well designed randomized control trials would try to solve this dilemma.

Micronutrient supplementation supporters have a standpoint that the potential benefits of routine supplementation overweigh any potential adverse reaction that can be attributed. In the other hand, the daily requirements are easily met in all individuals having a balanced diet. Although deficiency states are rare, several pharmaceutical companies produce over-the-counter vitamin – plus- mineral nutritional supplements, despite the lack of clear evidence to support their supplemental consumption.

Currently, micronutrient supplementation should be chosen on an individual basis. In the near future, the goal would be to estimate micronutrient status prior to conception or in the early pregnancy, in order to define patients who must receive appropriate micronutrient supplementation.

Chapter IV - A number of health disorders may find their cause in the formation, accumulation and damaging effect of endogenous toxins. The disorders appear to include the metabolic syndrome, diabetes, hypertension, cardiovascular disease, Alzheimer's disease, colorectal and possibly other epithelial cancers. The identification of the endogenous toxins and the development of preventive strategies is difficult, however, as the toxins cannot be readily isolated and identified. To surmount this problem the authors have developed cell systems that model *in vivo* tissue cytotoxicity associated with known endogenous toxins and tested the relative ability of micronutrients to mitigate their cytotoxic effects. The toxins evaluated were: 1) Oxidative stress, i.e. superoxide, hydrogen peroxide, hypochlorite and nitric oxide, that can result for example from inflammatory processes such as bacterial infection and from hypoxia:reoxygenation injury of endothelial and astrocyte cells; 2) Carbonyls from the autoxidation or metabolism of unsaturated fatty acids or phospholipids to form advanced lipid endproducts (ALE); 3) Dicarbonyls from the autoxidation or metabolism of glucose/ fructose to form advanced glycation endproducts; and 4) Fatty acids from fat and/or carbohydrate overload that can result in the metabolic syndrome and related disease processes. In studies of combined endogenous toxins the authors observed a marked synergism in the cytotoxicity of oxidative stress (H_2O_2) and exposure to carbonyls (associated with fructose) and increased cytotoxicity of fatty acids (polyunsaturated fatty acids). The micronutrients, evaluated and ranked for their ability to prevent cytotoxicity *in vitro*, included vitamins, minerals and plant-derived antioxidants and scavengers of reactive oxygen species (ROS). The results demonstrate marked differences in the ranking of the micronutrients with the different endogenous toxins. They thus suggest that mitigation studies with micronutrients could provide an assessment of the association of endogenous toxins with disease and a systematic strategy for testing the role of micronutrients on oxidative stress and disease prevention.

Chapter V - The high prevalence of research related to micronutrients (i.e. vitamins and minerals) warrants attention, especially when current scientific guidelines such as dietary reference intakes (DRIs) for micronutrient requirements are geared to healthy populations.

This poses a dilemma for health professionals who care for individuals with various diseases and medical conditions which are further complicated by treatments. Answers for many clinical queries about micronutrient supplementation remain ambiguous and health care recipients are caught in the middle while the media exacerbates the situation. Clinical efficacy for (safe) supplementation with micronutrients requires sufficient evidence, relevant to the specific clinical situation and tailored for a given individual. It requires weighing risks versus benefits. Since studies are not typically powered to assess risks, potential harm may be under-assessed or shared as anecdotal reports or singular case studies. Any purported benefits must translate into meaningful clinical outcomes, rather than endpoints (e.g. intermediate biochemical markers) of questionable significance. Megadoses of individual micronutrients require special consideration as they can cause relative deficiency of other micronutrients and result in detrimental health effects. Health professionals must ensure that their sources of evidence meet high standards of credibility because they are accountable for their micronutrient recommendations. Evidence for micronutrient supplementation must be sought from multiple perspectives, including disease etiology, treatment and prognosis. This chapter describes a learning journey, with five central goals: 1. constructing clinical queries related to micronutrients. 2. locating relevant and high quality evidence. 3. assessing whether there is sufficient evidence for micronutrient supplementation. 4. identifying and bridging gaps in the existing body of knowledge. 5. applying knowledge when counseling a patient about micronutrient supplements.

Chapter VI - Traditionally cattle were thought to be relatively tolerant of copper (Cu) accumulation, and cattle diets were regularly supplemented with Cu well above physiological needs. In recent years, however, an increasing number of episodes of Cu toxicity have been reported in cattle, in most cases associated with excessive Cu intake in the ration. It has also been reported that dietary supplements leading to Cu accumulation in the liver at concentrations only slightly above normal show negative effects on animal performance, in terms of reduced feed intake and average daily gain (subclinical toxicity). Identification of animals in the silent chronic phase of Cu accumulation is very important to avoid not only economic losses due to subsequent severe disease or death, but also to avoid subclinical disease. Currently available laboratory markers of Cu toxicity are mainly used for diagnostic purposes, i.e. to demonstrate changes associated with clinical manifestations already present. However, there is a clear need to identify markers of early changes, with a capacity to predict risk of Cu accumulation in the liver before actual tissue or functional damage occurs. In this chapter, the authors evaluate the suitability of some blood parameters as potential markers of hepatic Cu accumulation in cattle during the silent phase as well as the use of *in vivo* biopsies for evaluation of risk of chronic Cu toxicity.

The authors results indicate that under moderately high Cu exposure, none of the blood markers currently available accurately predicted hepatic Cu accumulation in cattle and analysis of Cu content in the liver is probably the best diagnostic tool available for assessing the risk of chronic Cu toxicity. However, the limit between safe-adequate Cu concentrations and those associated with toxicity is very narrow, and for this reason the total hepatic Cu concentration is not *per se* a good indicator of risk of toxicity in animals with marginal hepatic Cu concentrations. Studies of subcellular hepatic Cu accumulation indicate that the large-granule (lysosomal) fraction has a limited capacity for Cu sequestration and Cu content in this compartment tends to reach a plateau phase at relatively low Cu exposure levels, leading to higher Cu accumulation in the nucleus and cytosol. This pattern of Cu accumulation, as in sheep, may be due to the limited capacity for metallothionein binding of Cu and excretion in bile. Further research into the molecular basis of Cu homeostasis in cattle is essential to better understand the pathogenesis of chronic Cu hepatic accumulation and to validate the use of subcellular Cu parameters as potential markers of the risk of Cu toxicity in cattle.

Chapter VII - The role of trace elements in the pathogenesis of liver cirrhosis and its complications is still not clearly understood.

Zinc, copper, manganese and magnesium are essential trace elements whose role in liver cirrhosis and its complications is still a matter of research.

Zinc is associated with more than 300 enzymatic systems. Zinc is structured part of Cu-Zn superoxide dismutase, important antioxidative enzyme. Zinc acts as an antioxidant, a membrane and cytosceletal stabilizator, an anti-apoptotic agent, an important co-factor in DNA synthesis, an anti-inflammatory agent, etc. Copper is an essential trace element which participates in many enzymatic reactions. Its most important role is in redox processes. Reactive copper can participate in liver damage directly or indirectly, through Kupffer cell's stimulation. Scientists agree that copper's toxic effects are related to oxidative stress. Manganese is a structural part of arginase, which is an important enzyme in the urea metabolism. Manganese acts as an activator of numerous enzymes in Krebs cycle, particularly in the decarboxilation process.

Magnesium is important for the protein synthesis, enzyme activation, oxidative phosphorilation, renal potassium and hydrogen exchange etc.

Since zinc, copper, manganese and magnesium have a possible role in the pathogenesis of liver cirrhosis and cirrhotic complications, the aim of our study was to investigate the serum concentrations of mentioned trace elements in patients with liver cirrhosis and compare them with concentrations in controls.

Serum concentrations of zinc, copper, manganese and magnesium were determined in 105 patients with alcoholic liver cirrhosis and 50 healthy subjects by means of plasma sequential spectrophotometer. Serum concentrations of zinc were significantly lower (median 0.82 vs. 11.22 µmol/L, $p<0.001$) in patients with liver cirrhosis in comparison to controls. Serum concentrations of copper were significantly higher in patients with liver cirrhosis (median 21.56 vs. 13.09 µmol/L, $p<0.001$) as well as manganese (2.50 vs. 0.02 µmol/L, $p<0.001$). The concentration of magnesium was not significantly different between patients with liver cirrhosis and controls (0.94 vs. 0.88 mmol/L, $p=0.132$). There were no differences in the concentrations of zinc, copper, manganese and magnesium between male and female patients with liver cirrhosis. Only manganese concentration was significantly different between Child-Pugh groups ($p=0.036$). Zinc concentration was significantly lower in patients with hepatic encephalopathy in comparison to cirrhotic patients without encephalopathy (0.54 vs. 0.96 µmol/L, $p=0.002$). The correction of trace elements concentrations might have a beneficial effect on complications and maybe progression of liver cirrhosis. It would be recommendable to provide analysis of trace elements in patients with liver cirrhosis as a routine.

Chapter VIII - Diacylglycerol (DAG), which consists mainly of 1,3-DAG, is a naturally occurring oil present in low concentrations in vegetable oils that has a long history of use as food. Compared with conventional triacylglycerol (TAG) oil, DAG has beneficial effects in humans and rodents, with no adverse effects.

Long-term ingestion of DAG prevents body fat accumulation compared to TAG ingestion in humans and rodents. DAG and TAG with a similar fatty acid composition have similar energy values and are absorbed similarly in rats, suggesting that these properties are not associated with the anti-obesity effect of DAG. DAG stimulates β-oxidation gene expression in the liver, small intestine, and skeletal muscle, and decreases the postprandial respiratory quotient, suggesting that dietary DAG induces fat oxidation postprandially and chronically, which might be one of the mechanisms underlying the anti-obesity effect of DAG. Additionally, DAG protects against the development of glucose intolerance and impaired insulin resistance in animal models of metabolic abnormalities, suggesting that DAG helps to maintain appropriate carbohydrate metabolism in addition to appropriate fat metabolism.

A single oral administration of DAG decreases postprandial plasma triglyceride (TG) levels compared with those after TAG administration. A potential explanation for this difference was generated by studies in which the lymphatic transport of chylomicrons after 1,3-DAG ingestion was significantly delayed and reduced, presumably as a result of poor reesterification of fatty acids onto 1-monoacylglycerol (MAG) in the intestinal mucosa. Another mechanism was suggested by the results of a recent study in which DAG administration decreased TG levels, but increased MAG and 1,3-DAG levels in secreted chylomicrons compared with TAG administration, thus leading to a more rapid clearance of DAG-chylomicrons by lipoprotein lipase-mediated lipolysis than that of TAG-chylomicrons.

Plant sterols (PS) are cholesterol-lowering agents. A review of previous human studies indicates that the effective dose of PS is 0.4 g/day when dissolved in DAG, whereas that of PS dissolved in TAG is estimated to be at least 0.8 g/day. PS at 0.5 g/day dissolved in DAG oil, but not in TAG oil, has cholesterol-lowering effects, suggesting that PS act synergistically with DAG, or that DAG enhances the actions of PS. Further studies are needed, however, to clarify the mechanism.

In conclusion, DAG and PS/DAG are useful for the prevention of metabolic abnormalities, and are expected to decrease risk factors for disease when incorporated into human daily dietary habits.

Chapter IX - Vitamins are organic molecules which are required in small amounts to sustain life but which cannot be made by the organism. Most vitamins are coenzymes, molecules that facilitate the chemical reactions catalyzed by enzymes, while two are hormone precursors, which bind and activate transcription factors. However, both types of vitamins share some of the functions exhibited by the other: vitamin K_2, a coenzyme in γ-carboxylation, can also bind and activate the steroid and xenobiotic receptor (SXR); lipoic acid, a coenzyme in oxidative decarboxylation, can bind and activate the insulin receptor; and nicotinic acid, a component of NAD^+ which is involved with redox reactions, can signal through a G protein-coupled receptor. On the other hand, the active forms of vitamin D and vitamin A, which bind nuclear receptors (VDR and RAR, respectively), can have nongenomic effects by binding and activating enzymes through their receptors. For example, the VDR can bind and stimulate the phosphoinositide 3-kinase, while the RAR can bind and activate protein kinase Cδ. This review explores several of these multifunctional compounds and tries to provide a possible explanation for this double duty from an evolutionary perspective.

Chapter X - The *in vitro* cytomutagenetic study was carried out in intact and mutagen-treated (cadmium chloride, dioxidine, bleomycin) peripheral lymphocytes obtained in G_2 phase of the cell cycle from healthy donors within and after 14- and/or 30-day period of supplementation with vitamin and vitamin and mineral complexes.

It was established that the supplementation with complexes containing vitamins at total doses exceeding the daily allowances, does not increase the spontaneous mutagenesis and reduces the sensitivity of human cells to the chemical mutagens. Besides, the vitamin complexes of different quantity and quality contents were found able to induce *in vitro* the comutagenic modification of cell susceptibility to the effect of certain mutagens used in certain concentrations.

The revealed antimutagenic and comutagenic modifying effects were shown to depend upon the duration of consumption, amount and quality content of vitamin complexes used, the nature of mutagen and the level of induced cytogenetic damages.

Chapter XI - Using synchrotron radiation total-reflection X-ray fluorescence spectrometry (SRTXRF), it was possible to determine the concentration of several elements in lung, spleen, thymus, lymph nodes and liver samples of BALB/c mice infected with *Toxocara canis* nematode and in healthy group, as a control. The elements P, S, Cl, K, Ca, Ti, Cr, Mn, Fe, Ni, Cu, Zn, As, Rb, Ba and Pb were detected with concentration between 0.16 (Ni-liver) and 5091 (P-thymus) $\mu g.g^{-1}$. The measuring time was 100 seconds and detection limits varied from 0.20 $\mu g.g^{-1}$ for Ni to 25.88 $\mu g.g^{-1}$ for P. Moreover, inflammatory immune response was evaluated, by chemometric techniques, such as principal component and cluster analyses using the elemental concentrations data. Lung, spleen and thymus showed a characteristic pattern between 12 and 24 days post infection, whereas lymph nodes, between 24 and 48 days post infection; liver did not show remarkable features. Since spleen, thymus and lymph nodes have a significant role in immune response, these days could point out a peak of leukocytes activation for each organ.

In: Micronutrients and Health Research
Editor: Takumi Yoshida, pp. 1-9
ISBN: 978-1-60456-056-5
© 2008 Nova Science Publishers, Inc.

Expert Commentary

X-Ray Fluorescence Spectrometry and Its Variants in the Analysis of Trace Elements in Clinical, Pharmaceutical, Alimentary or Environmental Samples

O.L.A.D. Zucchi[1,*], V.F. Nascimento Filho[2] and M.J. Salvador[3,*]

[1]Faculdade de Ciências Farmacêuticas de Ribeirão Preto, Universidade de São Paulo (USP), Depto. Física e Química. CEP 14040-903, Ribeirão Preto (SP), Brasil;
[2]Centro de Energia Nuclear na Agricultura, Universidade de São Paulo (USP), Laboratório de Instrumentação Nuclear. CEP 13400-970, Piracicaba (SP), Brasil;
[3]Instituto de Pesquisa e Desenvolvimento, Universidade do Vale do Paraíba (UNIVAP). CEP 12244-000, São José dos Campos (SP), Brasil and Instituto de Biologia, Universidade Estadual de Campinas (UNICAMP), Curso de Farmácia, Caixa Postal 6109, CEP 13083-971, Campinas (SP), Brasil

ABSTRACT

In this work were reported analytical procedures applying X-ray spectrometry and its variants in the characterization of trace elements present in biological, environmental and food samples in an effort to better understand the participation of trace elements in bioinorganic and in the biologic processes.

Keywords: X-ray Fluorescence; Trace elements; Biological, environmental and food samples

---

* Correspondence concerning this article should be addressed to: olzucchi@fcfrp.usp.br or mjsalvador1531@yahoo.com.br.

INTRODUCTION

The optimization of chemical analysis systems has become more and more important in face of the current demands from different areas of knowledge (chemistry, biology, health, etc) for analytic procedures that are simple, cheap, fast, and robust and with adequate precision and accuracy.

Thus, the enhancement and application of complementary instrumental techniques and automation resources as well as the adequate treatment of the data obtained using, for example, chemiometric models and other statistical tools are current challenges to improve the analytical performance.

The increasing demand for analyses has determined the development of efficient, fast analytical methods that excel in precision and accuracy. Such demand is mainly for matrices in which the analite is found in small concentration (trace elements), in which the decrease of the concentration of the analyzed compound can lead to an increase in the systematic error, and in situations in which *in situ* analysis is required (Castro, 2002; Ullmann's, 1986).

Along the years the tendency in the development of analytical methods has been towards reaching a greater sensitivity with consequential improvement in the detection limits, regardless of the nature of the matrix to be analyzed. At present there is a growing demand for versatile analytical methods which offers the possibility of using sensitive equipment, with analyses that are close to the quantification limit (μgL^{-1} or ngL^{-1}), minimizing the spectral and/or chemical interference and also interference from components of the matrix (Skoog e Leary, 1992; Christian, 1986).

However, in a general way, the procedures related to the initial steps of preparation of samples have not followed the evolution of quantification techniques.

Therefore, the development of alternative methods that optimize the process of sample pre-treatment, making the analytic work more efficient and cheaper is necessary and of great importance. In this matter the use of separation and/or pre-concentration techniques, which transfer the analite of interest to a new stage with lower volume, can be an interesting alternative.

This strategy makes it possible to expand the potential relative to technical sensitivity, besides giving the possibility to improve the selectivity when needed and allowing to get the information regarding the chemical speciation. For this, it is desirable that the methods of analytical separation/pre-concentration show, for example, (Hoenig e Kersabiec, 1996): a) high separation factors; b) simultaneous separation of the greatest possible number of ions to be determined with absence of interelementary interference; c) final solution free from potential interfering species.

Many different techniques have been used in the separation and pre-concentration of samples such as the liquid-liquid extraction, the liquid-solid extraction, co-precipitation and eletro-analytic deposition. Among these, since 1985, the liquid-solid extraction has been used because it presents (Castro, 2002): a) speed; b) elevated factors of pre-concentration; c) possibility to reach good selectivity either for a specific element or for a group of elements; d) possibility of determining the absorbed element directly in the solid stage; e) easy to be automated.

Among the spectrometric techniques of analysis, the ones that use X-ray have proven highly qualified for the chemical characterization (Settle, 1999) of different samples, liquid or solid (food, medication, vegetable tissue, animal tissue, etc.). The X-ray fluorescence technique (Vives *et al.*, 2006; Zucchi *et al.,* 2005a,b) has been applied with success in many different fields, such as: animal nutrition, agronomy, environment pollution control, geology, metallurgy, food industry, etc. Some works can also be found in the biological and pharmaceutical areas, although this technique and its potential are not yet widely diffused and used.

This technique allows the identification and multielementary quantification of the inorganic compounds in different matrices, making it possible to accomplish a sequential or simultaneous analysis without the need for the chemical separation of elements and shows high detection sensitivity, in the order of parts per billion (Moreira *et al.*, 2006; Salvador *et al.*, 2004; Salvador *et al.*, 2002; Matsumoto *et al.*, 2002; De Jesus *et al.*, 2000; Simabuco *et al.*, 2000; Zucchi *et al.*, 2000; Zucchi e Salvador, 1998; Bennighoff *et al.*, 1997; von Czarnowski *et al.*, 1997; Wagner *et al.*, 1997; Zucchi *et al.*, 1995; Price e Major, 1990).

The X-ray fluorescence is based on the measure of the intensities of characteristic X-rays emitted by the elements that constitute the sample, and can be done through the dispersion of wave length (WDXRF) or energy (EDXRF). Fundamentally this technique consists of three stages: excitement of the elements that constitute the sample, dispersion and detection of characteristic x-rays emitted and measuring of these X-rays.

In a monoenergetic excitation the intensity of the characteristic radiation, K_α, produced by an element situated in a layer dx, at x depth under a surface of the sample (matrix), homogeneous and with D width, is the product of three probabilities:

P_1 : probability of the radiation of excitation (primary excitation) of energy E_0 to reach depth x ;

P_2 : probability of the radiation of excitation to produce vacancy in the atoms of the elements i of the layer dx and that this vacancy cause the emission of a photon K_α ;

P_3 : probability of the characteristic radiation produced in the layer dx to cross the width x and reach the detector producing an electric pulse.

This way the fluorescent intensity of the element i in the layer dx is proportional to these three probabilities, which means:

$$dI \; \alpha \; P_1 . P_2 \, P_3 \tag{1}$$

Introducing a probability constant, named geometry factor G, which depends on the geometry of the analyzing system, tension and current of the tube, we have:

$$dI = G.e^{-[\mu_M(E_0)/\text{sen}\,\phi 1 + \mu_M(E_i)/\text{sen}\,\phi 2].\rho_M x} . \tau_i(E_0).w_{Ki}.[1 - 1/j_{Ki}].f_i.\rho_i.\varepsilon(E_i).dx \tag{2}$$

$\mu_M(E_0), \mu_M(E_i)$: coefficient of mass absorption (cm^2.g^{-1}) of the matrix in the energy of the excitation photons (E_0) and in the energy of the characteristic photons (E_i) of element i, respectively:

$\phi1, \phi2$: angle of incidence between the direction of the incident beam and the surface of the sample and between the surface of the sample and the direction of the characteristic emerging photons, respectively;

$\rho_M x$: superficial density (g.cm^{-2}) of the matrix;

$\tau_i(E_0)$: mass absorption coefficient (cm^2.g^{-1}) to the photoelectric effect of the element in the excitation energy;

w_{Ki} : fluorescence yield for the element i in K layer;

j_{Ki} : proportion of the jump from layer K to L;

f_i : fraction of photons K emitted as K_α;

$\varepsilon(E_i)$: efficiency of energy detection of the element i and

$\rho_i dx$: superficial density (g.cm^{-2}) of the element i in the layer dx

Grouping the fundamental parameters that depend on the element for a specific excitation energy E_0 in a single term K_i, named constant of the fundamental parameters (eq. 3)

$$K_i = \tau_i(E_0).w_{Ki}.[1 - 1/j_{Ki}].f_i \qquad (3)$$

and defining the coefficient of absorption of total mass (χ_i) as being:

$$\chi_i = \mu_M(E_0)/\operatorname{sen}\phi1 + \mu_M(E_i)/\operatorname{sen}\phi2 \qquad (4)$$

Thus, equation one is now written as:

$$dI = G.\varepsilon(E_i).K_i.\rho_i.e^{-\chi_i.\rho_M x} dx \qquad (5)$$

Integrating these functions until a D width of the sample, we obtain the fluorescent intensity of a specific element i:

$$I_i = G.\varepsilon(E_i).K_i.\rho_i.[1 - e^{-\chi_i.\rho_M D}]/(\chi_i \rho_M) \qquad (6)$$

as ρ_i/ρ_M is the fraction in weight (W_i) of the element of interest and defining the elementary sensitivity S_i (sensitivity of the system to a specific element i, cps.cm^2.g^{-1}) as being:

$$S_i = G.\varepsilon(E_0).K_i \tag{7}$$

Substituting in equation 6 we obtain the fundamental equation for the fluorescence of X-rays with monoenergetic excitation (eq. 8).

$$I_i = S_i.W_i.[1 - e^{-\chi_i.\rho_M D}].1/\chi_i \tag{8}$$

For thin samples, in which the absorption of X-rays can be insignificant, we have $\chi_i.\rho_M D \rightarrow 0$ and $e^{-\chi_i.\rho_M D} \approx 1 - \chi_i\rho_M D$. Thus:

$$I_i = S_i.W_i\rho_M D = S_i.m_i \tag{9}$$

being m_i the superficial density of the element i

In the case of thick samples, in which there is partial absorption of characteristic X-ray by the sample, $\chi_i.\rho_M D \rightarrow \infty$ and equation 8 becomes:

$$I_i = S_i.W_i.(1/\chi_i) \tag{10}$$

were the coefficient of mass absorption of the matrix in the excitation energy or in the characteristic energy calculated as being the sum of the product of mass absorption coefficients by the respective fractions in weight of the elements present in the sample (eq. 11).

$$\mu_M(E) = \sum_{i=1}^{n} \mu_i(E).W_i \tag{11}$$

$\mu_M(E), \mu_i(E)$: mass absorption coefficient ($cm^2.g^{-1}$) of the sample and of element i in

E energy

W_i: fraction in weight of element i

EXPERIMENTAL PROCEDURE FOR QUANTIFICATION OF THE ELEMENTS PRESENT IN THIN SAMPLES

In the case of possessing certified thin standards as the ones produced by MicroMatter Co, after obtaining the I_i intensities, we determine the respective experimental sensitivities through equation 9, as the superficial densities ($\mu g.cm^{-2}$) for the element i in these standards are known with precision of $\pm 5\%$.

Knowing the physical parameters of the detector employed, usually of $Si(Li)$ (resolution of 165 eV to the energy of K_α from Mn), supplied by the maker of the spectrometer, we can estimate the efficacy of detection in the energy of element i. Through equation 3 we can obtain the constant of the fundamental parameters (K_i), once all the terms of this equation are charted.

Thus, with the help of equation 7 we determine the average geometry factor ($\overline{G}$) for the experimental arrangement adopted. Through the standard deviation and coefficient of variation of this number we can verify the dispersion of this geometry factor (obtained for each i element) in relation to the average and consequently the stability of the experimental arrangement, recalculating the sensitivity (eq. 7), now named calculated sensitivity (S_i^{calc}).

Once the sensitivity (S_i^{calc}) is also function of the atomic number of element i present in the standard deviation, through the analysis of the variance we obtain the equation:

$$\ln S_i = a_0 + a_1.Z_i + a_2.Z_i^2 + a.Z_i^3 \tag{12}$$

with significant parameters at the level of 5% of probability. So, through equation 12 we can determine the elementary sensitivity to any element present in the sample (as long as it has an atomic number within Z_i domain, used in the calibration curve).

Thus, the superficial density for element i in the sample can be obtained through equation 9 and consequently its fraction in weight will be:

$$W_i = \frac{(\rho_i D)_i}{(\rho_M D)} = \frac{I_i A}{S_i M} \tag{13}$$

being $\rho_M D$ the superficial density of the sample (mass of sample by irradiated area).

It must be emphasized that the samples must be deposited in support similar to the one used in the standard ("mylar"). Another way to obtain the function of the sensitivity would be the elaboration of 5 to 6 multielementary standards, obtained through a stock solution, which are deposited in a "mylar" support and dried (at 40°C).

The samples (vegetable extracts, water or even solid material that have gone through acid digestion) may be supported in membranes, as those of Nucleopore type (diameter of the pore of 0.45 μm). In this case, the standards must be also supported in these membranes. So after the adequately choosing the complex agent, which will depend on the elements we wish to dose, both the samples and the standard deviation must go through the same process (Zucchi et al., 2002).

EXPERIMENTAL PROCEDURE FOR QUANTIFICATION OF THE ELEMENTS PRESENT IN THICK SAMPLES

When working with this kind of sample, it's necessary to make the correction of the matrix effect. In the case of having standards we have, by the technique of fundamental parameters, that the coefficient of total mass absorption (χ_i) is given by equation (14), which means:

$$\chi_i = \mu_M(E_0)/sen\phi1 + \mu_i(E_i)/sen\phi2 \qquad (14)$$

being $\mu_M(E_0) = \sum_{i=1}^{n} \mu_i(E_0).W_i$ and $\mu_M(E_i) = \sum_{i=1}^{n} \mu_i(E_i).W_i$ where μ_i is charted for the excitation energy (E_0) and for the energy of the element i (E_i), the fraction in weight W_i of element i known, as well as the angles of incidence and emergence (ϕ_1, ϕ_2, respectively), we determine the coefficient of total mass absorption (eq.14). Thus, applying the equation we obtain the elementary sensitivity.

Therefore, for the dosing of the elements present in the sample both the coefficient of total mass absorption and the elementary sensitivity are known, obtaining, experimentally, the intensity I_i. So, the fraction in weight of this element can be estimated applying equation 10. If this element is not present in the standard used, we obtain the sensibility function ($\ln S_i = f(Z_i)$) with the help of standards.

If there were no standard-samples, one of the solutions would be the elaboration of these standards with composition similar to that of the samples as, for example, samples of mineral supplement for animals (Zucchi et al., 1995).

Another possible experimental situation would be dosing trace elements in raw materials to follow the process of production of a specific product.

In this case the composition of the sample is known, thus, after the irradiation of the samples the trace elements would be determined. Normalizing the data and applying the technique of fundamental parameters the fractions in weight of trace elements would be obtained.

The same procedure could be adopted to dose the microelements in biological tissues (liver, brain, blood etc.), as long as the weight fraction of macros composition is known.

With the increasing concern about environmental contamination, the procedure described before can be used in the detection of heavy metals in sweet water (contamination of phreatic zone) and sea water (oil extraction).

We can also dose the impurity in a certain sample as for example, commercially available medication. In this case the procedure described before does not apply, as the weight fraction composition of the pharmaceutical excipient does not supply of the responsible laboratory. So, we either digest the sample and chelated the elements of interest and analyze the sample like the thin sample or to elaborate from 4 to 5 standards using the sample plus a percentage of elements we wish to dose. Through the radiation spread (Compton effect) we can determine the multivariate model for the light-fraction. Assuming $\overline{Z}$ from the matrix to be the element oxygen (major constituent), the estimates of the concentrations of trace elements can be obtained with the procedure described before.

Thus, the development and validation of analytic procedures applying X-ray spectrometry and its variants in the characterization of trace elements present in biological, environmental and food samples in an effort to better understand the participation of trace elements in bioinorganic and in the biologic processes must be encouraged.

ACKNOWLEDGEMENTS

To Fundação de Amparo à Pesquisa do Estado de São Paulo (FAPESP) for the financial support.

REFERENCES

Bennighoff, L.; Von Czarnowski, D.; Denkhaus, E.; Lemke, K. Analysis of human tissues by total reflection X-ray fluorescence. Application of chemometrics for diagnostic cancer recognition. *Spectrochim. Acta Part B*, *v.52*, p.1039-1046, 1997.

Castro; M.T.P.O. Estudo analítico da extração líquido-sólido para pré-concentração de metais utilizando o sistema FEN/SDS/XAD-2 e determinação por espectrometria de absorção atômica com chama. 2002, S/N. Tese de Doutorado, IQ-UNICAMP – Campinas-SP.

Christian, G.D. In: *Analytical chemistry*. 4th ed, John Wiley & Sons, New York, 1986, 414p.

De Jesus, E.F.O.; Simabuco, S.M.; Lopes, R.T. Synchrotron Radiation X-ray fluorescence analysis of trace elements in *Nerium oleander* for pollution monitoring. *Spectrochim. Acta Part B*, *v.55*, p.1181-1187, 2000.

Hoenig, M.; Kersabiec, A.M. Sample preparation steps for analysis by Atomic Spectroscopy Methods: present status. *Spectrochim. Acta Part B*, *v.51*, p.1297-1307, 1996.

Matsumoto, E.; Simabuco, S.M.; Pérez, C.A.; Nascimento Filho, V.F. Atmospheric particulate analysis by synchrotron radiation total reflection (SR-TXRF). *X-Ray Spectrom.*, *v.31*, p.136-140, 2002.

Moreira, S.; Ficaris, M.; Vives, A.E.S.; Nascimento Filho, V.F.; Zucchi, O.L.A.D.; Barroso, R.C.; De Jesus, E.F.O. Heavy metals in groundwater using synchrotron radiation total reflection X-ray analysis. *Instrum. Sci. Technol.*, *v. 34*, n.5, p.567-585, 2006.

Price, B.J.; Major, H.W. X-ray fluorescence proves useful for quality control. Analyzers of elemental concentrations are now less expensive, easier to use, and rugged enough for outline quality testing. *Food Technol.*, *v.44*, p.66-69, 1990.

Salvador, M.J.; Dias, D.A.; Moreira, S.; Zucchi, O.L.A.D. Determination of trace elements in *Alternathera brasileira* and *Pfaffia glabrata* by SRTXRF: application in environmental pollution control. *Instrum. Sci. Technol.*, *v.32*, p.319-331, 2004.

Salvador, M.J.; Dias, D.A.; Moreira, S.; Zucchi, O.L.A.D. Analysis of medicinal plants by synchrotron radiation total reflection x-ray fluorescence. *J. Trace Microprobe Techn.*, *v.21*, p.377-388, 2003.

Salvador, M.J.; Lopes, G.N.; Nascimento Filho, V.F.; Zucchi, O.L.A.D. Quality control of commercial tea by X-ray fluorescence. *X-ray Spectrom.*, *v.31*, p.141-144, 2002.

Settle, F. *Handbook of instrumental techniques for analytical chemistry.* New York: Prentice Hall PTR, 1999. 995p.

Simabuco, S.M.; Matsumoto, E. Synchrotron radiation total reflection for rainwater analysis. *Spectrochim. Acta Part B*, *v.55*, p.1173-1179, 2000.

Skoog, D.A.; Leavy, J.L. *Principles of instrumental analysis.* 4th ed. Harcout Brace College. Publishers, New York, 1992, 218p.

Ullmanns´S, *Encyclopedia of industrial chemistry.* 5th ed. VCH, Weinhein, *v. B5*, p.18, 1966.

Vives, A.E.S.; Moreira, S.; Brienza, S.M.B.; Medeiros, J.G.D.; Tomazello Filho, M.; Zucchi, O.L.A.D.; Nascimento Filho, V.F. Monitoring of the environmental pollution by trace element analysis in tree-rings using synchrotron radiation total reflection X-ray fluorescence. *Spectrochim. Acta, Part B*, *v.61*, p.1170-1174, 2006.

von Czarnowski, D.; Denkaus, E.; Lemke, K. Determination of trace element distribution in cancerous and normal human tissues by total reflection X-ray fluorescence analysis. *Spectrochim. Acta Part B*, *v.52*, p.1047-1052, 1997.

Wagner, M.; Rostam-Khani, P.; Wittershagen, A.; Rittmeyer, C.; Kolbesen, B.O.; Hoffman, H. Trace element determination in drugs by total reflection X-ray fluorescence spectrometry. *Spectrochim. Acta Part B*, *v.52*, p.961-965, 1997.

Zucchi, O.L.A.D.; Dias, D.A.; Nascimento Filho, V.F.; Salvador, M.J. Characterization of two medicinal plants by X-ray spectrometry. *J. Trace Microprobe Tech.*, *v.18*, p.441-450, 2000.

Zucchi, O.L.A.D.; Moreira, S.; Salvador, M.J. Santos, L.L. Multielement analysis of soft drinks by X-ray fluorescence spectrometry. *J. Agr. Food Chem.*, *v.53*, p.7863-7869, 2005a.

Zucchi, O.L.A.D., Moreira, S.; De Jesus, E.F.O.; Sálvio Neto, H.; Salvador, M.J. Charaterization of hypogycemiant plants by total refection X-ray fluorescence spectrometry. *Biol. Trace Element Res.*, *v. 103*, n. 3, p.277-290, 2005b.

Zucchi, O.L.A.D.; Nascimento, V.F. Caracterização qualitativa e quantitativa de elementos, pela técnica de fluorescência de raios X, em suplementos minerais para animais. Parte I: Dispersão de comprimento de onda. *Pesq. Agropec. Bras.*, *v.30*, p.1427- 1439, 1995.

Zucchi, O.L.A.D.; Salvador, M.J. Análise elementar de cosméticos por fluorescência de raios X. *Cosmetics & Toiletries (edição em português)*, *v.10*, p.52-61, 1998.

Zucchi, O.L.A.D.; Schiavetto, I.A.; Salvador, M.J.; Moreira, S. SRTXRF analysis in different pharmaceutical forms of diclofenac sodium. *Instrum. Sci. Technol.*, *v. 33*, p. 223-235, 2005.

In: Micronutrients and Health Research
Editor: Takumi Yoshida, pp. 11-22

ISBN: 978-1-60456-056-5
© 2008 Nova Science Publishers, Inc.

Short Communication

INTERACTIONS BETWEEN DRUGS AND MICRONUTRIENTS

Uwe Gröber [*]

Essen, Germany.

Interactions between drugs and micronutrients have received only little or no attention in the medical and pharmaceutical world in the past. Since more and more pharmaceutics are used for the treatment of patients, this topic is increasingly relevant. As such interactions – depending on the duration of treatment and the status of micronutrients – impact the health of the patient and the action of the drugs, physicians and pharmacists should pay more attention to such interactions in the future. The following article intends to point out the relevance of mutual interactions between micronutrients and drugs, without claiming to be exhaustive.

Thanks to modern health care and the improvement of life quality, the average life expectancy of Europeans has almost doubled over the past 100 years. It is estimated that by 2010 more than 20% of the European population will be over 70 years of age. The increase in the mean age goes along with an increasing number of multimorbid patients, who suffer from nutrition-associated diseases and usually depend on complex pharmacotherapy.

Multimorbidity inevitably leads to polypharmacotherapy. Surveys on the prescription habits in German clinics reveal that a patient is given, on average, 3 to 6 different drugs during clinical treatment. Each additional medication, however, increases the risk of side effects or interactions. The problem of adverse effects has been confirmed by the results of a meta-analysis carried out by the Journal of the American Medical Association in 1998, which investigated the incidence of side-effects in clinical patients in the US. The analysis of 39 prospective studies showed that severe side-effects had occurred in 6.7% of patients, with a death rate of 0.32%. The authors estimated that in 1994 severe side effects had occurred in

---

[*] Correspondence concerning this article should be addressed to: Uwe Gröber, Rüttenscheider Strasse 66, D-45130 Essen, Germany.

2,216,000 clinical patients whereas 106,000 patients had died from such effects. Although the results of this analysis should not be overrated given the heterogeneity of the conducted studies, it becomes clear that adverse medical effects are of high clinical relevance and can take on critical dimensions.

INTERACTIONS BETWEEN DRUGS AND MICRONUTRIENTS

Only in very rare cases it is possible that drugs eliminate a pathological condition without interfering with physiological or metabolic functions. Side effects and interactions are therefore inevitable, when a drug impacts the same control-cycle or uses the same absorption mechanism as another substance. This not only applies to additional drugs, but also to essential micronutrients.

For the processing of absorption, digestion, and elimination, micronutrients and drugs use the same transportational and metabolic functions of the body respectively. When one or more drugs are taken, patients are exposed to the risk of interactions of the drugs with the nutrients' balance. As a consequence, the absorption of a drug may be disturbed by a micronutrient (e.g. calcium inhibits tetracyclines) or a medicament may inhibit the physiological function of a vitamin or mineral nutrient (e.g. folic acid antagonism of MTX).

Vitamins, mineral nutrients and trace elements have a considerable preventive medical and therapeutic potential in the prevention and therapy of nutrition-associated diseases. A disturbance of the micronutrient status can result in severe disorders of the metabolism, because almost every physiological process in the body involves one of these bio catalysts. In view of the frequency and steadily increasing number of drugs, the adverse effects of pharmacotherapy on micronutrients should be given far more consideration than in the past in order to minimize the potential risks for patients.

A number of drugs, for example, interfere with the physiological excretion of homocysteine, an angiotoxic and neurotoxic amino acid,

- acting as direct or indirect antagonists of cofactors and enzymes
- by interfering with the absorption or biotransformation of vitamins
- and/or enzyme modulation (e.g. Cytochrom-P450 enzyme induction)

which leads to hyperhomocysteinaemia. What should make us think is the fact that the list contains a number of drugs (see *table 1*) which are regularly used to treat cardiovascular diseases (e.g. dyslipoproteinaemia, hypertonia, diabetes mellitus) without the awareness that an increase of the homocysteine plasma level poses a high risk to health.

Next to the necessary medication, monitoring the homocysteine levels and the supplement of folic acid, vitamin B12 and B6, constitute further important elements in the pharmacotherapy of cardiovascular disease to decrease the individual cardiovascular risk!

Table 1. Drugs that may increase the level of homocysteine (Hcy)

Drug	Mechanism
a) Drugs frequently used for cardiovascular diseases	
Cholestyramine	Impairment of folic acid and cobalamin absorption
Fibrates (e.g. Fenofibrat)	PPARα activation, interference with renal function, reduced homocysteine excretion (alternatively: Gemfibrozil)
Diuretics (e.g. thiazide)	renal excretion↑ of folic acid, B12 and B6
HCT/Triamteren	renal excretion↑ of folic acid / folic acid antagonism
Metformin	binding of calcium, vitamin B12 absorption ↓, folic acid/ B12-plasma level ↓
Niacin (in pharmacological dosage: 0,5 – 3 g/d)	vitamin B6 antagonist, inhibits pyridoxal kinase
b) Further drugs	
Anti-epileptic drugs (e.g. carbamazepine, phenytoin, valproic acid)	folic acid antagonism, enzyme induction, inhibit folat absorption
Cyclosporin A	renal function ↓, renal excretion ↓ of homocysteine
Levodopa	substrate of SAM-dependent methylation
Isoniazid	vitamin-B_6 antagonist through complex formation
Oral Contraceptives	interference with folic acid
Laxatives	folic acid absorption ↓
L-Methionine	homocysteine precursor
Methotrexate (MTX)	folic acid antagonism, inhibits dihydrofolate reductase
Omeprazole	Impairment of vitamin B12 absorption
Sulfasalazine	folic acid absorption ↓
Theophylline	vitamin-B6 antagonist, inhibits pyridoxal kinase
Trimethoprim	inhibition of dihydrofolate reductase

CONSEQUENCES OF LATENT MICRONUTRIENT DEFICIENCIES

In the clinical context, it has to be assumed that the dark figure of drug-induced imbalances of micronutrients is quite high, although they only seldom appear as manifest deficiency symptoms (see *table 2*). They rather occur as unspecific disturbances due to latent micronutrient deficiency, which expresses through lack of appetite, general weakness, learning and concentration disturbances, headaches, nervousness and increased liability to infections or stress. In the medical and pharmaceutical practice, such symptoms are often disregarded, or accepted as metabolic imbalances due to age, environment or genetics, although they considerably impact the health and well-being of the patients.

Latent deficiencies can rapidly give way to clinically manifest deficiencies, when the organism is exposed to major strains (e.g. influenzal infection, physical or emotional stress, medication). Current surveys on consumption habits and nutrition reports diagnose latent nutrient deficiencies in almost all groups of people. School children, working women and men, athletes, pregnant women and elderly people are particularly affected. If we take into account that the activity of magnesium-dependent enzymes falls by 50% when the supply of magnesium to the cells decreases by 25%, we can hardly imagine the impact of long-lasting and latent micronutrient deficiencies on our health.

Table 2. Symptoms of marginal micronutrient deficiencies (selection)

Micronutrient	Symptoms
vitamin B_1	learning and concentration disorders
niacin	depression, fatigue, nervousness
vitamin B_6	headache, fatigue, nervousness
vitamin B_{12}	apathy, mental deficits, dementia
folic acid	apathy, mental deficits, dementia
vitamin C	reduced physical performance, episodes of depression, liability to infections
magnesium	tension headache, liability to stress, nervousness
iron	pallor, fatigue
zinc	liability to infections, poor wound healing

Physicians of Harvard University recently evaluated scientific studies stretching over a period from 1966 to 2002 and came to the conclusion that a latently existing undersupply of vitamins considerably increases the risk of chronic diseases. Reduced absorption of folic acid, vitamin B6 and B12 represents a risk factor for cardiovascular diseases, neural tube defects as well as breast and colon cancer. Suboptimal supply with vitamin D and K increases the risk of osteoporosis. The risk of contracting radicals-associated diseases such as arteriosclerosis, macula degeneration or cancer is increased by inadequate supply of anti-oxidative vitamins (e.g. vitamin A, E, C, lutein). As most people do not have the optimum quantity of all micronutrients, the Harvard physicians recommend that adults should daily take a food supplement containing multivitamins and mineral nutrients to prevent potential undersupply. Here they particularly stress the importance of folic acid, vitamin B6, B12 and vitamin D!

FACTORS INFLUENCING DRUG–MICRONUTRIENT INTERACTIONS

The administering of drugs that influence the metabolism of vitamins and minerals is not always associated with the risk of drug-induced micronutrient deficiencies. What is important is the duration of the therapy and the nutritional status before the treatment.

The status of micronutrients in a healthy man, who cares for a balanced nutrition, is usually not negatively affected by taking a drug over a short period of time. In case of a persistent undersupply of a particular micronutrient and a long-term therapy or polypharmacotherapy, interactions between micronutrients and drugs can become relevant and should be increasingly included in diagnostic and therapeutic considerations. Chronically ill patients (permanent medication) and elderly people (multimorbidity, polypharmacotherapy) as well as patients who treat themselves without consulting their pharmacist or physician are exposed to a higher risk in particular. The quality and intensity of interactions between a drug and a micronutrient depend on numerous influencing factors (see *table 3*). It specially includes the pharmacological and toxicological action profile of the drug, the duration of medication, as well as the dietary habits and the micronutrient status of the patient at the beginning of medication.

Table 3. Drug-micronutrient interactions & influencing factors

Drug
- indication, dosage and duration of medication
- absorption, distribution, biotransformation and elimination ($\rightarrow$ pharmacokinetics)
- pharmacological/toxicological action profile, site of action, mechanism of action and strength ($\rightarrow$ pharmacodynamics)
- physical and chemical properties ($\rightarrow$ application, pharmaceutical form, galenics)
- mono- or combination therapy
- substance-substance interactions

Micronutrient
- biochemical and physiological functions
- absorption, distribution, biotransformation, storage and elimination
- physical and chemical properties (e.g. fat soluble, water soluble, structure)

Patient
- age, gender, diseases
- status of micronutrients
- medication (even uncontrolled self-medication, supplements of vitamin preparations)
- food habits
- gastrointestinal integrity
- function of the liver and kidneys
- stimulants consumption (alcohol, smoking, sweets)

INTERACTION MECHANISMS

Interactions manifest when the effect and/or side-effect of a substance is qualitatively or quantitatively altered by a second substance which either impacts absorption, metabolism or elimination, or causes a synergistic or antagonistic effect in a different location. Based on the underlying mechanisms, interactions between remedies and nutrients can be categorized into

- *pharmacodynamic* and
- *pharmacokinetic*

interactions in analogy to the interaction of remedies.

PHARMACODYNAMIC INTERACTIONS

Pharmacodynamic interactions between drugs and micronutrients may occur, when the interacting substances have either an antagonistic or a synergistic effect on a particular site of action (e.g. enzyme) or in a closed loop. Since many micronutrients act as co-enzymes (e.g. folic acid) or co-factors (e.g. magnesium), interactions manifest especially on the enzymatic level.

The inhibition of micronutrient-specific effects on a physiological site of action (see *table 4*) is the therapeutic principle of specific drugs, including anticoagulants of the Dicoumarol-type, antibacterial folic-acid antagonists or cardiac glycosides.

Table 4. Micronutrient antagonists (selection)

Micronutrient	Antagonist	Enzyme (site of action)
Folic acid	Methotrexat, Tetroxoprim, Trimethoprim, Triamteren, Pyrimethamin	Dihydrofolat-reductase
Vitamin K	Phenprocoumon, Warfarin	Vitamin-K epoxide-reductase
Calcium	Magnesium	myocardial cell (competition for membrane calcium channels and bindings to Troponin)
Potassium	cardiac glycosides	Mg-dependent Na+/K+-ATPase

VITAMIN K AND DICOUMAROL DERIVATES

There is a great analogy in structure between the vitamin-K antagonist Phenprocoumon and the natural vitamin K. It inhibits (see *figure1*) vitamin K epoxide reductase in the so-called vitamin K cycle, thereby suppressing the carboxylation of vitamin-K-dependent clotting factors and reducing blood coagulation.

Vitamin K is not only essential for coagulation, but also for the gamma-carboxylation of osteocalcin, a bone protein which mainly occurs in the fast growing sections of the bones. Osteocalcin (Oc) is a non-collagen glycoprotein that is produced in the osteoblasts and stimulates the formation of bones. When, because of a lack of vitamin K or during a therapy with vitamin K–antagonists, gamma-carboxylation is blocked, the fraction of non-carboxylated osteocalcin (ucOc) in the plasma increases. Under-carboxylated osteocalcin is an important indicator for impairments in the bone metabolism. Thus it cannot be ruled out that patients undergoing a long-term therapy with anticoagulants of the Dicoumarol-type are not put to a higher risk for osteoporosis. However, as large quantities of vitamin K (e.g. vitamin K preparations, vegetables) may diminish the effectiveness of vitamin K antagonists, the dosage of vitamin K should be determined depending on the Cumarine-anticoagulants-therapy, and the coagulation parameters should be closely controlled.

POTASSIUM AND CARDIAC GLYCOSIDES

Depending on the concentration, cardiac glycosides bind magnesium-dependent Na+/K+-ATPase of myocardial cells and reduce the action of enzymes. This, in turn, leads to a reduced leakage of sodium ions out of the cell and influx of potassium ions into the cell. Increased intracellular sodium concentration leads to an increased calcium influx into the cell via plasma membrane Na+/Ca2+- exchanger, resulting in increased myocardial contraction (positive inotropic effect). One disadvantage of cardiac glycosides is their narrow therapeutic bandwidth, which becomes particularly manifest in potassium imbalances. Potassium depletion (e.g. caused by Thiazides or loop diuretics, laxatives) increases the effects of cardiac glycosides and thus the risk for cardiac dysrhythmia. Parenteral applied calcium salts increase toxicity as well. For this reason, injections of calcium-containing solutions are best avoided under glycoside therapy, whereas potassium (e.g. mineral nutrient preparations) or potassium-sparing diuretics (e.g. Spironolacton, Triamteren) reduce the therapeutic effect of cardiac glycosides.

The glycoside tolerance, however, can be enhanced with magnesium, because it regulates the potassium balance and, in terms of calcium antagonist, protects the myocardial cells from over-loading with calcium ions. It is therefore recommended to closely monitor the level of potassium and magnesium under cardiac glycoside therapy and, if necessary, use substitutes to regulate the system.

The antibacterial *folic-acid antagonists Trimethoprim* and *Tetroxoprim*, which are often used in combination with sulfonamide (*Sulfamethoxazol, Sulfadiazin*), inhibit the dihydrofolate-reductase in bacteria. Although the affinity to humane dihydrofolate-reductase is several decimal levels higher for the bacterial enzyme, patients treated with this drug showed impaired haematopoesis (megaloblastic anaemia) and homocysteine metabolism. The same interactions can occur under therapy with the *potassium-sparing diuretic Triamteren* or with the *Antiprotozoal drug Pyrimethamine.*

PHARMACOKINETIC INTERACTIONS

Pharmacokinetic interactions between drugs and micronutrients manifest, among other things, as absorption, biotransformation or excretion processes. They usually lead to a reduced bioavailability of a drug or micronutrient in the gastrointestinal tract, which is most closely associated with pharmacokinetic interactions.

INTERACTIONS WITH ABSORPTION

• Mineral Nutrients and Antibiotics (Tetracyclines, Gyrase inhibitors)

One of the most frequent causes for therapeutic failure among antibacterials is the intake of *Tetracyclines* (e.g. Doxycycline) or *Gyrase inhibitors* (e.g. Ciprofloxacin) together with calcium, magnesium, iron and/or zinc (e.g. milk products, mineral nutrients). The formation of poorly absorbable *mineral nutrient-drug-complexes* results in a partial or complete loss of efficiency of the antibiotic. For this reason, the second drug should be taken after a minimum interval of three hours.

• Fat-soluble Vitamins and Colestyramine

The anion-exchange resins *Colestyramine* and *Colestipol* – used to reduce high cholesterol levels – promote via the adsorption of bile acids the excretion of bile acids and reduce so the hepatic bile acid pool. The new synthesis of bile acids from cholesterol leads to a lower level of cholesterol in the blood. Disorders in the absorption and digestion of fats can result in a lack of *fat soluble vitamins* (A, D, E, K, Pro-Vitamin A).

In research studies carried out with healthy test persons who received 16 g Colestyramine on four consecutive days, the *vitamin B12* absorption dropped by 55 to 90%. Colestyramine becomes bound to the intrinsic factor (IF), thereby affecting the absorption of vitamin B12.

Moreover, the formation of poorly soluble complexes with *iron, calcium* or *magnesium* significantly lowers the bio-availability of mineral nutrients.

• Vitamin B12 and Ulcus Drugs (e.g. Omeprazole, Ranitidine)

Long-term therapies with *proton pump inhibitors* (e.g. Omeprazole) and *H2-blockers* (e.g. Ranitidine) can significantly lower the vitamin B12 serum levels due to reduced vitamin B12 absorption. In our food, *vitamin B12* is bound to proteins and is to be released from the binding in the stomach dependent from pH through hydrochloric acid and pepsin. Only then can it become bound to the intrinsic factor in the upper part of the small intestine and absorbed with the help of specific receptors. Up to 40% of elderly people (> 60) suffer from a lack of vitamin B12 as a consequence of atrophic gastritis. In regard to a sufficient supply with vitamin B12, such patients should be given proton pump inhibitors with utmost care.

The inhibition of the intrinsic factor through H2-blockers is of lesser importance for the bioavailability of vitamin B12. What is more important is the risk of pathogenic bacteria populating the gastric mucosa (e.g. Helicobacter pylori) as a consequence of a reduced bactericidal effect of the gastric juice. In addition to vitamin B12 absorption, antacids also decrease the pH-gradient stimulated intestinal absorption of folic acid and thus bioavailability.

BIOTRANSFORMATION AND METABOLISM

• Vitamin D and Anti-Epileptics

Anti-epileptics such as *Phenobarbital, Phenytoin, Primidone* or *Carbamazepine* induce Cytochrom-P450-containing mono-oxygenases in the liver, which catalyze the degradation and metabolism of vitamin D. This results in a significant decrease of the 25-(OH)- and 1.25-(OH)2 vitamin D3 level in the serum and, due to hypocalcaemia, to an increase of the Parathormone level (secondary hyper-parathyreoidism). The excretion of Pyridinoline crosslinks rises as an indicator for increased bone absorption. Decreasing bone density (lumbar spine L2–L4) and proliferation of osteocytes are associated with a significantly increased risk of fractures. Pharmacists should therefore inform patients, who regularly take anticonvulsants, about the importance of vitamin D and the individual risk of osteoporosis caused by a lack of vitamin D.

Table 5. Bone metabolism disorders caused by anticonvulsants – mechanisms

- activation (induction) of Cytochrom-P-450 containing mono-oxygenases in the liver that catalyze metabolism and degradation of vitamin D
- increased biliary vitamin D excretion (excretion with bile acids)
- reduced intestinal and renal Calcium absorption (e.g. Phenytoin)
- increased release of Parathormones due to drop of calcium and 25-hydroxy vitamin D3 levels in the serum *(secondary hyperparathyreoidism)*
- hypophosphataemia
- increased bone isoenzyme of alkaline phosphatase (bone AP) in the serum
- direct toxic effects (e.g. Carbamazepine, Phenytoin) on osteoblasts
- inhibition of Calcitonine secretion (especially Phenytoin)

Without adequate substitution of vitamin D, long-term medication with anticonvulsants frequently leads to a lack of vitamin D. Teens who do little physical exercise as well as multiple morbid patients with little exposure to UV light are particularly affected. More often than not epileptic patients consume lots of caffeine-containing drinks (e.g. coffee) due to the side-effects (fatigue) of the drugs, which, however, contribute to a further loss of micronutrients.

Patients with long-term medication of anticonvulsants should be advised to regularly visit their orthopaedist to measure bone density (DXA-measuring method) and take an adequate amount of bone-related micronutrients such as vitamin D (1,000 – 2,000 (4,000) i.u./d), calcium and vitamin K, especially during the winter months. Hypovitaminosis D is indicated by a 25-(OH)-Vitamin-D3-(Calcidiol) serum level of < 70 nmol/l.

• Grapefruit Juice and Drugs

Cytochrom-P-450-dependent enzymes catalyze the metabolism of numerous endogenous and exogenous substrates. The CYP3A4 iso-enzyme metabolises up to 70% of all drugs. CYP3A4 is expressed in the liver as well as in the epithelial cells of the small intestine. Secondary plant substances of grapefruit juice (e.g. Bergamottin, Naringenin) can reduce the CYP3A4-related intestinal first-pass effect of a number of orally applied drugs such as calcium channel blockers (e.g. Felodipine) or immunosuppressors (e.g. Ciclosporine,

Tacrolimus). When patients drink grapefruit juice, the bioavailability of these CYP3A4 substrates increases along with the risk of toxicologically relevant side-effects (e.g. increased nephrotoxicity of Ciclosporine). The consumption of large quantities of juice ($\geq$ 500 ml per day) leads to an increased absorption of substances responsible for the inhibition of CYP3A4 and the hepatic degradation of such drugs.

• Vitamin B6 and L-Dopa

The aim of Parkinson's drug therapy is to substitute the missing Dopamine in the central nervous system and mitigate the increased cholinergic activity. The most efficient anti-Parkinson drug to-date is Levodopa (L-Dopa) which improves all symptoms of the Parkinson's disease, in particular Akinesia and psychic disorders. Since 90% of the orally applied L-Dopa dose is degraded in the periphery so that only 10% is available for the CNS, L-Dopa is almost exclusively used in combination with the *decarboxylase inhibitors Benserazide* or *Carbidopa*. Benserazide and Carbidopa inhibit the peripheral decarboxylation of L-Dopa to Dopamine and increase the availability of Dopamine in the brain. Thanks to this combination, the dose of L-Dopa can be considerably lowered and the peripheral vegetative side-effects reduced.

Higher doses of vitamin B6 (e.g. supplements) can significantly affect the bioavailability and the effectiveness of L-Dopa. Vitamin B6 in the form of Pyridoxal-5'-phosphate is a coenzyme of numerous enzymes which play a role predominantly in the amino-acid metabolism. As coenzyme of L-amino acid decarboxylases the vitamin accelerates the peripheral decarboxylation of L-Dopa to Dopamine. Consequently, the dopaminergic nerve endings in the nigrostriatum have less L-Dopa available, which can be decarboxylated to the active substance Dopamine.

Parkinson symptoms such as rigor, akinesia and tremor intensify. Moreover, the un-physiologically high Dopamine levels in the periphery lead to gastrointestinal and cardiovascular disorders. Although the combination of L-Dopa with a Decarboxylase inhibitor (e.g. Carbidopa) mitigates the problematic interaction, patients should not take vitamin B6 in high pharmacological doses (> 10–20 mg/day, p.o.) without consulting their physician before!

EXCRETION

Diuretic therapy will in principle cause a multiple loss of micronutrients, especially of the water-soluble vitamins and mineral nutrients, due to renal hyper-excretion.

• Mineral Nutrients and Diuretics

Loop diuretics (e.g. Furosemide, Torasemide) and thiazides (e.g. Hydrochlorothiazide) lead to a loss of potassium, magnesium and zinc. As opposed to thiazides, loop diuretics also lead to an increased expulsion of calcium. A diuretic therapy should therefore include careful monitoring of the blood electrolytes and, if necessary, compensate with substitutes.

• Vitamin B1 and Furosemide

Long-term Furosemide therapy for patients suffering from chronic heart failure resulted in thiamine depletion as a consequence of extraordinarily high renal thiamine excretion. According to its physiological importance for energy metabolism, after absorption in the gastrointestinal tract vitamin B1 is quickly distributed to the organs and tissues depending on their individual metabolic rate. At 3–8 µg/g the myocardium holds the highest proportion of vitamin B1. Thiamine depletion may further deteriorate the cardiac pump function that is already affected by cardiac insufficiency. The thiamine status should be regularly controlled under Furosemide therapy (parameter: thiamine level in the blood, transketolase activity) and compensated through substitution with highly bioavailable thiamine derivates (e.g. Benfotiamin).

• Lithium and Diuretics

The excretion of lithium is closely related to the excretion of sodium. The absorption of hydrogen carbonate and larger quantities of sodium chloride increases the renal elimination of lithium, thereby reducing the effectiveness of the antidepressant. In contrast, diuretics (thiazides, potassium-saving diuretics and loop diuretics) reduce renal elimination thus increasing the level of lithium in the plasma and with it the danger of lithium intoxication.

• L-Carnitine and Valproic Acid

The kidneys play a key role in the homeostasis of the Carnitine metabolism. Over 95% of the ultra-filtered Carnitine are reabsorbed. The renal clearance of Acylcarnitine is significantly higher (> 3 times) than of free Carnitine. Valproic acid binds L-Carnitine (Valproyl-Carnitine) and may result in iatrogenic Carnitine depletion due to increased excretion of Valproyl-L-Carnitine esters. The beta-oxidation of fatty acids, i.e. fat burning and energy gain in the form of ATP, is thus disturbed, because fatty acids can only be transported in the form of Carnitine esters (Acylcarnitine) through the inner mitochondrial membrane. Valproic acids also affect the cellular Carnitine uptake by inhibiting the activity of membrane Carnitine transporters, such as e.g. Carnitine-Acylcarnitine translocase (CAT).

Long-term therapy with Valproic acid showed that adults, and children in particular, suffer from a lower L-Carnitine plasma level, elevated Acyl-Carnitine : total Carnitine ratio in the urine as well as from reduced tubular reabsorption of free L-Carntine in the kidneys. Factors contributing to Valproic-acid-induced Carnitine depletion are, besides long-term medication, also combination therapies with other anti-epileptics (Phenobarbital,

Phenytoine). Patients, who are treated with the anti-epileptic Valproic-acid over a long period, may benefit from Carnitine supplements (500 bis 1,000 mg/d, p.o.)

- **L-Carnitine and Pivalic-acid-containing antibiotics (e.g. Cefetamet-Pivoxil)**

After hydrolysis of Pivaloyloxymethyl esters from Beta-Lactam antibiotics, the Pivalic acid becomes bound to L-Carnitine and is excreted as Pivaloyl-L-Carnitine via the kidneys. Patients who receive therapy with antibiotics containing Pivalic-acid (including new Virustatica such as Adefovir Dipivoxil) may develop severe Carnitine depletion without adjuvant Carnitine substitution, which manifests as myopathia (e.g. amyasthenia), ketogenese disorders and/or hypoglycaemia.

Research studies on the influence of Cefetamet-Pivoxil on the L-Carnitine status and fat metabolism have shown that the standard dose of 2 x 500 mg/day of the ester prodrug leads to a drop of free L-Carnitine in the plasma level to 40% as compared to the original values, which comes back to normal only 7 days after antibiotic therapy.

It is therefore recommended to think in time of an adequate compensation for the iatrogenic loss of Carnitine in patients who undergo antiepileptic therapy with Valproic acid or Pivalic acid-containing antibiotics (including virustatica).

REFERENCES

Gröber, U., Arzneimittel und Mikronährstoffe. *Medikationsorientierte Supplementierung.* Wissenschaftliche Verlagsgesellschaft mbH, Stuttgart, 2007

Gröber, U., Interaktionen zwischen Arzneimitteln und Mikronährstoffen. *Medizinische Monatsschrift für Pharmazeuten (MMP),* 29(1), 26-35, 2006.

In: Micronutrients and Health Research
Editor: Takumi Yoshida, pp. 23-70

ISBN: 978-1-60456-056-5
© 2008 Nova Science Publishers, Inc.

Chapter I

ADVANCES OF ZINC IN HEALTH RESEARCH

Cuong D. Tran

Gastroenterology Unit, Children, Youth and Women's Health Service,
North Adelaide SA 5006, Australia;
Discipline of Physiology, School of Molecular and Biochemical Science, University of
Adelaide SA 5005, Australia.

ABSTRACT

The main focus of this chapter is to provide an overview of the significance of zinc in human health research. The following issues are discussed: (1) the history of our understanding of human zinc deficiency; (2) the biochemistry and biology of zinc with an emphasis on the relevance of zinc in human nutrition and the importance of human zinc deficiency; (3) the clinical spectrum of zinc deficiency; (4) the lack of biomarkers for milder zinc deficiency states to ascertain their prevalence and clinical outcomes, including growth retardation, diarrhoea, pneumonia, other infections and abnormalities in neuropsychological performance; (5) human zinc requirements with special focus on estimation of average dietary zinc requirements and zinc toxicity; (6) the causes of zinc deficiency, particularly in the developing world; and (7) potential strategies for the prevention and management of human zinc deficiency. The chapter concludes with an emphasis on the immediate need for expanded research on human zinc metabolism and homeostasis at a molecular, cellular, organ and whole body level.

INTRODUCTION

Evidence of zinc deficiency was first reported in the 1960s. Since then our understanding of the clinical importance of zinc deficiency has rapidly progressed. These advances occurred during the 1990s and at the beginning of the millennium when a series of well-designed, high quality randomised controlled studies of zinc supplementation took place. Results from recent meta-analyses and pooled analyses of multiple high-quality world-wide intervention studies have established zinc as a critical player in physical growth and normal functioning of the gastrointestinal tract and immune system of humans. More importantly is the reduction observed in the incidence and prevalence of diarrhoea and pneumonia with zinc supplementation programs. There are suggestions that daily zinc supplementation among full-term, small-for-gestational-age infants significantly reduces the mortality rate. These beneficial effects however, are likely to be dependent on existing zinc deficiency states. Accumulating data also suggest that zinc deficiency may be related to adverse outcomes of pregnancy and compromised neurobehavioral function in children. Insights to the importance of zinc were derived from studies evaluating individuals with acrodermatitis enteropathica and from studies assessing markers of zinc status and specific functions. Hospital and community-based interventions and animal model studies gave zinc credibility in improving human health. In this chapter we will review the impact of zinc supplementation on human health in terms of improving growth and development, preventing morbidity from common infections and reducing child mortality. To date, there are no simple quantitative biochemical or functional markers of zinc status sensitive enough to identify mild to moderate zinc deficiency in humans. Consequently, efforts to quantify the global prevalence of zinc deficiency have been thwarted. Resulting lack of information has hampered the development of specific intervention programs. Another aspect of this chapter is to review available methods for specific assessment of zinc status in individuals and populations. These include serum and plasma zinc concentrations, hair zinc concentrations, zinc fluorophores, and current specific measures of zinc metabolism using stable isotopes. A critical area for future investigation is the development of superior methods to assess zinc status of individuals. Given the diverse array of biological functions of zinc, it is not surprising that zinc plays critical roles in multiple physiological functions such as growth and development, immuno-competence, reproduction, and neuro-behavioural development. However, further information is needed on the mechanisms of the protective effects of zinc against infection. Information is also required to define the consequences of zinc deficiency on foetal development and foetal delivery, postpartum maternal health and infant health. Little is known about the magnitude of zinc deficiency on neuro-behavioural development and therefore studies are needed to define the range and magnitude of these effects.

HISTORICAL PERSPECTIVE OF HUMAN ZINC DEFICIENCY

The history of the importance of zinc in nutrition, clinical medicine and public health is considerably short. The first role of zinc in biology was observed in micro-organisms and was not reported until the late nineteenth century, centuries after the discovery of the biological role of iron and its importance in human health. [1]. It was not until the 20th century that researchers discovered zinc to be essential for growth and survival of higher plants, poultry, rodents and swine [2]. By the late 1950s abnormalities of human zinc metabolism had been observed and it was well accepted that zinc was a necessary micronutrient for humans. Despite these findings, many nutritionists doubted that zinc deficiency occurred because of the lack of obvious clinical signs in presumably high-risk human populations and because of the element's ubiquitous distribution in the environment.

The first major conceptual discovery came in 1961 [3] with the hypothesis linking a dietary deficiency of bioavailable zinc to the syndrome of "adolescent nutritional dwarfism" identified mainly and extensively in mid-Eastern countries. Due to the complexities of the multiple nutrient deficiency that contributed to this syndrome and the limited data derived from randomised controlled intervention studies, the impact of this hypothesis was diminished. However, the practical relevance of these findings was associated with a number of possible environmental/nutritional aetiological factors not apparent to western societies at the time. Nonetheless, this finding made an outstanding contribution to the recognition of zinc as an important micronutrient in human nutrition.

Approximately 10 years later, severe zinc deficiency had been identified in industrialised countries. The phenotypic expression of the rare autosomal recessive inherited disorder acrodermatitis enteropathica was attributed to a defect in zinc metabolism [4]. More importantly at the time and persisting beyond the 1970s, was iatrogenic severe zinc deficiency. This was attributed to the failure to add zinc to intravenous infusates of hospitalised patients who were totally dependent on intravenous feeding [5]. Our understanding of the clinical outcomes of zinc deficiency still owes a great deal to descriptions of the presentation of patients with inherited (acrodermatitis enteropathica) and acquired severe zinc deficiency states.

On the contrary, nutritional zinc deficiency has been well documented from a series of randomised controlled studies of dietary zinc supplementation in young children in Denver during the late 1970s and early 1980s. Results of these trials indicated the occurrence of growth retardation zinc deficiency in otherwise apparently normal infants and young children [6-9]. Eventually, these findings were eclipsed by advances during the 1990s and at the beginning of the millennium. These progresses were primarily attributed to a number of well designed clinical intervention trials of zinc supplementation in children within a wide range of populations throughout the world [9-11]. The critical role of zinc in physical growth and normal functioning of the gastrointestinal tract and immune system of humans was ascertained [4]. More importantly, the results of these trials confirmed that zinc supplementation increases growth among stunted children [9] and reduces the prevalence of common childhood infections such as diarrhoea and pneumonia [10]. In addition, these studies [9-10] have provided a significant impact on our understanding of the global public health importance of human zinc deficiency. [12].

THE BIOLOGICAL FUNCTIONS OF ZINC

Zinc is ubiquitous in biologic systems and has abundant and varied functions within these systems. These extraordinary characteristics are due to its unusually versatile physicochemical properties. That is, the zinc atom has the ability to participate in readily exchangeable ligand binding in addition to assuming a number of coordination geometries to provide functional needs to other ligands [13]. Furthermore, under physiologic conditions, zinc is not subject to oxido-reductive reactions, which, in contrast to iron and copper, allows its utilisation without the risk of oxidant damage [14-15].

The properties of zinc make it an ideal candidate to participate in catalytic, structural, and cellular regulatory functions. Zinc is required for the activity of > 300 enzymes, covering all six classes [oxidoreductases, transferases, hydrolases, lysases, isomerases, and ligases] of enzymes [16] including RNA polymerase, alcohol dehydrogenase, carbonic anhydrase, and alkaline phosphatase [13]. Zinc is an essential component of the catalytic site or sites of at least one enzyme in every enzyme classification [17].

The biologic role of zinc is now recognised in terms of structure and function of proteins, including enzymes, transcription factors, hormonal receptor sites and biologic membranes [13]. By facilitating the folding of proteins into three-dimensional configurations zinc enables their biologic activity. This folding often involves chelation of zinc with the amino acids cysteine and histidine and the formation of a tetrahedral arrangement finger-like motif, referred to as "zinc-fingers". A major progress in our understanding of the biology of zinc has been through the identification of proteins that contain a zinc-finger motif [18]. Hundreds of zinc-finger motifs have been and continue to be identified. Over 3% of all identified human genes contain zinc-finger domains [19]. Thus, zinc plays a broad role in gene expression. Although much remains to be learned about the extent of zinc's role as an intracellular regulatory ion, the potential importance of this role is attracting increasing attention [20].

Zinc has numerous central roles in DNA and RNA metabolism [21]. Zinc metalloenzymes and zinc-dependent enzymes have been identified and are involved in nucleic acid metabolism and cellular proliferation, differentiation and growth [22]. Zinc also plays a regulatory role in apoptosis [23], with cytoprotective functions that suppress major pathways leading to programmed cell death. A decline in intracellular zinc also directly influences apoptotic regulators. Zinc can modulate cellular signal recognition, second-messenger metabolism, protein kinase and protein phosphatase activities. In the brain, zinc is sequestered in the presynaptic vesicles of zinc-containing neurons and released into the cleft where it is recycled into the presynaptic terminal [24]. Zinc plays a role in modulation of brain excitability. Vesicular-rich regions such as the hippocampus are responsive to dietary zinc deprivation.

There are two aspects of the complex biology of zinc which need to be addressed to fully appreciate its significance in human nutrition. Firstly, it is the ubiquity and versatility of this metal. Secondly, it is the less understood central or complex combination of the roles zinc has in gene expression, cellular growth and differentiation. Some knowledge of the biology and ramifications of zinc is important in human zinc nutrition and deficiency. Even a partial understanding of the importance of zinc in cellular growth and differentiation alerts us to the effects of an inadequate supply of zinc on the rapidly growing embryo, foetus, infant and young child. The patient mounting an immune response or requiring tissue repair also requires zinc. An appreciation of the extraordinary effects of dietary zinc restriction of growth and differentiation in the animal model [25] alerts us to the special vulnerability to zinc deficiency of cells that are rapidly dividing and other systems that are not noted for rapid cell turnover such as the central nervous system [26].

TISSUE ZINC DISTRIBUTION AND STORAGE

Zinc is present in all organs, tissues, fluids, and secretions of the body. Most zinc is located in fat-free mass, with about 30 mg zinc/kg tissue, almost all of which (>95%) is intracellular. The zinc content of the adult human body ranges from 1.5 to 2.5 g, with higher average contents in men than in women. Due to the bulk of skeletal muscle and bone in the body, zinc in these tissues accounts for the majority of whole body zinc. The concentration and total zinc content of various tissues, and the proportion contributed to total body zinc are shown in Table 1.

When total body zinc content is reduced during depletion, the loss of zinc is not uniform across all tissue. Skeletal muscle, skin and heart zinc are maintained, while zinc levels decline in bone, liver, testes and plasma [27]. It is not clear what mechanisms allow certain tissues to release zinc during depletion while others retain zinc. There are no known tissue reserves of zinc that can be released or sequestered quickly in response to variations in dietary supply. Nonetheless, it has been proposed that bone may serve as a passive reserve because some zinc may become available during normal turnover of osseous tissue [28]. The release of zinc from bone does not increase during zinc deficiency. Interestingly, the skeleton sequesters zinc during normal turnover of bone when dietary supply is low [29]. The authors showed that the results support the existence of two zinc pools in the skeleton, one a small, rapid turning-over pool (10-20% in size), and the other a slow turning-over pool. When rats suffer marginal zinc restriction, zinc from the readily turning-over bone pool is utilized for soft tissue needs. This is followed by decreased growth rate in order to maintain zinc homeostasis. Furthermore, chicks fed on higher zinc-containing diets accumulated more skeletal zinc and were more resistant to growth failure during a period of very low zinc intake compared to animals fed a marginally adequate zinc diet [30]. This suggests that the risk of zinc deficiency among individuals with poor dietary zinc intakes may be reduced by zinc supplementation. These issues are considered further in a subsequent section.

Table 1. Approximate zinc content of major organs and tissues in normal adult man (70kg)

Tissue	Approx. zinc concentrations (μg/g wet wt)	Total zinc content (g)	Proportion of total body zinc (%)
Skeletal muscle	51	1.53	57 (approx)
Bone	100	0.77	29
Skin	32	0.16	6
Liver	58	0.13	5
Brain	11	0.04	1.5
Kidneys	55	0.02	0.7
Heart	23	0.01	0.4
Hair	150	<0.01	0.1 (approx)
Blood plasma	1	<0.01	0.1 (approx)

Table reproduced from M. J. Jackson (1989) Physiology of Zinc: General Aspect. In C. F. Mills (ed) Zinc in Human Biology. Springer-Verlag Berlin Heidelberg, pp 2.

ZINC METABOLISM

The body has developed sophisticated mechanisms to remove zinc from dietary constituents. The body can absorb it together with 30-40 other elements in amounts which prevent either depletion or excess. Other sophisticated mechanisms incorporate transporting the element to all tissues of the body, maintaining appropriate concentrations in tissues, turning over biological substances that bind zinc and excreting zinc in suitable quantities.

Zinc is released from food as free ions during digestion. These liberated ions may then bind to endogenously secreted ligands or to exogenous materials in the intestinal lumen, the glycocalyx. The subsequent transcellular uptake occurs in the distal duodenum and proximal jejunum [31-34] from the brush border membrane. The mechanisms of exogenous zinc uptake have not yet been entirely elucidated, although both saturable and unsaturable processes are involved [35]. The active transport process at the apical surface of the enterocyte has the greatest capacity of intake at physiologic levels. It is difficult to detect the low capacity of the paracellular linear passive diffusion route except with higher luminal levels than those required to achieve near maximal absorption by the active transport route [33].

The saturable process was demonstrated in experimental animals many years ago [34]. Recently we have characterised a detailed dose response of quantity absorbed zinc (AZ) versus various doses of aqueous zinc supplement (5-30 mg) in fasted healthy adults using zinc stable isotope techniques (discussed in a subsequent section). The data from this study were best fit by the Hill Equation [36] and supported a saturable transport process for zinc absorption. The results indicated that absorption of about 13 mg zinc is the maximum that can be achieved from a single administration of an aqueous solution of zinc sulfate in the post-absorptive state of healthy young adults [37]. Of greater practical relevance, 80% of the Amax (the predicted maximum absorption of zinc based on the Hill Equation model) was achieved with a dose of 20 mg zinc with relatively low uptake for increments in doses beyond this (Figure 1). When an aqueous zinc dose was given for multiple days before measuring absorption, AZ was also reduced by half in the fasting state.

Although our study [37] supports a saturable process for the absorption of zinc, it does not support the mechanism of absorption. Recently, the mechanism of zinc absorption has been well described through the identification and characterisation of zinc transporters. Zinc transporters belong to at least 6 different transporter families. Three of these, the ABC transporters, the RND transporters, and the CorA proteins have been implicated in bacteria only [38] and will not be considered here. Similarly, few P-type ATPase have been found to play roles in eukaryotes zinc transport. Known eukaryotic zinc transporters come mainly from two families, ZIP (SLC39) and CDF/ZnT (SLC30) proteins. These two families will be described briefly, for additional information refer to other recent reviews [39-43].

The ZIP (Zrt, Irt-like protein) family is named after the yeast Zrt1 protein and the Arabidposis Irt1 protein. Mammalian members of this family have been given the systematic designation "SLC39" [42]. A key feature of the ZIP family is the transport of zinc from the extracellular space or the lumen into the cytoplasm. Most ZIP proteins have eight predicted topologies with the N- and C-termini of the protein located on the extracytoplasmic face of the membrane [44]. Many members also have a long loop region located between transmembrane domain 3 and 4, and a histidine-rich sequence is frequently found in this TM3-4 loop. The mechanism of transport used by the ZIPs is not clear. Zinc transport by the yeast Zrt1 protein is energy dependent while the human ZIP2 [SLC39A2] transporter is driven by the gradient of HCO_3^- that exists across the membrane of cells [45].

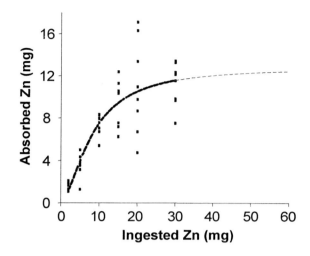

Figure 1. The absorbed zinc (AZ) vs. ingested zinc (IZ) and the fitted Hill Equation model (thick solid line) and extrapolated beyond the measurement range to demonstrate predicted absorption, approaching the Amax value of 13 mg [dashed line]. The Hill equation model is represented by the following equation; $AZ = Amax \times IZ^H / IZ^H + IA_{50}$ where the parameters Amax, IA_{50}, and H are the maximum absorbed zinc, the ingested zinc (IZ) that results in AZ of 50% of Amax, and the Hill (or sigmoidicity) coefficient, respectively with $R^2 = 0.73$.

The CDF designation stands for cation diffusion facilitator. Mammalian members of this zinc transporter family have been named "ZnT" and given the systematic name of SLC30 [43]. The key feature of this family is that they transport zinc from the cytoplasm into the lumen of intracellular organelles or to the outside of the cell. Thus the CDF proteins work in opposition to the ZIP transporters. Most members of this family have six predicted transmembrane domains [44]. Like the ZIP transporters, many CDF family members have histidine rich motifs, usually in the cytoplasmic loop between transmembrane domains 4 and 5. These domains may also bind to metal during transport. The mechanism of transport for many CDF proteins appears to be via zinc/H^+ or K^+ antiport [46]. Despite their name, CDF proteins do not serve as diffusion facilitators but rather as secondary active transporters using gradient of other ions to drive the transport of zinc [44].

The zinc transporters facilitate passage of zinc across the basolateral membrane of the enteroctyes into the portal circulation [47-48]. The portal system carries absorbed zinc directly to the liver, where it is taken up rapidly and released into the systemic circulation for delivery to other tissues [31]. About 70% of zinc in the circulation is bound to albumin, and any conditions that alter serum albumin concentration have a secondary effect on serum zinc levels. The circulation of zinc is reduced during pregnancy due to the expansion in plasma volume [49]. It is also reduced in hypoalbuminemia which accompanies the ageing process and protein-energy malnutrition [50]. Infections [51], acute trauma [52-53], and other stresses that increase secretion of cortisol and cytokines also affect the circulation of zinc. During fasting, serum zinc concentrations rise due to release of zinc by muscles. Following meals, serum zinc levels decline progressively in association with hormonal changes [54]. Although serum zinc represents only 0.1% of the whole body zinc, the circulating zinc turns over rapidly (~ 150 times per day) to meet tissue needs.

Loss of zinc through the gastrointestinal tract accounts for approximately half of all zinc eliminated from the body [55]. The pancreas secretes considerable amounts of zinc (~ 3-5 mg) into the intestine following each meal. Biliary and intestinal secretions also contain sizeable amounts of zinc [56]. The total endogenous gastrointestinal zinc secretion may well exceed the amount consumed in the diet. However, much of the zinc secreted into the intestine is reabsorbed. This process serves as an important point for zinc homeostasis regulation. Other routes of zinc excretion include the urine, which accounts for approximately 15% of total zinc losses, epithelial cell desquamation, sweat, semen, hair and menstrual blood, which together account for approximately 17% of total zinc loss [57]. The faecal loss of endogenous zinc from the body is less than 1 mg/d when a zinc-free diet is administered to healthy individuals [58]. The amount of endogenous zinc excreted in the faeces increases as the total absorbed increases. Faecal excretion of endogenous zinc declines when either dietary zinc intake is reduced or zinc needs are increased [59-60] due to growth or lactation [61]. When dietary zinc is decreased, the individual goes into negative zinc balance for a period of time before balance is re-established at the lower level of intake [28]. This transient negative zinc balance results in a small loss of zinc from the exchangeable zinc pool. This loss of exchangeable zinc could have a subtle effect on zinc function. However, functional consequences are generally not apparent until the capacity of these adaptive mechanisms is exceeded.

THE IMPORTANCE OF ZINC FOR HUMAN HEALTH

Given the functional diversity of zinc, it is not surprising that multiple physiologic and metabolic functions, such as physical growth, immuno-competence, reproductive function and neuro-behavioural development are all affected by zinc status. When supply of dietary zinc is inadequate to support these functions, biochemical abnormalities and clinical signs may develop. Evidence regarding the effects of zinc status on physiologic function has been derived from three types of studies in human subjects: (1) evaluations of individuals with acrodermatitis enteropathica; (2) the association between markers of zinc status and specific functions; and (3) clinical or community-based intervention trials. In addition, studies in experimental animal models also provide significant insight into the functional consequences of zinc deficiency [55].

Acrodermatitis enteropathica is a rare autosomal recessive genetic disorder that results in zinc malabsorption [62]. The clinical symptoms associated with this disease have provided much insight into the functional outcomes of zinc deficiency and the physiologic roles of zinc. The clinical manifestations include impairment of the dermal, gastrointestinal, neurologic, and immunologic systems [63].

The severity and manifestation of zinc deficiency may vary at different ages [64]. In infants up to 2 months of age, diarrhoea is a prominent symptom [65]. Early zinc deficiency leads to cognitive function impairment, behavioural problems, mood changes, memory impairment, problems with spatial learning, and neuronal atrophy [66]. Other manifestations of zinc deficiency include skin and gastrointestinal problems and anorexia [67]. Alopecia, growth retardation, blepharoconjuctivitis (inflammation of eyelids and conjunctiva), and recurrent infections are common [67].

Evidence for the global public health importance of zinc deficiency has been derived from a series of well-designed randomised controlled trials of zinc supplementation. These were undertaken primarily within the past 20 years, especially in infants and young children of low-income communities. In contrast to studies of acrodermatitis enteropathica where the various clinical symptoms are likely to reflect severe zinc deficiency, functional impairment identified in community-based trials may be more representative of mild or moderate deficiency. These intervention trials have established zinc deficiency as a major contributor to the prevalence of poor physical growth [9], immune function [68], and neurologic or behavioural function [69]. It is important to recognise that results of these studies may be affected by concurrent deficiency of other nutrients.

PUBLIC HEALTH SIGNIFICANCE OF HUMAN ZINC DEFICIENCY

Severe Zinc Deficiency

Organ systems known to be clinically affected by severe zinc deficiency include the epidermal, gastrointestinal, central nervous, immune, skeletal and reproductive systems [70]. It is likely that zinc-dependent metabolic functions are impaired in all tissues. Documented severe zinc deficiency states have ranged from the life-threatening inherited disease acrodermatitis enteropathica [70] and acquired states with similar clinical features to mild growth-limiting deficiency states, mainly in children [1].

The identification of humans with phenotypic presentation of the lethal milk mutation in mice suggest that the likelihood of acrodermatitis enteropathica is related to the inherited defects in zinc transport which may occur in multiple organs [71-72]. The specific biochemical correlates underlying the clinical features have not been readily ascertained. Elucidating the clinical features of severe zinc deficiency states and their biochemical correlates is of value in advancing our understanding of milder zinc deficiency states. Although less impressive in their clinical presentation the latter are of greater importance numerically. Moreover, most of the clinical features of acrodermatitis enteropathica were documented in milder zinc deficiency states.

The clinical and laboratory observations in acrodermatitis enteropathica have assisted us in the identification of parallel consequences of milder acquired zinc deficiency syndromes. Firstly, diarrhoea is prominent as a clinical feature of most cases of acrodermatitis enteropathica [73]. Secondly, a wide variety of immune defects (compromised T-cell function) have long been recognised in acrodermatitis enteropathica, with corresponding vulnerability to a wide range of viral, bacterial, and fungal infections. Thirdly, the central nervous system is affected; the initiation of zinc therapy in acrodermatitis enteropathica is followed by remarkable increases in hedonic tone, motivation, alertness, and responsiveness [74].

Milder Zinc Deficiency States

The recent rapid progress in the recognition of the public health significance of milder, but clinically important, zinc deficiency states, especially in the developing world, coupled with increasing knowledge of the biology of zinc, has given zinc recognition as an important and essential micronutrient in human nutrition. This section provides an overview of the challenges of detecting and determining the prevalence of milder zinc deficiency states and clinical effects and public health relevance.

Measurement of Zinc Status

The most obvious factors that have hampered our understanding of the prevalence of this micronutrient deficiency have been, and continue to be, the lack of adequate laboratory biomarkers [75-76] and the lack of obvious clinical features of zinc deficiency states. Though efforts have been made to determine the worldwide prevalence of zinc deficiency by indirect indicators [77], the lack of a single adequate biomarker [78] has confounded this task.

Serum and plasma zinc concentrations are the most widely used biochemical markers of zinc status. Plasma zinc concentrations remain the best biomarker available and normal ranges have recently been proposed in the US depending on age, gender and time of sample collection [79]. The confounding factor of hypozincemia is the acute phase response to infection [51] as well as the lack of sensitivity necessary to give plasma zinc a strong endorsement as a biomarker of zinc status.

The application of other indices, for example, hair zinc concentrations capable of yielding interesting and useful data [80], have been even less defined [81]. Furthermore, other theoretically more appealing putative biomarkers, notably indices relating to zinc-dependent functions such as activity of a zinc-dependent enzyme, have also been vague. In general, initial enthusiasm has not been followed by convincing application. Typically there has been a lack of independent confirmation of the usefulness of these proposed indices.

Intracellular free zinc is thought to be the pool of zinc utilised for biological function. Intracellular free zinc ions are often confused for "available zinc" which is a component of several intracellular pools. This includes transient free zinc pool and zinc loosely-bound to ligands, including proteins and other compounds that freely donate zinc. It has been proposed that intracellular free zinc is a marker of zinc status. The tools currently available to measure total intracellular zinc include atomic absorption spectrometry (flame and graphite furnace), X-ray microanalysis [82] and nuclear magnetic resonance (NMR). These methods have varying sensitivities to zinc and can be used to quantitatively measure zinc in cellular compartments. However, they say little about the regional distribution and localisation of zinc within the cell. Reports of histochemical visualisation and semi-quantification in singe cells and tissues have become prevalent in recent years primarily because of the development of zinc sensitive fluorimetric probes.

Zinc-sensitive quinoline sulfonamide fluorescent probes were developed in the early 1960s but were not fully evaluated and commercially available until the mid-1980s [83]. Two other quinoline derivatives have been developed; N-(6-methoxy-8-quinolyl-carboxybenzoylsulfonamide) and Δ-methyl-8-p-toluenesulphonamido-6-quinlyloxyacetic acid (Zinquin), which have higher sensitivities to zinc. Zinquin has been used to quantify zinc in thymocytes, human CLL cells, pancreatic islet cells, and hepatocytes [84-87]. Zinquin is an ethyl ester derivative of quinoline and is mainly specific for zinc with cadmium causing weak fluorescence among many metals tested [84]. Zinc binds to Zinquin by either one or two nitrogen atoms to form complexes in a ratio of 1:1 and/or 1:2 (zinc: zinquin) [84]. A unique property of Zinquin is its retention in living cells as the ethyl ester cleaved by cytosolic esterase imparts a negative charge that impedes its efflux across the plasma membrane. However this may also impede its entry into the nucleus and cytoplasmic vesicles [84, 86]. We [88] have used Zinquin to localise zinc in small intestinal sections (Figure 2) but had limited success in measuring the intracellular free zinc pool.

Zinquin is a unique tool that provides high-resolution images of zinc in tissues (Figure 2) and single cells (Figure 3). It is a rapid, inexpensive, and reproducible method with high selectivity for zinc. This method can be used for visualisation and semi-quantitative estimation of zinc pool(s) that can be sequestered by the quinoline sulfonamide moiety [89].

Zinc stable isotope techniques have been implicated in the assessment of zinc status. Specifically, techniques using these isotopes can provide information on how effective the intestine absorbs exogenous dietary zinc and conserves endogenous zinc. Isotopes can estimate the quantity of readily exchangeable zinc in the body [90]. There are 5 naturally occurring stable isotopes of zinc, three of which (^{67}Zn, ^{68}Zn and ^{70}Zn) are present in concentrations low enough to allow enriched preparations in tracer studies of human zinc metabolism [91]. Stable-isotope techniques are safe to use. Other potential advantages over zinc radioisotope techniques include the availability of multiple tracers that can be administered on the same day. These isotopes can be used to track the metabolic fate of zinc, including absorption, retention, excretion of endogenous mineral and turnover rates [92]. Data derived from tracer kinetic techniques based on zinc stable isotopes can provide extensive information on zinc status and bioavailability of dietary zinc, allowing researchers to relate zinc intake to physiologic and pathologic conditions [93].

With a lack of biomarkers deemed adequate to provide reliable estimates of the prevalence and clinical effects of milder zinc deficiency states, information has been dependent to a very large extent on results of well-designed and well-executed randomised intervention studies with dietary zinc supplements. These studies have made a significant contribution to recent progress in impaired physical and neuropsychological development and to the prevalence of gastrointestinal and respiratory infection of many developing communities.

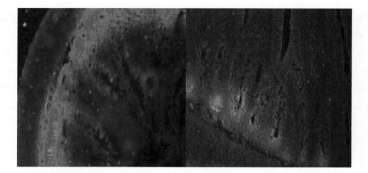

Figure 2. Localisation of zinc mainly in the base of the crypts (in the Paneth cells region) of the jejunum (left panel) and ileum (right panel) in the small intestine of rats as determined by Zinquin fluorescence intensity.

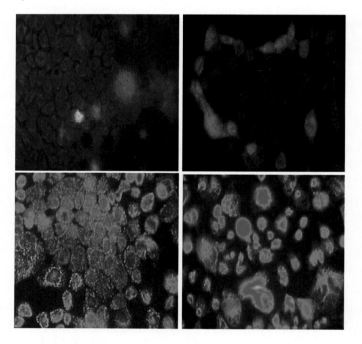

Figure 3. Application of Zinquin in live Caco-2 cells which was incubated with 20 μM ZnSO₄ in the presence of increasing pryrithione concentrations of a zinc ionophore shows increasing Zinquin fluorescence. This demonstrates that zinc concentration within cells can be manipulated. Top left panel; Caco-2 cells with 0 μM pryrithione (auto fluorescence). Top right panel; Caco-2 cells with 0.1 μM pryrithione (low fluorescence). Bottom left panel; Caco-2 cells with 1 μM pryrithione (moderate fluorescence). Bottom right panel; Caco-2 cells with 10 μM pryrithione (high fluorescence).

GROWTH AND DEVELOPMENT

One clinical feature studied mostly is the impairment of physical growth. Given the roles of zinc in DNA replication, RNA transcription, endocrine function and metabolic pathways, it is not surprising that the state of zinc nutrition affects growth and development. As with other features of zinc deficiency, physical growth has been well investigated, although the primary mechanism(s) whereby zinc influences growth is uncertain [55]. The most definitive investigations of zinc deficiency and physical growth have been the Colorado studies in the 1970s and 1980s. Apparently healthy infants [8] and older infants, toddlers or young children with non-organic failure to thrive presented with similar features to mild growth-limiting zinc deficiency states. Subsequently, many studies of zinc supplementation have included growth measurement. As it turned out, these advances were eclipsed by extraordinary progress during the 1990s and the beginning of the millennium. This was primarily attributed to the execution of rigorous and repeated meta-analyses and pooled analyses [9] of multiple high-quality world-wide intervention studies. The confirmation of zinc supplements increasing the height and weight velocity in young children [94] was determined. In some instances, effects have been observed on body composition rather than on weight or linear growth velocity [95-97]. These different responses serve as a reminder of what remains to be learned about variations of zinc deficiency and factors responsible.

Low-Birth Weight Infants

Low birth weight infants (<2500 g at birth) may be vulnerable to zinc deficiency [98]. Studies of low birth weight infants in lower-income countries have demonstrated that weight gain increased among those who received the zinc supplement [99-100]. However, the responses in linear growth have been less consistent. One study reported increased growth among low birth weight Chilean infants [100] but this was not seen in the study in Brazil [99], possibly due to the low zinc supplement (5 mg zinc/day) given for a short period (8 weeks). In a study of low birth weight in premature infants in Canada, a significant increase in linear growth was reported in zinc supplemented female infants only [101].

Severely Malnourished Infants and Children

Studies carried out in Jamaica with severely malnourished hospitalised children revealed increases in weight and lean tissue synthesis with zinc supplementation (~ 2-10 mg zinc/kg body weight/day for 2 weeks) compared to unsupplemented children [102-103]. Subsequent trials in Bangladesh [104-105] have likewise found greater weight gain among severely malnourished inpatients who received supplemented zinc (10 mg zinc/kg body weight/day up to a maximum of 50 mg zinc/day, for 3 weeks) during the course of nutritional rehabilitation. Interestingly, one study [106] demonstrated that severely malnourished inpatients who received 6 mg zinc/kg body weight/day for 15 or 30 days starting immediately after hospital admission had increased mortality compared with similar patients who received 1.5 mg zinc/kg body weight/day. This suggests that excessive zinc may increase the risk of severe complications.

Infants and Children

The effects of zinc supplementation on children's growth were examined in a recently completed meta-analysis of 33 randomised intervention trials conducted in pre-pubertal children [9]. Zinc supplementation significantly increased linear growth and weight gain, but had no effect on weight-for-height indices. Growth responses were greater in children with low initial weight-for-age or height-for-age Z-scores. Thus, the beneficial effect of zinc on children's growth may be limited to a population with evident pre-existing growth failure. The magnitude of the zinc-induced growth impact tended to be greater in studies with younger children, but these age-related differences were not statistically significant, possibly because of the limited number of studies available for analysis. In some studies, zinc supplementation had greater impact in males than in females [107-108]. This may be because males have higher body weight percentages and higher growth rates than females therefore requiring more zinc. This finding however was not consistent in all trials.

Adolescents

The first cases of human zinc deficiency described in the 1960s were reported in male adolescents from the Middle East [3, 109-110]. In this group, zinc deficiency was characterised by delayed sexual development, short stature, anaemia, enlargement of the liver and spleen, and abnormalities in skeletal maturation. Zinc supplementation resulted in significantly increased height, weight, bone development and sexual maturation [111-112]. Decreased sperm count and testosterone levels were also observed during experimental zinc depletion among adolescent males [113]. Zinc supplementation (10 mg zinc /day as zinc sulphate) over 12 months significantly increased height-for-age Z-scores in boys, but not in girls, compared with their unsupplemented counterparts. This was observed in a study of Chilean adolescents with idiopathic short stature [114]. Not many studies have been performed in this age group since these early reports.

DIARRHOEA

It is estimated that diarrhoeal disease causes over three million children's deaths in the developing world each year and contributes substantially to malnutrition in surviving children [115]. The first study for the therapeutic use of oral zinc in acute diarrhoea was conducted by Sachdev et al. [116] in India. Children were between the ages of six months and 18 months. The study found children with low concentrations of rectal mucosal zinc treated with 40 mg elemental zinc had a significant reduction in diarrhoea duration (33%) and severity (18%) compared to those receiving placebo. Early studies in India [117] and Bangladesh [118] demonstrated that children receiving zinc supplements had a 23% and 14% reduction in the duration of diarrhoea, respectively, and the number of watery stools was reduced by 39% and 36%, respectively, compared to unsupplemented children.

Two well documented determinants of diarrhoeal duration are low weight-for-age and decreased cell-mediated immunity [119-120]. A common determinant for both of these factors is zinc deficiency [94, 121]. Zinc deficiency is now known to make a major contribution to the incidence, severity and duration of diarrhoea [115]. Diarrhoea results in increased faecal losses of zinc [122] thereby increasing the risk and severity of zinc deficiency. Infectious diarrhoea has been recognised as a serious public health problem that many developing countries face, particularly among infants and young children. Zinc supplementation in young children during management of acute diarrhoea is not limited to reduced severity and duration of that episode compared with their placebo-treated counterparts [116, 123-125]. In two cases [99, 126] the beneficial effects of zinc supplementation on the incidence of diarrhoea extended beyond the actual period of zinc administration. Furthermore, when zinc was administered (20 mg zinc/day) with each episode of diarrhoea over the course of approximately one year in a controlled, cluster-randomised intervention study, it was found to be associated with a significant reduction in the incidence and duration of acute diarrhoea over the entire year [127]. These results suggest that short-term top-ups of accessible zinc stores are effective in maintaining improved zinc status over a period of several weeks, sufficient to significantly reduce the overall incidence and/or severity of morbidity related to diarrhoea. Similarly, the World Health Organization (WHO/UNICEF) has endorsed a strategy of supplementing 20 mg zinc/day to hospitalised children with diarrhoea [128]. However, the dose chosen is based on an arbitrary choice of dose for major randomized controlled trials.

Recently, a pooled analysis of randomised, controlled trials of zinc supplementation performed in nine lower-income countries (Latin America, the Caribbean, South and Southeast Asia, and the western Pacific) indicated that supplemented zinc led to an 18% reduction in the incidence of diarrhoea and a 25% reduction in diarrhoeal prevalence [10]. Additional zinc supplementation trials in Africa [129-130] also demonstrated significant reductions in the incidence of diarrhoea. The evidence reviewed here regarding the therapeutic or preventive effect of zinc supplementation is based on a substantial number of randomised controlled trials with results being more applicable to the developing world. The mechanisms of the effects of zinc on diarrhoea are unclear. Zinc deficiency is associated with many immunologic deficits. Zinc supplementation has been shown to improve immune function, leading to increased clearance of pathogens in children of developing countries [121, 131]. This issue is considered further in a subsequent section. Other possible mechanisms include effects of zinc deficiency on intestinal permeability [132-134] and intestinal epithelial tissue repair [134-135]. Improved absorption of water and electrolytes by the intestine and increased levels of enterocyte brush-border enzymes have been suggested as possible mechanisms for the beneficial effect of zinc treatment [136].

The use of zinc adjunctive therapy in diarrhoeal disease control strategies in the developing world has the potential to improve the management of diarrhoea and increase survival rates in children. Furthermore, the benefits continue to emerge from epidemiologic and clinical trials. However, information on the dosing regimen and whether zinc should be administered as a separate supplement or as part of a micronutrient mix is yet to be defined. Our published preliminary studies [37] show that ingestion of two doses of 20 mg zinc on consecutive days in the post absorptive state of healthy adults resulted in a 40% reduction in fractional absorption of zinc (FAZ) from 0.56 on day 1 to 0.34 on day 2. In addition, data from a single subject showed that ingestion of a 20 mg zinc oral dose over six consecutive days in the post absorptive state resulted in a 50% reduction in FAZ from 0.49 (day 1) to 0.24 (day 6). However, FAZ (0.53) was unchanged when 20 mg zinc was orally administered with a 6 day interval. These results indicate that FAZ and AZ from single doses are much lower when a 20 mg zinc dose has been administered on previous or several previous days, a circumstance likely to occur in practice with the administration of zinc supplements. In utilising adults for this study [37] we are aware that we cannot extrapolate quantitatively to young children, thus a separate study will need to be conducted in healthy children.

Diarrhoea and Indigenous Australian Children

Infectious diarrhoea among Aborigines of Australia has been recognised as a serious public health problem. For more than three decades it continues to be one of the main causes of under nutrition and widespread failure to thrive [137]. More specifically, Lee et al., [138] investigated the frequency of recurrent gastroenteritis among infants during their first year of life in Western Australia. The authors showed that the proportion of patients with the recurrent disease was also significantly higher for Aborigines (39%) than for non-Aborigines (15%). Childhood hospitalisation patterns in 10 rural Aboriginal community health centres in the Northern Territory of Australia showed the mean admission rates for Aboriginal children aged 0-1 year were two to three times the national average. There was a fourfold excess in the number of days spent in hospital and in the number of deaths before the age of five years for Aboriginal infants and children [137]. Kukuruzovic and Brewster [139] demonstrated that the severity of diarrhoeal disease in Aboriginal children in tropical Australia has a direct influence on the underlying small intestinal mucosal damage which is associated with an intestinal permeability lactulose-rhamnose (L/R) ratio measure. A recent study by Valery et al., [140] demonstrated that there was no clinical benefit of vitamin A, zinc or the two combined in hospitalised young Indigenous Australians in Alice Springs. An increase in the readmission rate for zinc supplemented children was also reported. This may be due to the fact that these children had less disease severity evidenced by absence of hypoxia. Most were over 12 months of age and the majority were not significantly malnourished.

PNEUMONIA

Pneumonia is one of the ancient diseases recognised in both adults and children. In the 1950s bacteria had been recognised as responsible for some causes of pneumonia and despite the development of antibiotics, morbidity and mortality remained high. From 2000 to 2003, it has been reported globally that pneumonia caused approximately 2.0 million (19.6%) of 10.6 million deaths among children younger than 5 years [141]. More than 90% occurred in less developed countries [142]. Pneumonia is responsible for 1-3% of deaths in children aged <5 years in developed countries, and for 10-25% aged <5 years in developing countries [143]. Pooled-analyses of community zinc supplementation studies in children of developing countries have demonstrated a very substantial statistically significant reduction in the prevalence of pneumonia [10]. Pooled-analyses of trials conducted in India, Jamaica, Peru and Vietnam indicate that daily zinc supplementation can reduce incidence of pneumonia by 41% [10].

In a recent study in Bangladesh, zinc together with antimicrobial therapy in young children with pneumonia was associated with significant reduction in the duration of pneumonia compared with control children who received the same antimicrobial therapy without zinc [144]. Comparable benefits of zinc supplementation were reported from a study in Kolkarta, India but for male children only [145]. Other studies [146-147] have reported no benefits of zinc supplements in the management of pneumonia in young children in India. Although Bose et al. [146] have been thorough in reviewing factors that may have accounted for the negative result, no apparent explanation has been forthcoming. Though a pharmacologic effect of zinc is plausible [144], it is widely accepted that the beneficial effects of zinc supplements in the prevention and treatment of diarrhoea and pneumonia are attributed to prevention/correction of zinc deficiency.

In contrast to drug therapy, beneficial effects of zinc supplements in acute management of pneumonia are not expected unless the infant/child is zinc deficient. The mean baseline serum zinc in Bose et al's study [146] was higher than the two studies giving positive results [144-145]. However a wide range of mean baseline serum/plasma zinc has been reported in studies where zinc supplements had a positive effect in preventing diarrhoea and pneumonia [10] or in treating diarrhoea [115]. The study of Bose et al. [146] had cast doubts on the general benefits derived from routine administration of zinc as adjuvant therapy for pneumonia in young children of the developing world. The authors indicate a priority need for additional studies in representative populations.

Pneumonia and Indigenous Australian Children

The incidence of pneumonia in Australian children (<18 years of age) is about 5-8 per 1000 persons per year and is a major cause of hospital admissions in children less than 5 years of age [148]. Indigenous children are at a 10-20 fold higher risk of hospitalisation compared to non-Indigenous children [148]. In a study of all Western Australia live births in 1986, 5% of non-Indigenous and 17% of Indigenous children were admitted to hospital with a diagnosis of pneumonia in the first two years of life [149]. 11% of the Indigenous children had repeated admissions with pneumonia. Another study showed that out of 200 consecutive patients admitted to Cairns Hospital, Australia, during 1992 with a diagnosis of pneumonia, half were Indigenous patients [150]. Furthermore, in an early retrospective study [151] surveying all children in the district of Bourke, New South Wales, Australia, and carried out over a three year period to determine the frequency of pneumonia in the first years of life, 25.2% of Indigenous children had one or more episodes of pneumonia, compared with 3% of non-Indigenous children. These data reveal that Indigenous children have a very high rate of pneumonia. Effective treatment strategies are required if admissions and deaths are to decrease.

A recent study by Chang et al. [152] in hospitalised young Indigenous Australians with pneumonia reported similar findings to Bose et al. [146], that zinc and/or vitamin A supplementation showed no clinical benefit. The authors concluded that the effect of supplementation may depend on the prevalence of deficiency of these micronutrients in the population. The negative results from these studies [146, 152] compared to the meta-analysis in developing countries demonstrate the importance of further studies. Interestingly, it has been demonstrated that rural Aboriginal children in the Northern Territory, Australia, that were involved in a pilot study have a very low zinc absorption capacity consistent with underlying environmental enteropathy (unpublished data).

Bose et al. [146] suggested that more studies are needed in a variety of populations before rational policy recommendations can be made on the role of zinc in the treatment of severe pneumonia. Currently, there are 4 studies in progress, two in Africa and two in Nepal. As in the trial of Bose et al. the possibility exists that the study groups may not be zinc deficient and therefore show no benefit from zinc supplementation [153].

MALARIA

Malaria is a major cause of morbidity and mortality in tropical and subtropical regions. Malaria often occurs in populations that are both impoverished and malnourished with a large burden falling on the most vulnerable within the population; children, and pregnant women [154].

Randomised, placebo-controlled studies in Gambia [155] and Papua New Guinea [156] suggest that zinc supplementation reduces the morbidity of *Plasmodium falciparum* infections. The trial conducted in Gambia demonstrated a 32% reduction in clinic visits due to *P. falciparum* infections among those given 70 mg zinc twice weekly for 18 months [155]. Similarly, the trial in Papua New Guinea showed a 38% reduction in clinic visits attributable to *P. falciparum* parasitemia among pre-school children when 10 mg zinc daily was administered [156]. Furthermore, zinc supplementation resulted in a 69% reduction in clinical based malarial episodes (with high densities of *P. falciparum* parasites in the blood). In contrast a study conducted in Africa did not find any reduction in episodes of *falciparum* malaria among children who received 10 mg zinc daily for 6 months [129]. In a recent randomised, placebo-controlled clinical trial [157] daily supplementation of iron and zinc provided protection against *Plasmodium vivax* malaria in younger children, suggesting there may be a potential role of zinc in the prevention of malaria.

IMMUNE FUNCTION AND RISK OF INFECTION

The defenses against infection are particularly sensitive to disturbances in zinc status. Zinc is known to play a central role in the immune system, where zinc deficient persons experience increased susceptibility to a variety of pathogens [121].The mechanism by which zinc effects the immune system is multifactorial; from the barrier of the skin to gene regulation within lymphoctyes. Zinc deficiency decreases all kinds of immune cell function.

In monocytes, all functions are impaired, in natural killer cells, cytotoxicity is decreased, and in neutrophil granulocytes, phagocytosis is reduced [158].

Zinc effects both non-specific and specific immune functions at a variety of levels. The effects of zinc on immune functions are mediated via its possible antioxidant properties, via release of glucocorticoids and via a decrease in thymulin activity, [55, 121]. In terms of non-specific immunity, zinc affects the integrity of the epithelial barrier. It has been proposed that zinc has a protective role in airway epithelium against oxyradicals and other noxious agents [159], and this may have important implications in inflammatory diseases where the physical barrier is compromised. Zinc deficiency also compromises the function of neutrophils, natural killer cells, macrophages, polymorphonuclear leukocytes, and complement activity [121]. Zinc plays a specific role in the signal transduction of monocytes, in particular, activation and inhibition of signalling pathways interacting with signal transduction of pathogen sensing receptors, eventually leading to secretion of pro-inflammatory cytokines [160].

With regards to specific immunity, lymphopoenia and declined T and B lymphocyte function occur in zinc deficiency, as do alterations in the balance of T helper cell population (Th1 and Th2) and cytokine production [55]. More specifically, zinc deficiency effects development of acquired immunity by preventing both the outgrowth and functions of T lymphocytes such as activation, Th1 cytokine production, and B lymphocyte help. Likewise, B lymphocyte development and antibody production, particularly immunoglobulin G, is compromised. The macrophage, a pivotal cell in many immunologic functions, is adversely affected by zinc deficiency which may dysregulate intracellular killing, cytokine production and phagocytosis [121]. The effects of zinc on these key immunologic mediators is not surprising given its numerous roles in basic cellular function such as DNA replication, RNA transcription, cell division, and cell activation. Furthermore, given the ubiquitous involvement of zinc in cellular functions, ranging from gene expression and membrane stability [13], it is difficult to explain the effect of zinc on immunity solely on changing cell number. The specific links between zinc-related aspects of immune function and the incidence and severity of different infections are not well understood. The documented changes in immune function are clinically important because decreased rates of infection such as diarrhoea, pneumonia and malaria have been observed following zinc supplementation in population-based studies as described above.

Most knowledge of the effect of zinc on immune function has been derived from experimental animals or *in vitro* models. Several studies have shown that perturbations of zinc status can affect immune competence in adult human subjects [161-165]. Elderly subjects who received zinc supplements demonstrated improvements in delayed cutaneous hypersensitivity [165-166], improvements in the number of circulating T cells, and serum IgG antibody response to tetanus toxoid [166]. Studies involving induced mild zinc deficiency states in human subjects, reduced serum thymulin and IL-2 activity, and reductions in specific subpopulations of lymphocytes occurred [160, 167]. Impaired immune functions due to zinc deficiency are shown to be reversed by an adequate zinc supplementation, which is adapted to the actual requirements of the patient. High dosages of zinc evoke negative effects on immune cells and show alterations that are similar to those observed with zinc deficiency [158].

NEUROPSYCHOLOGICAL PERFORMANCE

There have been limited studies of zinc supplementation examining the effects on activity or development among infants and children. Some studies have provided evidence that zinc deficiency contributes to compromised neuro-behavioural function among infants and children [168]. A study [101] among very low birth weight infants showed improved developmental scores when they received supplemental zinc in formula. Evidence of improved brain development attributed to improved zinc status has been derived from studies in young children in India [169] and Guatemala [170]. Furthermore, improvements in neuropsychological performance have been reported with zinc supplementation in young Chinese children when other micronutrients were given [171-172].

In contrast, other studies concluded that zinc supplementation in infants and young children failed to improve mental development. In a randomised, double-blind, placebo-controlled trial of zinc supplementation in children aged between 12-18 months, zinc did not affect the mental or psychomotor development index scores in a setting where zinc deficiency is common [173]. In another trial in which full term infants were supplemented with zinc for 5 months, mental development scores were lower compared to the placebo, although the effects were small [174]. The improvement in motor development and behaviour with zinc supplementation is also consistent with other studies [175-176] in particular in low birth weight infants.

The exact mechanism of how zinc may influence cognition and motor functioning is still unclear. However, it is postulated that in the central nervous system, zinc is concentrated in the synaptic vesicles of specific glutaminergic neurons [26]. During synaptic events, zinc is released and passed into postsynaptic neurons, serving as a neurotransmitter. Zinc is considered to be essential for nucleic acid and protein synthesis. Zinc deficiency may interfere with these processes and compromise subsequent development [177]. Furthermore, zinc deficiency may be particularly relevant to early development because it plays fundamental roles in cell division and maturation, and in the growth and function of many organ systems, including the central nervous system [26].

The evidence linking zinc supplementation to early cognition and motor development is inconclusive. However, there are suggestions that zinc supplementation may promote activity and perhaps motor development in the most vulnerable infants. This in turn is thought to promote cognitive development by enabling children to be more independent to explore their surroundings [177]. Although initial findings provide some convincing evidence linking zinc deficiency to compromises in activity and motor development, additional research is needed to examine the impact of timing and severity of zinc deficiency, its reversibility and its long-term consequences.

RELEVANCE TO CHILDHOOD
MORBIDITY AND MORTALITY RATES

In a recent review [178] it has been reported that more than 10 million children under the age of 5 years die each year. In addition, zinc has been ranked number four in effectiveness out of all biological agents or actions that can reduce mortality. It was calculated that this agent alone could save a minimum of 350,000 young children from death each year. Furthermore, its use as a treatment intervention would avert an additional 400,000 deaths per year, i.e. a total of three-quarters of a million lives saved [179]. The majority of child deaths are caused by neonatal disorders (34%), diarrhoea (23%), pneumonia (21%) and malaria (10%). Additionally, zinc deficiency increases the risk of mortality from diarrhoea, pneumonia and malaria by 13-21% [180].

It has been estimated that the beneficial effects of zinc supplementation for diarrhoea prevention are of the same magnitude as those achieved by cleaning the water supply and providing quality sanitation in appropriate areas. In one study involving full-term, small-for-gestational-age infants in north India, daily zinc supplementation of 1-5 mg zinc/day, from 15-30 days of age, followed by 5 mg zinc/day, from 30 days of age til 269 days of age, significantly reduced mortality by 67% compared with the control group that did not receive zinc supplements [181]. Another smaller trial of older children in Africa [130] found that mortality from all causes was reduced by more than 50% among those who received zinc supplements, although this difference was not statistically significant.

A study by Sazawal and colleagues [182] reported an overall non-significant 7% reduction in mortality in a randomised trial of daily zinc supplementation in children aged 1-48 months residing in Zanzibar. More specifically, a significant reduction in mortality was noted in children aged 12-48 months. Furthermore, the authors suggest that a meta-analysis of all studies of mortality and morbidity will help to make evidence-based recommendations for the role of zinc supplementation in public health policy that would improve mortality, morbidity, growth, and development in young children.

The sum of recent evidence indicates that maintenance of optimal zinc nutrition, even if only partial, is perhaps the most effective preventive measure that can be undertaken to reduce morbidity rates in young children in the developing world. Moreover, the recent experience with reduced infectious disease morbidity and mortality in well designed randomized controlled trials of zinc supplements administered to young children has high-lighted zinc deficiency as a public health problem of global proportions [178]. This applies especially to diarrhoea and pneumonia, the most prevalent causes of infectious disease mortality in young children world wide. Furthermore, zinc supplements as a preventive modality notably for pneumonia has been associated with decreased mortality [182].

MATERNAL HEALTH AND PREGNANCY OUTCOMES

Reproductive functions have been examined in relation to zinc status during pregnancy. The outcomes include foetal growth, timing, sequencing and efficiency of labour and delivery, the incidence of stillbirths and congenital malformations. Early studies have indicated that poor maternal zinc status in pregnancy can have adverse effects on foetal brain development [183]. Adverse outcomes associated with zinc status in zinc supplementation trials during pregnancy include intrauterine growth retardation, low birth weight, poor foetal neuro-behavioural development and increased neonatal morbidity. Adverse maternal outcomes include preterm delivery and pregnancy-induced hypertension. Other possible consequences of maternal zinc deficiency on pregnancy have been suggested. These suggestions were made from clinical observations of women with acrodermatitis enteropathica and from cross-sectional studies of maternal zinc status. Most of the zinc supplementation trials have measured only a subset of the possible outcomes described above.

Of the randomised, placebo-controlled zinc supplementation trials there were a handful conducted in developing countries: South Africa [184], India [185], Peru [186], and Bangladesh [187]. Some of the trials reported no effect on pregnancy outcomes. Two studies found significantly improved foetal growth, as measured by birth weight. One of these studies was carried out in the US among African American women with below average plasma zinc concentrations [188] and the other was conducted among poor urban Indian women [185]. Significant reductions in preterm deliveries were reported in three of the zinc supplementation trials [185, 188-189]. Two studies observed reductions in the incidence of maternal complications [190-191], in particular reduction in pregnancy-induced hypertension in Hispanic Californian women [190]. However, a similar study conducted among Hispanic adolescents in California did not show any effect of zinc supplementation on blood pressure [192].

A study in Peru [183] involving the addition of zinc with iron and folate during pregnancy resulted in greater foetal heart rate and foetal movements, indicators of foetal neurobehavioral development, compared with those receiving only iron and folate. One study [194] showed that zinc supplementation during pregnancy had no effect on birth weight. However, a follow-up study found that the risks of acute diarrhoea, dysentery and impetigo at 6 months were lower among infants whose mothers had received zinc supplements during pregnancy. Furthermore, another follow-up study on the same infants at 13 months of age did not show an effect on mental development or behaviour [195].

The results of zinc supplementation trials during pregnancy have been inconsistent. Several reasons may account for these discrepancies including; small sample sizes, varying degrees of underlying zinc deficiency, differing levels and periods of supplementation and differing measures used for pregnancy outcome. Failure to account for confounding factors, including concurrent nutrient deficiencies also contributed to discrepancies. In some cases, the studies were conducted in unselected women who were unlikely to be zinc deficient [196-197]. However, there is considerable information from animal studies, human observational studies and intervention trials that indicate maternal zinc nutrition influence several aspects of reproductive function and pregnancy outcomes. More double-blind, placebo-controlled trials among pregnant women are needed in developing countries where an elevated risk of zinc deficiency is evident and poor foetal growth is prevalent. Studies in the developing world are beginning to give needed attention to pregnancy and the effects of maternal zinc status on both prenatal and postnatal development [186].

HUMAN ZINC REQUIREMENTS

Theoretically, there are at least six strategies that could be used to assist in the estimation of dietary zinc requirements. These include, estimating habitual intakes in populations without evidence of zinc deficiency, using biomarkers of zinc status, utilising functional indices of zinc deficiency, combining baseline dietary intake data with results of zinc supplementation, using zinc balance data, and utilising the factorial approach [198]. Despite the limited data available, the latter approach offers the most useful strategy for estimating requirements. The WHO, Food and Agriculture Organisation (FAO), International Atomic Energy Association (IAEA) and the Food and Nutrition Board (FNB) of the US Institute of Medicine (IOM) have convened expert committees to develop estimates of human zinc requirements and propose corresponding dietary intakes needed to satisfy these requirements [55, 57, 199-200].

For most age and physiologic groups, the committee used a factorial method to estimate the average physiologic zinc requirement. It is defined as the amount of zinc that must be absorbed in order to offset the amount of endogenous zinc lost from both intestinal and non-intestinal sites [55]. Non-intestinal sources of zinc loss include urine, desquamated skin, hair, nails, sweat, and in adolescents and adults, semen and menstrual flow [57]. Two groups of special concern are young children and pregnant women, where the amount of zinc retained in newly accrued tissue is factored into total physiologic needs. In lactating women the zinc transferred in breast milk is also added to the requirements [198]. The estimation of average physiologic zinc requirement assumes that the amount of zinc lost from non-intestinal sites is fixed, because the losses are generally constant across a wide range of zinc intakes [57]. In contrast, intestinal excretion of endogenous zinc varies considerably in relation to the amount of zinc absorbed. Therefore, the figure used for intestinal loss of endogenous zinc is appropriately estimated as the level that occurs when total absorbed zinc is adequate to meet the theoretical physiologic needs.

Adult Men

The FNB/IOM committee estimated mean urinary zinc excretion by adult males to be 0.63 mg zinc/day, based on 17 previously published studies of individuals whose zinc intake (4 to 25 mg zinc/day) was within the range at which urinary concentrations are not influenced by zinc intake [57]. The figure derived from the FNB/IOM committee was reliable because a large number of studies were reviewed; including studies where zinc intakes had fallen within the range urinary excretion is constant. The figure is thus likely to include true physiologic requirement. The committee also provided extensive documentation of the analytic processes [55].

The FNB/IOM report also considered one study of integument and sweat loss of zinc [201], carried out in 11 adult males whose mean zinc losses of 0.54 mg zinc/day did not change in response to different levels of dietary zinc intakes (1.4 to 10.3 mg zinc/day) during periods of 28-35 days. Thus, the figure was used as surface losses of endogenous zinc can be translated to per kg body weight i.e., 6.5 µg/kg, as derived from Johnson et al. [201]. Therefore, a 65 kg adult man will lose 0.42 mg zinc/day via integument.

The FNB/IOM report also considered zinc loss in semen. The information was derived from two studies [201-202] where the concentration of zinc in semen and ejaculate volume was assessed in 11 volunteers. The men's semen zinc concentration (0.11 mg zinc/ml) did not change with restricted dietary zinc intake. However the ejaculate volume decreased at the lowest level of zinc intake (1.4 mg zinc/day). Thus, a figure of 0.10 mg zinc loss/day in semen was used, considering a mean ejaculate volume of 2.8 ml and a mean number of 2.45 ejaculations per week.

To estimate the intestinal loss of endogenous zinc, the FNB/IOM committee analysed 10 studies from 7 published articles [203-209]. The studies measured total absorbed zinc and intestinal excretion of endogenous zinc using radio- or stable-isotope techniques, where absorbed zinc was estimated from a whole day's dietary intake [55]. Studies that were conducted in North America or Europe involving a mean 19-50 years of age were accepted in the analysis. From the analysis it was concluded that excretion of endogenous zinc via the intestine is a major variable in the maintenance of zinc homeostasis and is strongly correlated with absorbed zinc [205-206]. Also, to estimate the physiologic requirement for absorbed zinc, it would be necessary to consider the amount of intestinal losses of endogenous zinc that would occur when the absorbed zinc is just sufficient to offset the sum of all sources of endogenous zinc lost from both intestinal and non-intestinal sites. Using the factorial approach, the FNB/IOM committee estimated that 2.57 mg zinc/day of endogenous zinc would be excreted in faeces when the amount of absorbed zinc is equivalent to the total losses of endogenous zinc from all sources. The physiologic requirement for absorbed zinc in adult men is therefore 3.84 mg zinc/day, with endogenous losses of 0.63 mg zinc/day from urine, 0.54 mg zinc/day from integument and sweat, 0.10 mg zinc/day from semen, and 2.57 mg zinc/day in faeces [55]. The estimate of the physiologic requirement for absorbed zinc derived from these data is illustrated in Figure 4.

Another committee, the International Zinc Nutrition Consultative Group (IZiNCG) suggested that an internationally relevant estimate of zinc requirement would be more appropriate [55]. Thus the IZiNCG committee expanded the database used in this analysis to include all available studies of apparently healthy men and women, regardless of age and race. The committee identified nine new studies (from 5 published articles) to include the new regression analysis of intestinal excretion of endogenous zinc and absorbed zinc [60, 210-213]. Prior to analysis, the relationship between total absorbed zinc and faecal losses of endogenous zinc was explored to determine whether there were any differences between the new set of studies added and to those used previously by the FNB/IOM. There were no significant differences in the slopes and intercepts of the respective best-fit lines. Furthermore, no significant difference in absorbed zinc and endogenous faecal losses of zinc was found with common food, semi-purified or formula diets. In addition, there were no significant differences in this relationship between men and women. The relationship between total absorbed zinc and endogenous faecal zinc of the 19 studies from 12 published studies [60, 203-213] is shown in Figure 5. Based on the combined data set derived from the IZiNCG committee, 1.54 mg zinc/day of endogenous zinc would be excreted in faeces when the amount of absorbed zinc is equivalent to the total losses of endogenous zinc from all sources, and the physiologic requirement for absorbed zinc in adult men is 2.69 mg zinc/day. That is, with endogenous losses of 0.63 mg zinc/day from urine, 0.42 mg zinc/day from integument and sweat, 0.10 mg zinc/day from semen, and 1.54 mg zinc/day in faeces, it would be necessary to replace a total of 2.69 mg zinc/day [55].

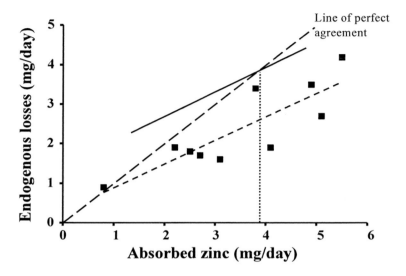

Figure 4. The model used by FNB/IOM [57] to estimate intestinal endogenous losses of zinc and total endogenous losses of zinc, when the amount of absorbed zinc is sufficient to offset all losses. The data points represent mean data from 7 published studies [203-209] of zinc absorption and intestinal losses of endogenous zinc in adult men (19-50 years of age). The regression dashed line represents the relationship between intestinal excretion of endogenous zinc and absorbed zinc. The parallel solid line represents the total endogenous losses of zinc after adding losses through urine, integument, and semen. The dashed line of perfect agreement indicates where total endogenous losses would be equal to the amount of absorbed zinc. The vertical dashed line is derived from the point where the total endogenous losses of zinc crosses with the line of perfect agreement, indicating the physiologic requirement for absorbed zinc in adult men (3.84 mg zinc/day).

Adult Women

The FNB/IOM and IZiNCG committees estimated women's surface losses of zinc by adjusting for differences in body surface area to extrapolate from the data available from men [55]. The same urinary losses of zinc for men, after adjusting for body size, were adopted for adult women (i.e., 0.0065 mg zinc/kg body weight/day × 55 kg = 0.36 mg zinc/day). There is limited information on endogenous losses in menstrual fluid. In a study [214], the average excretion of menstrual fluid during a single period was 60g, and the mean zinc content was 2.8 μg/g menstrual fluid or 154 μg during each menstrual period. This equates to an average daily zinc loss of 5 μg zinc/day. The IZiNCG reported [55] that loss of zinc by this route is negligible and can be ignored in estimates of zinc requirements. Using the regression analysis model (Figure 5), the amount of intestinal losses of endogenous zinc that occur in women is 1.06 mg zinc/day when the amount of absorbed zinc is just sufficient to offset the sum of all sources of endogenous zinc loss (1.86 mg zinc/day) from both intestinal and non-intestinal sites [55].

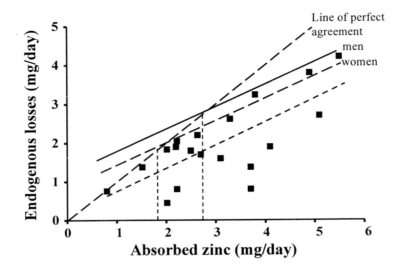

Figure 5. The model used by IZiNCG [55] to estimate intestinal endogenous losses of zinc and total endogenous losses of zinc, when the amount of absorbed zinc is sufficient to offset all losses. The data points represent mean data from 12 published studies [60, 203-213] of zinc absorption and intestinal losses of endogenous zinc in adult men (19-50 years of age). The regression dashed line represents the relationship between intestinal excretion of endogenous zinc and absorbed zinc. The parallel solid line and dashed line represents the total endogenous losses of zinc for men and women, respectively. The dashed line of perfect agreement indicates where total endogenous losses would be equal to the amount of absorbed zinc. The vertical dashed lines are derived from the point where the total endogenous losses of zinc crosses with the line of perfect agreement, indicating the physiologic requirement for absorbed zinc for adult men is 3.84 mg zinc/day and adult women is 1.86 mg zinc/day, respectively This is based on the assumption that the average body weight of adult men and women are 71 and 61 kg, respectively.

Children

Infants 0-6 Months

There is limited information available on physiologic requirement for absorbed zinc in infants less than 6 months of age. However, there is evidence that young infants may acquire a portion of their zinc needs by mobilising hepatic reserves accumulated during gestation [215].

Due to little empirical information on zinc homeostasis in this age group, the FNB/IOM committee did not estimate physiologic requirement of zinc. Instead, they made presumptions about the adequate intakes, based on the content of zinc in breast milk at different ages and the average amount of milk consumed. It is important to note that total zinc transferred through milk falls from 2.5 mg zinc/day at one month to approximately 0.8 mg zinc/day at six months [57]. Based on the average figures for zinc transfer in breast milk from 0-5 months post-partum, the FNB/IOM decided that 2.0 mg zinc/day was the adequate intake for infants in this age range [55, 198].

Another committee from WHO developed estimates of physiologic zinc requirements for young infants by extrapolating from adult data. Using this approach, the WHO committee suggested that the requirement for absorbed zinc from 0-5 months of age ranged from 0.7-1.3 mg zinc/day, depending on age and sex. The IZiNCG committee with the available information suggested that breast milk is a sufficient source of zinc for exclusively breastfed, normal-birth weight term infants until six months of age [55, 216]. However, in for non-exclusively breastfed infants the requirement is to absorb approximately 1.3 mg zinc/day during the first three months of life and 0.7 mg zinc/day during months 3-5.

Children 6 months to 18 years

The estimation of physiologic requirements of zinc in older infants and children were based on extrapolations from adults per unit body weight. Losses of endogenous zinc from non-intestinal sites (urinary and surface losses) were estimated at 0.014 mg zinc/kg/day [55]. Faecal excretion of endogenous zinc was estimated at 0.050 mg zinc/kg/day for infants 6-11 months of age (based on data obtained from breastfed infants) and 0.034 mg zinc/kg/day for older children (as extrapolated from adult data) [55]. In applying a factorial approach to children, retention required for growth has to be considered. The best estimate available is derived from chemical analysis of the whole body [217], which gives an average figure of approximately 20 mg per kg of new tissue. Therefore to determine the physiologic requirements of zinc in infants and older children, the faecal excretion of endogenous losses were added to the amount of zinc required for growth, which is estimated to be 0.020 mg zinc/g of tissue gained [198]. This was then multiplied by the reference body weight and the expected rate of weight gain at different ages. For male adolescents aged between 14-18 years, an additional 0.1 mg zinc/day was included in the estimated physiologic requirements to account for losses in semen. The total endogenous zinc losses are calculated at 0.064 mg zinc/kg/day for infants 6-11 months of age and 0.034 mg zinc/kg/day for children one year and older (urinary losses 0.0075 mg zinc/kg/day, surface losses 0.0065 mg zinc/kg/day, and intestinal losses of 0.05 mg zinc/kg/day for infants 6-11 months or 0.02 mg zinc/kg/day for children one year and older [55]).

For children 6-11 months of age who have a reference body weight of 9 kg and expected weight gain of 13 g/day, 0.576 mg zinc/day (i.e. 9 kg × 0.064 mg zinc/day) is needed to replace endogenous losses and 0.260 mg zinc/day (13 g/day × 0.020 mg zinc/day) for tissue accrual, thus resulting in total physiologic requirement of 0.84 mg zinc/day. The total physiologic requirements of zinc in children 1-3, 4-8, 9-13 and 14-18 years of age are 0.53, 0.83, 1.53, 2.52 (males) is 1.98 mg zinc/day (females) respectively [55].

Pregnancy

Accumulation of zinc in newly formed foetal and maternal tissue during pregnancy imposes an additional physiologic requirement for zinc. The FNB/IOM committee estimated these additional zinc needs as 0.16 mg zinc/day during the first trimester of pregnancy, 0.39

mg zinc/day during the second trimester and 0.63 mg zinc/day during the third trimester [218]. Similarly, WHO provided comparable estimates, 0.1 mg zinc/day during the first trimester, 0.3 mg zinc/day during the second trimester and 0.7 mg zinc/day for the third trimester [219]. For convenience the IZiNCG committee provided a single figure of 0.7 mg zinc/day, which covers the amount of additional zinc that needs to be absorbed during pregnancy [55].

Lactation

The amount of zinc transferred from mother to infant in breast milk must be added to lactating women's physiologic requirement for absorbed zinc. This amount was calculated by multiplying the average volume of milk transferred to the infant by the zinc concentration of human milk at different periods of post-partum. The FNB/IOM committee applied milk volume (0.78 L/day) that was measured in US women during the first year post-partum [57] as well as summarising the results of 12 studies to provide age-specific information on zinc concentration of human milk (2.75 mg zinc/L at 4 weeks, 2.0 mg zinc/L at 8 weeks, 1.5 mg zinc/L at 12 weeks and 1.2 mg zinc/L at 24 weeks). From this information a single estimate of 1.35 mg zinc/day for the average additional amount of absorbed zinc is needed to support lactation [55].

It was noted by the IZiNCG committee that women from developing countries typically breast feed for longer periods compared to US women, and breast milk volume changes with infant age. The committee decided to estimate zinc transfer in breast milk using data on milk output from women in developing countries [219]. The additional zinc needs imposed by lactation are considerable, especially during the early months of breastfeeding. Thus, on average about 1 mg of additional zinc must be absorbed during lactation [55].

ESTIMATES OF AVERAGE DIETARY ZINC REQUIREMENTS

Two committees developing dietary reference values were the FAO/WHO/IAEA Expert Consultation [199-200] and the US FNB/IOM Standing Committee on Evaluation of Dietary Reference Intakes [57]. Each committee extracted data from studies of zinc absorption and plotted the mean amount of absorbed zinc against the total zinc ingested. A regression equation was derived from the data and used to determine the amount of total zinc needed for ingestion so that the amount of absorbed zinc would be equivalent to the physiologic requirement. This amount of total zinc ingested represents the daily "estimated average requirement" (EAR) from the diet [55].

The IZiNCG committee reviewed the methods used by the two committees to estimate zinc absorption. Methodology used to measure absorption, the types of diets and subjects from which data were derived as well as the models used were taken into account [55]. The IZiNCG committee considered studies that used total-diet studies (multiple meals consumed over one day) to estimate dietary zinc requirement for two main reasons. Firstly, these studies were able to estimate true zinc absorption for each individual by correcting for simultaneous intestinal losses of endogenous zinc that occur during digestion. Secondly, there is evidence from these studies that the percentage iron absorption measured from a single meal differs significantly from that measured from a total diet [220-221]. Furthermore, the IZiNCG committee felt it was important to consider differences in zinc absorption based on diet type and dietary content of known inhibitors (eg. phytate) of zinc absorption [222]. In addition, to ensure the absorption estimate to be internationally representative, the IZiNCG committee discarded studies that included semi-purified zinc or diets that included exogenous sources of zinc in the form of salts [55]. The regression curve used to derive the zinc absorption estimate included both men and women.

Initially, 17 data points from 11 published articles meeting the IZiNCG committee's criteria were identified [55]. Zinc and phytate contents of study diets were available for 15 studies derived from nine separate published articles [60, 203, 209-213, 223-224]. The data were log transformed and a logit regression model was used to describe the relationship between absorbed zinc and total zinc intake. The final model (r^2 = 0.413, p<0.001) includes zinc and the phytate:zinc molar ratio, both of which are significant predictors of zinc absorption [55]. The range of phytate:zinc molar ratios were divided into two categories; 4-18 which represents mixed or refined vegetarian diets and 18-30, which represents unrefined, cereal-based diets. The midpoint of the range of the phytate:zinc molar ratios was used, that is 11 and 24 for each category. Finally, a curve is generated showing the relationship between total zinc intake and absorbed zinc for the two diet categories (Figure 6). Using the curves and the physiologic requirement for absorbed zinc of adult men (2.69 mg zinc/day) and women (1.86 mg zinc/day), the amount of total zinc intake needed to meet this requirement was determined for each diet type. This amount represents the average dietary zinc requirement (Figure 6).

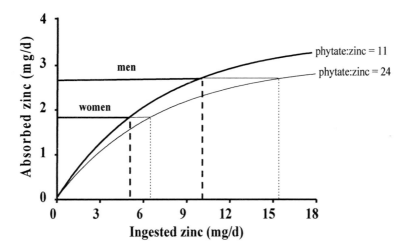

Figure 6. Derivation of the estimated average requirement of zinc for men and women of zinc absorption for mixed/refined vegetarian diets (phytate:zinc = 11) and unrefined cereal-based diets (phytate:zinc = 24), using the relationship between total zinc intake and absorbed zinc for each type of diet and physiologic requirement [55].

The IZiNCG committee felt there was no justification assuming different levels of zinc absorption for different age groups. Therefore the mean absorption figures for adult men and women from each diet type were applied to children 1-18 years of age (31% absorption from mixed/ refined vegetarian diets and 23% from unrefined, cereal-based diets) [55]. Zinc absorption is not increased during pregnancy [61]. Therefore, zinc absorption estimates being the same for pregnant and non-pregnant women were applied to each diet type [55]. In contrast, zinc absorption increases significantly during lactation [61, 225]. As there is insufficient data to determine whether lactating women were meeting their zinc requirement, it is preferable to assume the figure of 10% increased absorption as determined by Fung et al. [61].

ZINC TOXICITY

Animals, including humans, exhibit considerable tolerance to high intakes of zinc. Zinc is not mutagenic and has little, if any, clastogenic properties. It does not represent a carcinogenic risk to man, and is not teratogenic [226]. However, manifestations of overt toxicity symptoms such as nausea, vomiting, epigastric pain, lethargy, and fatigue will occur with extremely high zinc intakes, corresponding to 225-450 mg of zinc [227]. Longer term studies have suggested that lower supplemental doses may compromise the immune system [228] and *in vitro* studies have indicated adverse effects of excessive zinc on the function of the central nervous system [26]. One study has reported adverse effects on cognitive development with the administration of 20 mg zinc supplements to toddlers in Bangladesh [229]. There are mutual interactions between zinc and iron and zinc and copper in doses of zinc that are given as supplements to young children [230-231]. Doses of 25-35 mg zinc/day in adults do not appear to pose a health hazard. While the overall toxicity of zinc may be relatively low, it is undesirable, even if only as a general principal to administer excessive quantities.

The WHO/FAO/IAEA derived the upper limits of zinc intakes [199-200] based on the observation that 60 mg of supplemental zinc/day resulted in adverse interactions with other nutrients. It considered intakes not to exceed this amount. After accounting for a 25% possible variation in population intakes, the upper limit for males was set at 45 mg/day. The upper limits for adult males were extrapolated to other age and sex groups based on differences in metabolic rates [55].

CAUSES OF ZINC DEFICIENCY

The aetiology of zinc deficiency can be attributed to at least five general causes occurring either in isolation or in combination. These include inadequate intake, increased requirements, malabsorption, increased losses and impaired utilisation [232]. Dietary factors are a major contributor to zinc deficiency. Breast milk is an excellent source of zinc in early infancy, but by 6 months of age intake from breast milk is very limited [233] and early complementary foods are typically low in zinc worldwide. Meat, the major source of bioavailable zinc in the diet is not a common early complementary food and is typically lacking from the diet of older infants and young children in developing populations. Whole cereal grains and beans contain considerable amounts of zinc but also phytic acid which reduces the bioavailability of this micronutrient.

Several estimates of dietary zinc intakes indicate that inadequacy is widespread, occurring across a wide variety of geographical areas and dietary patterns [234]. Low intakes of absorbable zinc are further exacerbated by physiologic or pathologic conditions that lead to greater requirement for zinc, which in turn increases the risk of zinc deficiency.

Malabsorption of zinc may result in a number of different conditions. Acrodermatitis enteropathica is a rare genetic defect that specifically affects zinc absorption. Inflammatory bowel disease may result in poor absorption and/or losses of zinc from the body. Excess losses of zinc occur in diarrhoeal disease [65]. These are sufficient to increase the physiologic requirement for zinc threefold, i.e. the quantity of zinc that the body needs to absorb making diarrhoea a major aetiological factor in populations where early childhood diarrhoea is common.

Impaired utilisation of zinc may occur as a result of administration of certain drugs (ethambutol, halogenated 8-hydroxyquinolines, penacillamine) that chelate zinc systematically and make it less available for use by tissues [235]. The presence of infection results in the sequestration of zinc in the liver [236] with circulating levels decreasing. In response to infection-induced secretion of interleukin-1 and tumour necrosis factor-alpha, by monocytes and activated macrophages, there is increased hepatic synthesis of metallothionein, an intracellular metal-binding ligand [237]. Subsequently increased hepatic uptake of zinc and reduction of serum zinc concentration occurs. It is not known whether these alterations in zinc metabolism may benefit the host by making more zinc available in the liver or by reducing zinc availability in the peripheral blood.

PREVENTION AND MANAGEMENT OF ZINC DEFICIENCY

As is the case for all nutrients, the challenge is to achieve intakes of bioavailable zinc and tissue levels within a physiological range. It has become more apparent that there is a cost for intakes and levels above this range. Currently the level commonly considered is a total of 50 mg elemental zinc per day for adults, with a level of intake for children less clear. It is important to be aware of the upper limit, even if a decision is made to temporarily exceed this for anticipated pharmacological benefits.

The use of zinc, as a single micronutrient supplement, for research purposes has proved invaluable, and such studies will continue to have a significant impact on our understanding of the prevalence and effects of human zinc deficiency. The role of multi-nutrient supplements has proven to be important in improving mineral bioavailability. This could be a strategy applied at a local community level or global level. Currently, the use of zinc supplementation either as a single micronutrient or as a component of a multi-micronutrient mix is, at best, a stop gap measure [238]. The gap between successful zinc intervention trials for research purposes and long-term use of such supplements for zinc deficiency prevention is closing. There are practical issues, however, that need to be addressed. These include long-term acceptability, compliance, safety, and whether supplements are the best choice.

Any intervention designed to provide a sustainable strategy for the prevention of zinc deficiency in any population should commence with a detailed evaluation of the habitual dietary intake of zinc and, if possible, of phytate in the target population. Predominantly plant-based diet strategies that do not affect the overall dietary adequacy can be devised to enhance the content and bioavailability of zinc that may be sustainable at a community level [239]. When it is a food-based strategy, the same information is required for that food staple and for the one it is replacing. With current limitations of biomarkers of zinc status and uncertainties about zinc requirements, measurement of the increase in zinc absorption should be regarded as the logical first stage in efficacy testing. That is, it should precede any large scale study designed to measure public health outcomes [240].

Another promising strategy to improve zinc nutrition in vulnerable groups of developing countries is plant breeding. A low-cost and sustainable improvement in the intake of bioavailable zinc in populations would be to increase the concentrations of minerals in plants. Plant breeding techniques have improved, particularly crop genotypes ability to take up trace minerals from trace mineral deficient soils [241]. The nutrients emphasised are zinc, iron and vitamin A and the food crops are wheat, maize, rice, beans and cassava [242]. In addition, this ongoing plant breeding research can be used to increase the intake of bioavailable zinc from food staple crops in populations of developing countries or populations at risk of zinc deficiency [243].

CONCLUSION

Zinc has risen in importance and is on par with vitamin A, iodine and iron in terms of deficiency problems being addressed. It has been a general belief that zinc deficiencies are rare and predominantly confined to young children in few developing countries. However, the likelihood of the prevalence of global zinc deficiency remains high. The serious range of complications associated with this condition requires public health programs to prevent low zinc intake and absorption.

There are no generally accepted biomarkers of zinc status and the quantitative estimate of the percentage of the global population at risk of inadequate zinc nutrition and specific information on the prevalence of this micronutrient deficiency are still lacking. This lack has been a major hindrance in developing policy and programs to reduce the rate of zinc deficiency. Zinc deficiency may induce a number of critical functional abnormalities, such as impaired reproductive performance and depressed immune function with secondary increases in the incidence and severity of infections. Growth failure and secondary nutritional stunting and abnormalities of neuro-behavioural development are also attributable to zinc deficiency. Although some studies have reported that zinc supplementation did not show any significant outcomes, this may be because the study population was not sufficiently growth restricted or zinc deficient to begin with. Nevertheless, it is conceivable that children could benefit functionally from zinc supplementation.

There is sufficient evidence about the clinical and public health importance of zinc deficiency for the practical relevance of this micronutrient in human nutrition. In addition, the parallel progress in basic research has served to emphasise the ubiquity of zinc in biology and the dependence of a wide range of vital metabolic processes on an adequate supply of zinc has further emphasised the fundamental importance of zinc. According to Hambidge [238] concurrent progress should serve as a stimulus and cornerstone for expanded research in the following areas: (1) to accelerate the elucidation of the biology of zinc, (2) achieve better understanding of the pathophysiology and clinical significance of zinc deficiency, (3) unravel the complexities of zinc metabolism, (4) clarify the intricacy of zinc homeostasis and nutritional requirements, (5) identify adequate biomarkers of zinc status and finally (6) to develop optimal strategies for the management and prevention of zinc deficiency. In the long-term, we need measures to improve zinc intake in children, such as improvement in the overall diet, supplementation and food fortification. Sub-selection of crops with improved zinc content need to be explored and assessed.

There is now evidence that zinc supplementation can improve the outcomes of acute and persistent diarrhoea, as well as malaria. It is important to confirm these findings, especially for pneumonia and malaria where results from diverse settings are limited. Furthermore, it is important to evaluate the effects of zinc supplementation on childhood mortality in susceptible populations. The benefits of zinc use either therapeutically or preventively for public health applications are clearly evident.

ACKNOWLEDGEMENTS

I would like to extend my appreciation to Prof. Anne B Chang for providing me with the opportunity to write this article. I would like to thank Prof. Anne B Chang, Ms Pat Westin and Rosa Katsikeros for the proofreading of this work.

REFERENCES

[1]   Hambidge M. Human zinc deficiency. *J Nutr*. 2000;130(5S Suppl):1344S-9S.
[2]   Prasad AS. Discovery of human zinc deficiency and studies in an experimental human model. *Am J Clin Nutr*. 1991;53[2]:403-12.
[3]   Prasad AS, Halsted JA, Nadimi M. Syndrome of iron deficiency anemia, hepatosplenomegaly, hypogonadism, dwarfism and geophagia. *Am J Med*. 1961;31:532-46.
[4]   Moynahan EJ. Letter: Acrodermatitis enteropathica: a lethal inherited human zinc-deficiency disorder. *Lancet*. 1974;2(7877):399-400.
[5]   Kay RG, Tasman-Jones C. Letter: Zinc deficiency and intravenous feeding. *Lancet*. 1975; 2:605-6.
[6]   Walravens PA, Krebs NF, Hambidge KM. Linear growth of low income preschool children receiving a zinc supplement. *Am J Clin Nutr*. 1983;38(2):195-201.

[7]   Walravens PA, Hambidge KM, Koepfer DM. Zinc supplementation in infants with a nutritional pattern of failure to thrive: a double-blind, controlled study. *Pediatrics*. 1989;83(4):532-8.

[8]   Walravens PA, Hambidge KM. Growth of infants fed a zinc supplemented formula. *Am J Clin Nutr*. 1976;29(10):1114-21.

[9]   Brown KH, Peerson JM, Rivera J, Allen LH. Effect of supplemental zinc on the growth and serum zinc concentrations of prepubertal children: a meta-analysis of randomized controlled trials. *Am J Clin Nutr*. 2002;75(6):1062-71.

[10] Bhutta ZA, Black RE, Brown KH, Gardner JM, Gore S, Hidayat A, Khatun F, Martorell R, Ninh NX, Penny ME, Rosado JL, Roy SK, Ruel M, Sazawal S, Shankar A. Prevention of diarrhea and pneumonia by zinc supplementation in children in developing countries: pooled analysis of randomized controlled trials. Zinc Investigators' Collaborative Group. *J Pediatr*. 1999;135(6):689-97.

[11] Hotz C, Brown KH. Identifying populations at risk of zinc deficiency: the use of supplementation trials. *Nutr Rev*. 2001;59(3 Pt 1):80-4.

[12] Black RE. Therapeutic and preventive effects of zinc on serious childhood infectious diseases in developing countries. *Am J Clin Nutr*. 1998;68(2 Suppl):476S-479S.

[13] Vallee BL, Falchuk KH. The biochemical basis of zinc physiology. *Physiol Rev*. 1993;73(1):79-118.

[14] Williams RJP. An introduction to the biochemistry of zinc. In: Mills CF ed. *Zinc in Human Biology*. Berlin, Germany: Springer-verlag; 1989; pp15-31.

[15] Cousins RJ. Zinc. In: Ziegler EE, Filer LJ Jr, eds. *Present Knowledge in Nutrition*, 7th ed. Washington, DC; ILSI Press; 1996 pp

[16] McCall KA, Huang C, Fierke CA. Function and mechanism of zinc metalloenzymes. *J Nutr*. 2000;130(5S Suppl):1437S-46S.

[17] Fierke CA. Function and metabolism of zinc. *J Nutr*. 2000; 130:1437S-1446S.

[18] Miller J, McLachlan AD, Klug A. Repetitive zinc-binding domains in the protein transcription factor IIIA from Xenopus oocytes. *EMBO J*. 1985;4(6):1609-14.

[19] Maret W. Zinc biochemistry, physiology, and homeostasis – recent insights and current trends. *Biometals*. 2001; 14:187-90.

[20] Cousins RJ. A role of zinc in the regulation of gene expression. *Proc Nutr Soc*. 1998;57(2):307-11.

[21] MacDonald RS. The role of zinc in growth and cell proliferation. *J Nutr*. 2000;130(5S Suppl):1500S-8S.

[22] Chesters JK. Biochemical functions of zinc in animals. *World Rev Nutr Diet*. 1978;32:135-64.

[23] Zalewski PD, Forbes IJ, Seamark RF, Borlinghaus R, Betts WH, Lincoln SF, Ward AD. Flux of intracellular labile zinc during apoptosis (gene-directed cell death) revealed by a specific chemical probe, Zinquin. *Chem Biol*. 1994;1(3):153-61.

[24] Frederickson CJ, Bush AI. Synaptically released zinc: physiological functions and pathological effects. *Biometals*. 2001;14(3-4):353-66.

[25] Chester JK. Metabolism and biochemistry of zinc. In: *Clinical Biochemistry of nutritional aspects of trace elements*. Prasad A. ed. Alan R. Liss Inc., NY; 1982 pp. 221-234.

[26] Frederickson CJ, Suh SW, Silva D, Frederickson CJ, Thompson RB. Importance of zinc in the central nervous system: the zinc-containing neuron. *J Nutr.* 2000;130(5S Suppl):1471S-83S.

[27] Jackson MJ, Jones DA, Edwards RH. Tissue zinc levels as an index of body zinc status. *Clin Physiol.* 1982;2(4):333-43.

[28] King JC, Shames DM, Woodhouse LR. Zinc homeostasis in humans. *J Nutr.* 2000;130(5S Suppl):1360S-6S.

[29] Zhou JR, Canar MM, Erdman JW Jr. Bone zinc is poorly released in young, growing rats fed marginally zinc-restricted diet. *J Nutr.* 1993;123(8):1383-8.

[30] Emmert JL, Baker DH. Zinc stores in chickens delay the onset of zinc deficiency symptoms. *Poult Sci.* 1995;74(6):1011-21.

[31] Cousins RJ. Absorption, transport, and hepatic metabolism of copper and zinc: special reference to metallothionein and ceruloplasmin. *Physiol Rev.* 1985;65(2):238-309.

[32] Weigand E. Absorption of trace elements: zinc. *Int J Vitam Nutr Res Suppl.* 1983;25:67-81.

[33] Lonnerdal B. Intestinal absorption of Zn. In: Mill C, ed. *Zn in human biology.* Berlin: Springer-Verlag, 1989: pp 33-55.

[34] Davies NT. Studies on the absorption of Zn by rat intestine. Br J Nutr. 1980;43:189-203.

[35] Krebs NF. Overview of zinc absorption and excretion in the human gastrointestinal tract. *J Nutr.* 2000;130(5S Suppl):1374S-7S.

[36] Gabrielsson J, Weiner D. *Pharmacokinetic and Pharmacodynamic Data Analysis: concepts and applications.* 2nd ed. Stockholm, Sweden: Apotekarsocieteten, 1997.

[37] Tran CD, Miller LV, Krebs NF, Lei S, Hambidge KM. Zn absorption as a function of the dose of Zn sulfate in aqueous solution. *Am J Clin Nutr.* 2004;80:1570-3.

[38] Hantke K. Bacterial zinc transporters and regulators. Biometals. 2001;14(3-4):239-49.

[39] Liuzzi JP, Cousins RJ. Mammalian zinc transporters. *Annu Rev Nutr.* 2004;24:151-72.

[40] Taylor KM, Nicholson RI. The LZT proteins; the LIV-1 subfamily of zinc transporters. *Biochim Biophys Acta.* 2003;1611(1-2):16-30.

[41] Guerinot ML. The ZIP family of metal transporters. *Biochim Biophys Acta.* 2000;1465(1-2):190-8.

[42] Eide DJ. The SLC39 family of metal ion transporters. *Pflugers Arch.* 2004;447(5):796-800.

[43] Palmiter RD, Huang L. Efflux and compartmentalization of zinc by members of the SLC30 family of solute carriers. *Pflugers Arch.* 2004;447(5):744-51.

[44] Eide DJ. Zinc transporters and the cellular trafficking of zinc. *Biochim Biophys Acta.* 2006;1763(7):711-22.

[45] Gaither LA, Eide DJ. Functional expression of the human hZIP2 zinc transporter. *J Biol Chem.* 2000;275(8):5560-4.

[46] Guffanti AA, Wei Y, Rood SV, Krulwich TA. An antiport mechanism for a member of the cation diffusion facilitator family: divalent cations efflux in exchange for K^+ and H^+. *Mol Microbiol.* 2002;45(1):145-53.

[47] McMahon RJ, Cousins RJ. Mammalian zinc transporters. *J Nutr.* 1998;128(4):667-70.

[48] McMahon RJ, Cousins RJ. Regulation of the zinc transporter ZnT-1 by dietary zinc. *Proc Natl Acad Sci U S A*. 1998;95(9):4841-6.

[49] Campbell DM, MacGillivray I. The importance of plasma volume expansion and nutrition in twin pregnancy. *Acta Genet Med Gemellol (Roma)*. 1984;33(1):19-24.

[50] Sunderman FW. Current status of zinc deficiency in the pathogenesis of neurological, dermatological and musculoskeletal disorders. *Ann Clin Lab Sci*. 5(2):132-45.

[51] Brown KH. Effect of infections on plasma zinc concentration and implications for zinc status assessment in low-income countries. *Am J Clin Nutr*. 1998;68(2 Suppl):425S-429S.

[52] McClain C, Cohen D, Phillips R, Ott L, Young B. Increased plasma and ventricular fluid interleukin-6 levels in patients with head injury. *J Lab Clin Med*. 1991;118(3):225-31.

[53] Boosalis MG, Solem LD, McCall JT, Ahrenholz DH, McClain CJ. Serum zinc response in thermal injury. *J Am Coll Nutr*. 1988;7(1):69-76.

[54] Tran CD, Butler RN, Philcox JC, Rofe AM, Howarth GS, Coyle P. Regional distribution of metallothionein and zinc in the mouse gut: comparison with metallothionien-null mice. *Biol Trace Elem Res*. 1998;63(3):239-51.

[55] C Hotz. Brown KH. Rivera JA, Bhutta Z, Gibson RS, King JC, Lonnerdal B, Ruel MT, Sandstrom B, Wasantwisut E, Lopez de Romana D, Peerson JM. Assessment of the risk of zinc deficiency in populations and options for its control. International Zinc Nutrition Consultative Group (IZiNCG) Technical Document #1. Food Nutr Bull. 2004; 25:1 (suppl 2).

[56] Rofe AM, Winters N, Hinskens B, Philcox JC, Coyle P. The role of the pancreas in intestinal zinc secretion in metallothionein-null mice. *Pancreas*. 1999;19(1):69-75.

[57] Dietary Reference Intakes for Vitamin A, K, Arsenic, Boron, Chromium, Copper Iodine, Iron manganese, Molybdenum, Nickel, Silicon, Vanadium, and Zinc. Food and Nutrition Board Institute of Medicine. National Academy Press 2001, Washington, D.C.

[58] King JC, Keen Cl. Zinc. In: Shil ME, Olson JA, Shike M, Ross AC eds. *Modern Nutrition in Health and Disease*, 9th ed. Philadelphia: Lea & Febiger, 1999.

[59] Lee DY, Prasad AS, Hydrick-Adair C, Brewer G, Johnson PE. Homeostasis of zinc in marginal human zinc deficiency: role of absorption and endogenous excretion of zinc. *J Lab Clin Med*. 1993;122(5):549-56.

[60] Sian L, Mingyan X, Miller LV, Tong L, Krebs NF, Hambidge KM. Zinc absorption and intestinal losses of endogenous zinc in young Chinese women with marginal zinc intakes. *Am J Clin Nutr*. 1996;63(3):348-53.

[61] Fung EB, Ritchie LD, Woodhouse LR, Roehl R, King JC. Zinc absorption in women during pregnancy and lactation: a longitudinal study. *Am J Clin Nutr*. 1997;66(1):80-8.

[62] Neldner KH, Hambidge KM, Walravens PA. Acrodermatitis enteropathica. *Int J Dermatol*. 1978;17(5):380-7.

[63] Van Wouwe JP. Clinical and laboratory diagnosis of acrodermatitis enteropathica. *Eur J Pediatr*. 1989;149(1):2-8.

[64] Hambidge KM. Zinc deficiency in the weanling--how important? *Acta Paediatr Scand Suppl*. 1986;323:52-8.

[65] Hambidge KM. Zinc and diarrhea. *Acta Paediatr Suppl.* 1992;381:82-6.

[66] Penland JG. Behavioral data and methodology issues in studies of zinc nutrition in humans. *J Nutr.* 2000;130(2S Suppl):361S-364S.

[67] Prasad AS. Clinical manifestations of zinc deficiency. *Annu Rev Nutr.* 1985;5:341-63.

[68] Chandra S, Chandra RK. Nutrition, immune response, and outcome. *Prog Food Nutr Sci.* 1986;10(1-2):1-65.

[69] Grantham-McGregor SM, Ani CC. The role of micronutrients in psychomotor and cognitive development. *Br Med Bull.* 1999;55(3):511-27.

[70] Hambidge KM, Walravens PA. Disorders of mineral metabolism. *Clin Gastroenterol.* 1982;11(1):87-117.

[71] Atkinson SA, Whelan D, Whyte RK, Lönnerdal B. Abnormal zinc content in human milk. Risk for development of nutritional zinc deficiency in infants. *Am J Dis Child.* 1989;143(5):608-11.

[72] Zimmerman AW, Hambidge KM, Lepow ML, Greenberg RD, Stover ML, Casey CE. Acrodermatitis in breast-fed premature infants: evidence for a defect of mammary zinc secretion. *Pediatrics.* 1982;69(2):176-83.

[73] Hambidge KM. Zinc and diarrhea. *Acta Paediatr Suppl.* 1992;381:82-6.

[74] Walravens PA, Van Doorninck WJ, Hambidge KM. Metals and mental function. *J Pediatr.* 1978;93(3):535.

[75] Hambidge M, Krebs N. Assessment of zinc status in man. *Indian J Pediatr.* 1995;62(2):169-80.

[76] Wood RJ. Assessment of marginal zinc status in humans. *J Nutr.* 2000;130(5S Suppl):1350S-4S.

[77] International Zn Nutrition Consultative Group. Assessment of the risk of Zn status in populations and options for the control of Zn deficiency. Boston: International Nutrition Foundation for United Nations University Press, 2004.

[78] Hambidge M. Biomarkers of trace mineral intake and status. *J Nutr.* 2003;133 Supp3:948S-55S.

[79] Hotz C, Peerson JM, Brown KH. Suggested lower cutoffs of serum Zn concentrations for assessing Zn status: reanalysis of the second National Health and Nutrition Examination Survey data (1976-1980). *Am J Clin Nutr.* 2003;78:756-64.

[80] Ferguson EL, Gibson RS, Opare-Obisaw C, Ounpuu S, Thompson LU, Lehrfeld J. The zinc nutriture of preschool children living in two African countries. *J Nutr.* 1993;123(9):1487-96.

[81] Bradfield RB, Hambidge KM. Problems with hair zinc as an indicator of body zinc status. *Lancet.* 1980;1(8164):363.

[82] Kvist U, Bjorndahl L, Roomans GM, Lindholmer C. Nuclear zinc in human epididymal and ejaculated spermatozoa. *Acta Physiol Scand* 1985; 125(2):297-303.

[83] Frederickson CJ, Kasarskis EJ, Ringo D, Frederickson RE. A quinoline fluorescence method for visualizing and assaying the histochemically reactive zinc (bouton zinc) in the brain. *J Neurosci Methods* 1987; 20(2):91-103.

[84] Zalewski PD, Forbes IJ, Betts WH. Correlation of apoptosis with change in intracellular labile Zn(II) using zinquin [(2-methyl-8-p-toluenesulphonamido-6-

quinolyloxy)acetic acid], a new specific fluorescent probe for Zn(II). *Biochem J* 1993; 296 (Pt 2):403-408.

[85] Zalewski PD, Millard SH, Forbes IJ, Kapaniris O, Slavotinek A, Betts WH, Ward AD, Lincoln SF, Mahadevan I. Video image analysis of labile zinc in viable pancreatic islet cells using a specific fluorescent probe for zinc. *J Histochem Cytochem* 1994; 42(7):877-884.

[86] Coyle P, Zalewski PD, Philcox JC, Forbes IJ, Ward AD, Lincoln SF, Mahadevan I, Rofe AM. Measurement of zinc in hepatocytes by using a fluorescent probe, zinquin: relationship to metallothionein and intracellular zinc. *Biochem J* 1994;303 (Pt 3):781-786.

[87] Brand IA, Kleineke J. Intracellular zinc movement and its effect on the carbohydrate metabolism of isolated rat hepatocytes. *J Biol Chem* 1996;2 71(4):1941-1949.

[88] Tran CD, Butler RN, Howarth GS, Philcox JC, Rofe AM, Coyle P. Regional distribution and localization of zinc and metallothionein in the intestine of rats fed diets differing in zinc content. *Scand J Gastroenterol.* 1999;34(7):689-95.

[89] Keen CL, Jue T, Tran CD, Vogel J, Downing RG, Iyengar V, Rucker RB. Analytical methods: improvements, advancements and new horizons. *J Nutr.* 2003;133(5 Suppl 1):1574S-8S.

[90] Hambidge KM, Krebs NF, Miller L. Evaluation of zinc metabolism with use of stable-isotope techniques: implications for the assessment of zinc status. *Am J Clin Nutr.* 1998;68(2 Suppl):410S-413S.

[91] Krebs NE, Hambidge KM. Zinc metabolism and homeostasis: the application of tracer techniques to human zinc physiology. *Biometals.* 2001;14(3-4):397-412.

[92] Turnlund JR. The use of stable isotopes in mineral nutrition research. *J. Nutr.* 1989; 119:7-14.

[93] Fairweather-Tait SJ, Dainty J. Use of stable isotopes to assess the bioavailability of trace elements: a review. *Food Addit Contam.* 2002;19(10):939-47.

[94] Brown KH, Peerson LM, Allen LH. Effect of zinc supplementation on children's growth: a meta-analysis of intervention trials. *Bibl Nutr Dieta.* 1997;54:543-8.

[95] Bates CJ, Evans PH, Dardenne M, Prentice A, Lunn PG, Northrop-Clewes CA, Hoare S, Cole TJ, Horan SJ, Longman SC. A trial of zinc supplementation in young rural Gambian children. *Br J Nutr.* 1993;69(1):243-55.

[96] Cavan KR, Gibson RS, Grazioso CF, Isalgue AM, Ruz M, Solomons NW. Growth and body composition of periurban Guatemalan children in relation to zinc status: a longitudinal zinc intervention trial. *Am J Clin Nutr.* 1993;57(3):344-52.

[97] Kikafunda JK, Walker AF, Allan EF, Tumwine JK. Effect of zinc supplementation on growth and body composition of Ugandan preschool children: a randomized, controlled, intervention trial. *Am J Clin Nutr.* 1998;68(6):1261-6.

[98] Friel JK, Andrews WL. Zinc requirement of premature infants. *Nutrition.* 1994;10(1):63-5.

[99] Lira PI, Ashworth A, Morris SS. Effect of zinc supplementation on the morbidity, immune function, and growth of low-birth-weight, full-term infants in northeast Brazil. *Am J Clin Nutr.* 1998;68(2 Suppl):418S-424S.

[100] Castillo-Duran C, Rodriguez A, Venegas G, Alvarez P, Icaza G. Zinc supplementation and growth of infants born small for gestational age. *J Pediatr*. 1995;127(2):206-11.

[101] Friel JK, Andrews WL, Matthew JD, Long DR, Cornel AM, Cox M, McKim E, Zerbe GO. Zinc supplementation in very-low-birth-weight infants. *J Pediatr Gastroenterol Nutr*. 1993;17(1):97-104.

[102] Golden BE, Golden MH. Plasma zinc, rate of weight gain, and the energy cost of tissue deposition in children recovering from severe malnutrition on a cow's milk or soya protein based diet. *Am J Clin Nutr*. 1981;34(5):892-9.

[103] Golden MH, Golden BE. Effect of zinc supplementation on the dietary intake, rate of weight gain, and energy cost of tissue deposition in children recovering from severe malnutrition. *Am J Clin Nutr*. 1981;34(5):900-8.

[104] Khanum S, Alam AN, Anwar I, Akbar Ali M, Mujibur Rahaman M. Effect of zinc supplementation on the dietary intake and weight gain of Bangladeshi children recovering from protein-energy malnutrition. *Eur J Clin Nutr*. 1988;42(8):709-14.

[105] Simmer K, Khanum S, Carlsson L, Thompson RP. Nutritional rehabilitation in Bangladesh--the importance of zinc. *Am J Clin Nutr*. 1988;47(6):1036-40.

[106] Doherty CP, Sarkar MA, Shakur MS, Ling SC, Elton RA, Cutting WA. Zinc and rehabilitation from severe protein-energy malnutrition: higher-dose regimens are associated with increased mortality. *Am J Clin Nutr*. 1998;68(3):742-8.

[107] Hambidge KM, Hambidge C, Jacobs M, Baum JD. Low levels of zinc in hair, anorexia, poor growth, and hypogeusia in children. *Pediatr Res*. 1972;6(12):868-74.

[108] Ruz M, Castillo-Duran C, Lara X, Codoceo J, Rebolledo A, Atalah E. A 14-mo zinc-supplementation trial in apparently healthy Chilean preschool children. *Am J Clin Nutr*. 1997;66(6):1406-13.

[109] Prasad AS, Miale A Jr, Farid Z, Sandstead HH, Schulert AR. Zinc metabolism in patients with the syndrome of iron deficiency anemia, hepatosplenomegaly, dwarfism, and hypognadism. *J Lab Clin Med*. 1963;61:537-49.

[110] Halsted JA, Ronaghy HA, Abadi P, Haghshenass M, Amirhakemi GH, Barakat RM, Reinhold JG. Zinc deficiency in man. The Shiraz experiment. *Am J Med*. 1972;53(3):277-84.

[111] Ronaghy HA, Reinhold JG, Mahloudji M, Ghavami P, Fox MR, Halsted JA. Zinc supplementation of malnourished schoolboys in Iran: increased growth and other effects. *Am J Clin Nutr*. 1974;27(2):112-21.

[112] Ronaghy H, Fox MR, Garnsm, Israel H, Harp A, Moe PG, Halsted JA. Controlled zinc supplementation for malnourished school boys: a pilot experiment. *Am J Clin Nutr*. 1969;22(10):1279-89.

[113] Abbasi AA, Prasad AS, Rabbani P, DuMouchelle E. Experimental zinc deficiency in man. Effect on testicular function. *J Lab Clin Med*. 1980;96(3):544-50.

[114] Castillo-Durán C, García H, Venegas P, Torrealba I, Panteón E, Concha N, Pérez P. Zinc supplementation increases growth velocity of male children and adolescents with short stature. *Acta Paediatr*. 1994;83(8):833-7.

[115] Bhutta ZA, Bird SM, Black RE, Brown KH, Gardner JM, Hidayat A, Khatun F, Martorell R, Ninh NX, Penny ME, Rosado JL, Roy SK, Ruel M, Sazawal S, Shankar A. Therapeutic effects of oral Zn in acute and persistent diarrhea in children in

developing countries: pooled analysis of randomized controlled trials. *Am J Clin Nutr*. 2000;72:1516-22.

[116] Sachdev HP, Mittal NK, Yadav HS. Oral zinc supplementation in persistent diarrhoea in infants. *Ann Trop Paediatr*. 1990;10(1):63-9.

[117] Sazawal S, Black RE, Bhan MK, Bhandari N, Sinha A, Jalla S. Zinc supplementation in young children with acute diarrhea in India. *N Engl J Med*. 1995;333(13):839-44.

[118] International centre for Diarrhoeal Disease Research, Dhaka, Bangladesh. Zinc supplementation in the treatment of childhood diarrhoea. *Indian J Pediatr*. 1995; 62:181-93.

[119] Black RE, Brown KH, Becker S. Malnutrition is a determining factor in diarrheal duration, but not incidence, among young children in a longitudinal study in rural Bangladesh. *Am J Clin Nutr*. 1984;39(1):87-94.

[120] Baqui AH, Sack RB, Black RE, Chowdhury HR, Yunus M, Siddique AK. Cell-mediated immune deficiency and malnutrition are independent risk factors for persistent diarrhea in Bangladeshi children. *Am J Clin Nutr*. 1993;58(4):543-8.

[121] Shankar AH, Prasad AS. Zinc and immune function: the biological basis of altered resistance to infection. *Am J Clin Nutr*. 1998;68(2 Suppl):447S-463S.

[122] Kukuruzovic R, Robins-Browne RM, Anstey NM, Brewster DR. Enteric pathogens, intestinal permeability and nitric oxide production in acute gastroenteritis. *Pediatr Infect Dis J*. 2002;21(8):730-9.

[123] Ruel MT, Rivera JA, Santizo MC, Lonnerdal B, Brown KH. Impact of zinc supplementation on morbidity from diarrhea and respiratory infections among rural Guatemalan children. *Pediatrics*. 1997;99(6):808-13.

[124] Sazawal S, Black RE, Bhan MK, Jalla S, Sinha A, Bhandari N. Efficacy of zinc supplementation in reducing the incidence and prevalence of acute diarrhea--a community-based, double-blind, controlled trial. *Am J Clin Nutr*. 1997;66(2):413-8.

[125] Sazawal S, Black RE, Bhan MK, Bhandari N, Sinha A, Jalla S. Zinc supplementation in young children with acute diarrhea in India. *N Engl J Med*. 1995;333(13):839-44.

[126] Behrens RH, Tomkins AM, Roy SK. Zinc supplementation during diarrhoea, a fortification against malnutrition? *Lancet*. 1990;336(8712):442-3.

[127] Baqui AH, Black RE, El Arifeen S, Yunus M, Chakraborty J, Ahmed S, Vaughan JP. Effect of zinc supplementation started during diarrhoea on morbidity and mortality in Bangladeshi children: community randomised trial. *BMJ*. 2002;325(7372):1059.

[128] World Health Organization/UNICEF. *Clinical management of acute diarrhoea*. 2004. Geneva: WHO.

[129] Muller O, Becher H, van Zweeden AB, Ye Y, Diallo DA, Konate AT, Gbangou A, Kouyate B, Garenne M. Effect of zinc supplementation on malaria and other causes of morbidity in west African children: randomised double blind placebo controlled trial. *BMJ*. 2001;322(7302):1567.

[130] Umeta M, West CE, Haidar J, Deurenberg P, Hautvast JG. Zinc supplementation and stunted infants in Ethiopia: a randomised controlled trial. *Lancet*. 2000;355(9220):2021-6.

[131] Sazawal S, Jalla S, Mazumder S, Sinha A, Black RE, Bhan MK. Effect of zinc supplementation on cell-mediated immunity and lymphocyte subsets in preschool children. *Indian Pediatr.* 1997;34(7):589-97.

[132] Moran JR, Lewis JC. The effects of severe zinc deficiency on intestinal permeability: an ultrastructural study. *Pediatr Res.* 1985;19(9):968-73.

[133] Roy SK, Behrens RH, Haider R, Akramuzzaman SM, Mahalanabis D, Wahed MA, Tomkins AM. Impact of zinc supplementation on intestinal permeability in Bangladeshi children with acute diarrhoea and persistent diarrhoea syndrome. *J Pediatr Gastroenterol Nutr.* 1992;15(3):289-96.

[134] Bettger WJ, O'Dell BL. A critical physiological role of zinc in the structure and function of biomembranes. *Life Sci.* 1981;28(13):1425-38.

[135] Tran CD, Howarth GS, Coyle P, Philcox JC, Rofe AM, Butler RN. Dietary supplementation with zinc and a growth factor extract derived from bovine cheese whey improves methotrexate-damaged rat intestine. *Am J Clin Nutr.* 2003;77(5):1296-303.

[136] Hoque KM, Binder HJ. Zinc in the treatment of acute diarrhea: current status and assessment. *Gastroenterology.* 2006;130(7):2201-5.

[137] Munoz E, Powers JR, Mathews JD. Hospitalisation patterns in children from 10 aboriginal communities in the Northern Territory. *Med J Aust.* 1992;156:524-8.

[138] Lee AH, Flexman J, Wang K, Yau KK. Recurrent gastroenteritis among infants in Western Australia: a seven-year hospital-based cohort study. *Ann Epidemiol.* 2004;14(2):137-42.

[139] Kukuruzovic RH, Brewster DR. Small bowel intestinal permeability in Australian aboriginal children. *J Pediatr Gastroenterol Nutr.* 2002;35:206-12.

[140] Valery PC, Torzillo PJ, Boyce NC, White AV, Stewart PA, Wheaton GR, Purdie DM, Wakerman J, Chang AB. Zinc and vitamin A supplementation in Australian Indigenous children with acute diarrhoea: a randomised controlled trial. *Med J Aust* 2005;182(10):530-5.

[141] Bryce J, Boschi-Pinto C, Shibuya K, Black RE; WHO Child Health Epidemiology Reference Group. WHO estimates of the causes of death in children. *Lancet.* 2005;365(9465):1147-52.

[142] Williams BG, Gouws E, Boschi-Pinto C, Bryce J, Dye C. Estimates of world-wide distribution of child deaths from acute respiratory infections. *Lancet Infect Dis.* 2002;2(1):25-32.

[143] Rodriguez A, Hamer DH, Rivera J, Acosta M, Salgado G, Gordillo M, Cabezas M, Naranjo-Pinto C, Leguisamo J, Gomez D, Fuenmayor G, Jativa E, Guaman G, Estrella B, Sempertegui F. Effects of moderate doses of vitamin A as an adjunct to the treatment of pneumonia in underweight and normal-weight children: a randomized, double-blind, placebo-controlled trial. *Am J Clin Nutr.* 2005;82(5):1090-6.

[144] Brooks WA, Yunus M, Santosham M, Wahed MA, Nahar K, Yeasmin S, Black RE. Zinc for severe pneumonia in very young children: double-blind placebo-controlled trial. *Lancet.* 2004;363:1683-8.

[145] Mahalanabis D, Lahiri M, Paul D, Gupta S, Gupta A, Wahed MA, Khaled MA. Randomized, double-blind, placebo-controlled clinical trial of the efficacy of treatment

with zinc or vitamin A in infants and young children with severe acute lower respiratory infection. *Am J Clin Nutr* 2004;79:430-6.

[146] Bose A, Coles CL, Gunavathi , John H, Moses P, Raghupathy P, Kirubakaran C, Black RE, Brooks WA, Santosham M. Efficacy of zinc in the treatment of severe pneumonia in hospitalized children <2 y old. *Am J Clin Nutr*. 2006;83(5):1089-96.

[147] Mahalanabis D, Chowdhury A, Jana S, Bhattacharya MK, Chakrabarti MK, Wahed MA, Khaled MA. Zinc supplementation as adjunct therapy in children with measles accompanied by pneumonia: a double-blind, randomized controlled trial. *Am J Clin Nutr*. 2002;76(3):604-7.

[148] Burgner D, Richmond P. The burden of pneumonia in children: an Australian perspective. *Paediatr Respir Rev*. 2005;6(2):94-100.

[149] Read AW, Gibbins J, Stanley FJ. Hospital admissions for lower respiratory tract illness before the age of two years in western Australia. *Paediatr Perinat Epidemiol*. 1996;10(2):175-85.

[150] Thompson JE. Community acquired pneumonia in north eastern Australia; a hospital based study of aboriginal and non-aboriginal patients. *Aust N Z J Med*. 1997;27(1):59-61.

[151] Harris MF, Nolan B, Davidson A. Early childhood pneumonia in Aborigines of Bourke, New South Wales. *Med J Aust*. 1984;140(12):705-7.

[152] Chang AB, Torzillo PJ, Boyce NC, White AV, Stewart PM, Wheaton GR, Purdie DM, Wakerman J, Valery PC. Zinc and vitamin A supplementation in Indigenous Australian children hospitalised with lower respiratory tract infection: a randomised controlled trial. *Med J Aust*. 2006;184(3):107-12.

[153] Howie S, Zaman SM, Omoruyi O, Adegbola R, Prentice A. Severe pneumonia research and the problem of case definition: the example of zinc trials. *Am J Clin Nutr*. 2007;85(1):242-3.

[154] Caulfield LE, Richard SA, Black RE. Undernutrition as an underlying cause of malaria morbidity and mortality in children less than five years old. *Am J Trop Med Hyg*. 2004;71(2 Suppl):55-63.

[155] Bates CJ, Evans PH, Dardenne M, Prentice A, Lunn PG, Northrop-Clewes CA, Hoare S, Cole TJ, Horan SJ, Longman SC, Sterling D, Aggett PJ. A trial of zinc supplementation in young rural Gambian children. *Br J Nutr*. 1993;69:243-55.

[156] Shankar AH, Genton B, Baisor M, Paino J, Tamja S, Adiguma T, Wu L, Rare L, Bannon D, Tielsch JM, West KP Jr, Alpers MP. The influence of zinc supplementation on morbidity due to Plasmodium falciparum: a randomised trial in preschool children in Papua New Guinea. *Am J Trop Med Hyg*. 2000;62:663-9.

[157] Richard SA, Zavaleta N, Caulfield LE, Black RE, Witzig RS, Shankar AH. Zinc and iron supplementation and malaria, diarrhea, and respiratory infections in children in the Peruvian Amazon. *Am J Trop Med Hyg*. 2006;75(1):126-32.

[158] Ibs KH, Rink L. Zinc-altered immune function. J Nutr. 2003;133(5 Suppl 1):1452S-6S.

[159] Truong-Tran AQ, Carter J, Ruffin R, Zalewski PD. New insights into the role of zinc in the respiratory epithelium. *Immunol Cell Biol*. 2001;79(2):170-7.

[160] Haase H, Rink L. Signal transduction in monocytes: the role of zinc ions. *Biometals*. 2007;20(3-4):579-85.

[161] Beck FW, Prasad AS, Kaplan J, Fitzgerald JT, Brewer GJ. Changes in cytokine production and T cell subpopulations in experimentally induced zinc-deficient humans. *Am J Physiol*. 1997;272(6 Pt 1):E1002-7.

[162] Bogden JD, Oleske JM, Lavenhar MA, Munves EM, Kemp FW, Bruening KS, Holding KJ, Denny TN, Guarino MA, Krieger LM. Zinc and immunocompetence in elderly people: effects of zinc supplementation for 3 months. *Am J Clin Nutr*. 1988;48(3):655-63.

[163] Bogden JD, Oleske JM, Munves EM, Lavenhar MA, Bruening KS, Kemp FW, Holding KJ, Denny TN, Louria DB. Zinc and immunocompetence in the elderly: baseline data on zinc nutriture and immunity in unsupplemented subjects. *Am J Clin Nutr*. 1987;46(1):101-9.

[164] Chandra R. Nutrition and immunity in the elderly: clinical significance. *Nutr Rev*. 1995;53(4 Pt 2):S80-5.

[165] Bogden JD, Bendich A, Kemp FW, Bruening KS, Shurnick JH, Denny T, Baker H, Louria DB. Daily micronutrient supplements enhance delayed-hypersensitivity skin test responses in older people. *Am J Clin Nutr*. 1994;60(3):437-47.

[166] Duchateau J, Delepesse G, Vrijens R, Collet H. Beneficial effects of oral zinc supplementation on the immune response of old people. *Am J Med*. 1981;70(5):1001-4.

[167] Prasad AS, Meftah S, Abdallah J, Kaplan J, Brewer GJ, Bach JF, Dardenne M. Serum thymulin in human zinc deficiency. *J Clin Invest*. 1988;82(4):1202-10.

[168] Black MM. Zinc deficiency and child development. *Am J Clin Nutr*. 1998;68(2 Suppl):464S-469S.

[169] Sazawal S, Bentley M, Black RE, Dhingra P, George S, Bhan MK. Effect of zinc supplementation on observed activity in low socioeconomic Indian preschool children. *Pediatrics*. 1996;98(6 Pt 1):1132-7.

[170] Bentley ME, Caulfield LE, Ram M, Santizo MC, Hurtado E, Rivera JA, Ruel MT, Brown KH. Zinc supplementation affects the activity patterns of rural Guatemalan infants. *J Nutr*. 1997;127(7):1333-8.

[171] Sandstead HH, Penland JG, Alcock NW, Dayal HH, Chen XC, Li JS, Zhao F, Yang JJ. Effects of repletion with zinc and other micronutrients on neuropsychologic performance and growth of Chinese children. *Am J Clin Nutr*. 1998;68(2 Suppl):470S-475S.

[172] Penland JG, Sandstead HH, Alcock NW, Dayal HH, Chen XC, Li JS, Zhao F, Yang JJ. A preliminary report: effects of zinc and micronutrient repletion on growth and neuropsychological function of urban Chinese children. *J Am Coll Nutr*. 1997;16(3):268-72.

[173] Taneja S, Bhandari N, Bahl R, Bhan MK. Impact of zinc supplementation on mental and psychomotor scores of children aged 12 to 18 months: a randomized, double-blind trial. *J Pediatr*. 2005;146(4):506-11.

[174] Hamadani JD, Fuchs GJ, Osendarp SJ, Khatun F, Huda SN, Grantham-McGregor SM. Randomized controlled trial of the effect of zinc supplementation on the mental development of Bangladeshi infants. *Am J Clin Nutr*. 2001;74(3):381-6.

[175] Ashworth A, Morris SS, Lira PI, Grantham-McGregor SM. Zinc supplementation, mental development and behaviour in low birth weight term infants in northeast Brazil. *Eur J Clin Nutr*. 1998;52(3):223-7.

[176] Black MM, Sazawal S, Black RE, Khosla S, Kumar J, Menon V. Cognitive and motor development among small-for-gestational-age infants: impact of zinc supplementation, birth weight, and caregiving practices. *Pediatrics*. 2004;113(5):1297-305.

[177] Black MM. The evidence linking zinc deficiency with children's cognitive and motor functioning. *J Nutr*. 2003;133(5 Suppl 1):1473S-6S.

[178] Jones G, Steketee RW, Black RE, Bhutta ZA, Morris SS; Bellagio Child Survival Study Group. How many child deaths can we prevent this year? *Lancet*. 2003;362(9377):65-71.

[179] Black RE, Morris SS, Bryce J. Where and why are 10 million children dying every year? *Lancet*. 2003;361(9376):2226-34.

[180] Sazawal S, Black RE, Menon VP, Dinghra P, Caulfield LE, Dhingra U, Bagati A. Zinc supplementation in infants born small for gestational age reduces mortality: a prospective, randomized, controlled trial. *Pediatrics*. 2001;108(6):1280-6.

[181] Sazawal S, Black RE, Ramsan M, Chwaya HM, Dutta A, Dhingra U, Stoltzfus RJ, Othman MK, Kabole FM. Effect of zinc supplementation on mortality in children aged 1-48 months: a community-based randomised placebo-controlled trial. *Lancet*. 2007;369(9565):927-34.

[182] Brooks WA, Santosham M, Naheed A, Goswami D, Wahed MA, Diener-West M, Faruque AS, Black RE. Effect of weekly zinc supplements on incidence of pneumonia and diarrhoea in children younger than 2 years in an urban, low-income population in Bangladesh: randomised controlled trial. *Lancet*. 2005;366(9490):999-1004.

[183] Merialdi M, Caulfield LE, Zavaleta N, Figueroa A, DiPietro JA. Adding zinc to prenatal iron and folate tablets improves fetal neurobehavioral development. *Am J Obstet Gynecol*. 1999;180(2 Pt 1):483-90.

[184] Ross SM, Nel E, Naeye RL. Differing effects of low and high bulk maternal dietary supplements during pregnancy. *Early Hum Dev*. 1985;10:295-302.

[185] Garg hk, Singhal KC, Arshad Z. A study of the effect of oral zinc supplementation during pregnancy on pregnancy outcome. *Indian J Physiol Pharmacol*. 1993;37:276-84.

[186] Caulfield LE, Zavaleta N, Figueroa A, Leon Z. Maternal zinc supplementation does not affect size of birth or pregnancy duration in Peru. *J Nutr*. 1999;129:1563-8.

[187] Osendarp SJ, van Raaij JM, Arifeen SE, Wahed M, Baqui AH, Fuchs GJ. A randomized placebo-controlled trial of the effect of zinc supplementation during pregnancy on pregnancy outcome in Bangladeshi urban poor. *Am J Clin Nutr*. 2000;71:114-9.

[188] Goldenberg RL, Tamura T, Neggers Y, Copper RL, Johnston KE, DuBard MB, Hauth JC. The effects of zinc supplementation on pregnancy outcome. *JAMA* 1995;274:463-8.

[189] Cherry FF, Sandstead HH, Rojas P, Johnson LK, Batson HK, Wang XB. Adolescent pregnancy: association among body weight, zinc nutriture, and pregnancy outcome. *Am J Clin Nutr*. 1989;50:945-54.

[190] Hunt IF, Murphy NJ, Cleaver AE, Faraji B, Swendseid ME, Coulson AH, Clark VA, Browdy BL, Cabalum T, Smith JC Jr. Zinc supplementation during pregnancy: effects on selected blood constituents and on progress and outcome of pregnancy in low-income women of Mexican descent. *Am J Clin Nutr.* 1984;40:508-21.

[191] Jameson S. Zinc status in pregnancy: the effect of zinc therapy on perinantal mortality, prematurity, and placental ablation. *Ann N Y Acad Sci.* 1993;678:178-92

[192] Hunt IF, Murphy NJ, Cleaver AE, Faraji B, Swendseid ME, Browdy BL, Coulson AH, Clark VA, Settlage RH, Smith JC Jr. Zinc supplementation during pregnancy in low-income teenagers of Mexican descent: effects on selected blood constituents and on progress and outcome of pregnancy. *Am J Clin Nutr.* 1985;42:815-28.

[193] Merialdi M, Caulfield LE, Zavaleta, Figueroa A, DiPietro JA. Addaing zinc to prenatal iron and folate tablets improves fetal neurobehavioral development. *Am J Obstet Gynecol.* 1999;180:483-90.

[194] Osendarp SJM, van Raaji JMA, Darmstadt GL, Baqui AH, Hautvast JG, Fuchs GJ. Zinc supplementation during pregnancy and effects on growth and morbidity in low birthweight infants: a randomised placebo controlled trial. *Lancet* 2001;357:1080-5.

[195] Hamadani JD, Fuchs GJ, Osendarp SJ, Huda SN, Grantham-McGregor SM. Zinc supplementation during pregnancy and effects on mental development and behaviour of infants: a follow up study. *Lancet* 2002;360:290-4.

[196] Mahomed K, James DK, Golding J, McCabe R. Zinc supplementation during pregnancy: a double blind randomised controlled trial. *BMJ.* 1989;299(6703):826-30.

[197] Jønsson B, Hauge B, Larsen MF, Hald F. Zinc supplementation during pregnancy: a double blind randomised controlled trial. *Acta Obstet Gynecol Scand.* 1996;75(8):725-9.

[198] Hambidge M, Krebs NF. Zinc metabolism and requirements. *Food Nutr Bull.* 2001;22(2):126-32.

[199] World Health Organization, Food and Agriculture Organization, International Atomic Energy Association. *Trace Element in human health and nutrition,* 2nd ed. Geneva: World Health Organization, 1996.

[200] World Health Organization, Food and Agriculture Organization, International Atomic Energy Association. *Trace Element in human health and nutrition,* 2nd ed. Geneva: World Health Organization, 2002.

[201] Johnson PE, Hunt CD, Milne DB, Mullen LK. Homeostatic control of zinc metabolism in men: zinc excretion and balance in men fed diets low in zinc. *Am J Clin Nutr.* 1993;57(4):557-65.

[202] Hunt CD, Johnson PE, Herbel J, Mullen LK. Effects of dietary zinc depletion on seminal volume and zinc loss, serum testosterone concentrations, and sperm morphology in young men. *Am J Clin Nutr.* 1992;56(1):148-57.

[203] Hunt JR, Mullen LK, Lykken GI. Zinc retention from an experimental diet based on the US FDA Total Diet Study. *Nutr Res.* 1192;12:1335-44.

[204] Jackson MJ, Jones DA, Edwards RH Swainbank IG Coleman ML. Zinc homeostasis in man: studies using a new stable isotope-dilution technique. *Br J Nutr.* 1984;51;199-208.

[205] Lee DY, Prasad AS, Hydrick-Adair, Brewer G, Johnson PE. Homeostasis of zinc in marginal human zinc deficiency: Role of absorption and endogenous excretion of zinc. *J Lab Clin Med*. 1993;122:549-556.

[206] Taylor CM, Bacon JR, Aggett PJ, Bremner I. Homeostatic regulation of zinc absorption and endogenous losses in zinc-deprived men. *Am J Clin Nutr*.1991;53:755-763.

[207] Turnlund JR, Durin N, Costa F, Margen S. Stable isotope studies of zinc absorption and retention in young and elderly men. *J Nutr*. 1986;116:1239-47.

[208] Turnlund JR, King JC, Keyes WR, Gong B, Michel MC. A stable isotope study of zinc absorption in young men: effects of phytate and alpha-cellulose. *Am J Clin Nutr*. 1984;40;1071-7.

[209] Wada L, Turnlund JR, King JC. Zinc utilization in young men fed adequate and low zinc intakes. *J Nutr*. 1985;115(10):1345-54.

[210] Knudsen E, Sandstrom B, Solgaard P. Zinc, copper and magnesium absorption from a fibre-rich diet. *J Trace Elem Med Biol*. 1996;10(2):68-76.

[211] Hunt JR, Matthys LA, Johnson LK. Zinc absorption, mineral balance, and blood lipids in women consuming controlled lactoovovegetarian and omnivorous diets for 8 wk. *Am J Clin Nutr*. 1998;67(3):421-30.

[212] Hunt JR, Gallagher SK, Johnson LK, Lykken GI. High- versus low-meat diets: effects on zinc absorption, iron status, and calcium, copper, iron, magnesium, manganese, nitrogen, phosphorus, and zinc balance in postmenopausal women. *Am J Clin Nutr*. 1995;62(3):621-32.

[213] Lowe NM, Shames DM, Woodhouse LR, Matel JS, Roehl R, Saccomani MP, Toffolo G, Cobelli C, King JC. A compartmental model of zinc metabolism in healthy women using oral and intravenous stable isotope tracers. *Am J Clin Nutr*. 1997;65(6):1810-9.

[214] Hess FM, King JC, Margen S. Zinc excretion in young women on low zinc intakes and oral contraceptive agents. *J Nutr*. 1977;107(9):1610-20.

[215] Zlotkin SH, Cherian MG. Hepatic metallothionein as a source of zinc and cysteine during the first year of life. *Pediatr Res*. 1988;24(3):326-9.

[216] Abrams SA, Wen J, Stuff JE. Absorption of calcium, zinc, and iron from breast milk by five- to seven-month-old infants. *Pediatr Res*. 1997;41(3):384-90.

[217] Widdowson EM, Dickerson JWT. Chemical composition of the human body. In: Comar CL, Bronner F, ed. *Mineral metabolism. An advanced treatise*. Vol 2: The elements, Part A. New York: Academic Press, 1964:1-220.

[218] Swanson CA, King JC. Zinc and pregnancy outcome. *Am J Clin Nutr*. 1987;46(5):763-71.

[219] Brown KH, Dewey KG, Allen LH. Complementary feeding in young children in developing countries: a review of current scientific knowledge, WHO/NUT/98.1. Geneva: World Health Organization, 1998.

[220] Cook JD, Dassenko SA, Lynch SR. Assessment of the role of nonheme-iron availability in iron balance. *Am J Clin Nutr*. 1991;54(4):717-22.

[221] Tidehag P, Hallmans G, Wing K, Sjostrom R, Agren G, Lundin E, Zhang JX. A comparison of iron absorption from single meals and daily diets using radioFe (55Fe, 59Fe). *Br J Nutr*. 1996;75(2):281-9.

[222] Lonnerdal B. Dietary factors influencing zinc absorption. *J Nutr.* 2000;130(5S Suppl):1378S-83S.

[223] Adams CL, Hambidge M, Raboy V, Dorsch JA, Sian L, Westcott JL, Krebs NF. Zinc absorption from a low-phytic acid maize. *Am J Clin Nutr.* 2002;76(3):556-9.

[224] Pinna K, Woodhouse LR, Sutherland B, Shames DM, King JC. Exchangeable zinc pool masses and turnover are maintained in healthy men with low zinc intakes. *J Nutr.* 2001;131(9):2288-94.

[225] Sian L, Krebs NF, Westcott JE, Fengliang L, Tong L, Miller LV, Sonko B, Hambidge M. Zinc homeostasis during lactation in a population with a low zinc intake. *Am J Clin Nutr.* 2002;75(1):99-103.

[226] Leonard A, Gerber GB, Leonard F. Mutagenicity, carcinogenicity and teratogenicity of Zn. *Mutat Res.* 1986;168:343-53.

[227] Fosmire GJ. Zn toxicity. Am J Clin Nutr. 1990;51(2):225-7.14. Barceloux DG. Zn. *J Toxicol Clin Toxicol.* 1999;37:279-92.

[228] Fraker PJ, King LE, Laakko T, Vollmer TL. The dynamic link between the integrity of the immune system and zinc status. *J Nutr.* 2000;130:1399S-406S.

[229] Hamadani JD, Fuchs GJ, Osendarp SJ, Khatun F, Huda SN, Grantham-McGregor SM. Randomized controlled trial of the effect of Zn supplementation on the mental development of Bangladeshi infants. *Am J Clin Nutr.* 2001;74:381-6.

[230] Sandstrom B. Micronutrient interactions: effects on absorption and bioavailability. *Br J Nutr.* 2001;85 Supp2:S181-5.

[231] Wieringa FT, Berger J, Dijkhuizen MA, Hidayat A, Ninh NX, Utomo B, Wasantwisut E, Winichagoon P; for the SEAMTIZI (South-East Asia Multi-country Trial on Iron and Zinc supplementation in Infants) Study Group. Combined iron and zinc supplementation in infants improved iron and zinc status, but interactions reduced efficacy in a multicountry trial in southeast Asia. *J Nutr.* 2007;137(2):466-71.

[232] Solomons NW, Cousins RJ. Zinc. In: Solomons NW, Rosenberg IH eds. *Absorption and malabsorption of minerals nutrients.* New York: Alan R. Liss, 1984.

[233] Krebs NF, Westcott J. Zn and breastfed infants: if and when is there a risk of deficiency? *Adv Exp Med Biol.* 2002;503:69-75.

[234] Gibson RS. Zinc nutrition in developing countries. *Nutr Res Rev.* 1994;7:151-73.

[235] Aggett PJ, Harries JT. Current status of zinc in health and disease states. *Arch Dis Child.* 1979;54(12):909-17.

[236] Cousins RJ, Leinart AS. Tissue-specific regulation of zinc metabolism and metallothionein genes by interleukin 1. *FASEB J.* 1988;2(13):2884-90.

[237] Schroeder JJ, Cousins RJ. Interleukin 6 regulates metallothionein gene expression and zinc metabolism in hepatocyte monolayer cultures. *Proc Natl Acad Sci U S A.* 1990;87(8):3137-41.

[238] Hambidge KM. Zinc and health: current status and future direction. *J. Nutr.* 2000;130:1344S-49S.

[239] Gibson RS, Yeudall F, Drost N, Mtitimuni B, Cullinan T. Dietary interventions to prevent zinc deficiency. *Am J Clin Nutr.* 1998;68(2 Suppl):484S-487S.

[240] Hambidge KM, Miller LV, Tran CD, Krebs NF. Measurements of zinc absorption: application and interpretation in research designed to improve human zinc nutriture. *Int J Vitam Nutr Res.* 2005;75(6):385-93.

[241] Graham RD, Welch RM. Breeding for staple food crops with high micronutrient density. Working papers on agricultural strategies for micronutrients, no. 3. Washington, DC: International Food Policy Research Institute, 1996.

[242] Bouis H. Enrichment of food staples through plant breeding: a new strategy for fighting micronutrient malnutrition. *Nutr. Rev.* 1996; 54:131-7.

[243] Ruel MT, Bouis HE. Plant breeding: a long-term strategy for the control of zinc deficiency in vulnerable populations. *Am. J. Clin. Nutr.* 1998; 68(suppl):488S-94S.

In: Micronutrients and Health Research
Editor: Takumi Yoshida, pp. 71-106

ISBN: 978-1-60456-056-5
© 2008 Nova Science Publishers, Inc.

Chapter II

THE EFFECT OF NUTRITION ON MATERNAL-NEONATAL RETINOL AND FOLATE SERUM CONCENTRATIONS IN TWO ETHNIC GROUPS

Kleopatra H. Schulpis[1], George D. Vlachos[2], Kelly Michalakakou[3], George A. Karikas[4], Dimitrios G. Vlachos[1], Antonia Gounaris[5], Katerina Skenderi[6] and Ioannis Papassotiriou[3,*

[1]Institute of Child Health, Research Centre, Athens, Greece;
[2]First Department of Obstetrics and Gynecology,
Athens University Medical School, Greece;
[3]Department of Clinical Biochemistry, "Aghia Sophia"
Children's Hospital, Athens, Greece;
[4]Department of Medical Laboratories, Technological and
Educational Institute of Athens, Athens, Greece;
[5]"G. Papanikolaou" Research Center, "Saint Savas"
Regional Oncological Hospital of Athens, Athens, Greece;
[6]Laboratory of Nutrition and Clinical Dietetics, Harokopio University, Athens, Greece.

ABSTRACT

Background

Vitamin A is fundamentally required in physiological processes and growth and low folate level is implicated with neural tube defects.

---

* Correspondence concerning this article should be addressed to: Ioannis Papassotiriou, Ph.D. Department of Clinical Biochemistry, "Aghia Sophia" Children's Hospital, 115 27 Athens, Greece. Tel +30-210-7467931; Fax +30-210-7467171; e-mail: biochem@paidon-agiasofia.gr, jpapasotiriou@ath.forthnet.gr.

Aim

To evaluate retinol and folate serum levels in mothers and their newborns of two ethnic group.

Methods

Data concerned 710 Greeks and 686 Albanian mothers along with their newborns. Immediately after delivery blood from the umbilical cord and from the mothers were collected into light-protected tubes. Retinol serum level was measured with a reversed-phase HPLC method and serum folate with Bayer Advia-Centaur System. A 60d dietetic diary was kept by each woman during the last two months of pregnancy.

Results

Retinol values (0.9±0.1 and 18.5±3.47 μmol/L) were considered to be normal in Greek mothers and most of their newborns, respectively, whereas in Albanian mothers the lipid soluble vitamin was found low (0.6±0.1 μmol/L) $p<0.001$ and in 1/3 significantly low (< 0.45 μmol/L). Consequently retinol was found to be very low in their newborns (0.4±0.1 μmol/L) and in half cases extremely low. However, in 12% of the Albanian cord blood samples, retinol levels were dectected higher, than those of their mothers. Folate serum concentration in mothers and newborns were similar (18.7±9.1 and 26.5±15.2 nmol vs 18.1±8.6 and 24.6±14.7 nmol) in the two ethnic groups. Vitamin A intake was found extremely low in the group of immigrants.

Conclusions

The decreased vitamin A intake and their low blood status in the immigrant mothers may be due to their low socio-economic and nutritional status. In contrast, normal folate levels in the mothers of the two ethnic groups could be due to their normal intake of this vitamin. Immigrant programs for the elevation of the socio-economic status, along with a close follow up of the immigrant-pregnant women should be planned in Greece.

Keywords: vitamin A, retinol, folate, pregnancy, newborns.

INTRODUCTION

The measurement of specific micronutrient status indices links estimates of intakes of food and supplements (and hence nutrient intakes) and evidence of health status as well as the outcome of physiological processes, including those of pregnancy, lactation and early development in infancy are always of great importance.

Vitamin A is known to regulate diverse cellular activities such as cell proliferation, differentiation, morphogenesis, and tumorigenesis [1]. In physiological conditions, hepatic stellate cells (HSCs) store 80% of the total vitamin A in the whole body as retinyl palmitate in lipid droplets in the cytoplasm, and regulate both transport and storage of vitamin A.

The concentration of vitamin A in the bloodstream is regulated within the physiological range by these HSCs. By receptor-mediated endocytosis, the cells take up retinol, active form of vitamin A, from the blood, where it circulates as a complex of retinol and a specific binding protein called-retinol-binding protein (RBP) [2]. Once inside the cell, free retinol has several fates, one of which is reformation of the complex with RBP and returns to the bloodstream [3]. Thus, the HSCs are important for the regulation of homeostasis of vitamin A.

When [^{3}H] retinal, was injected via a portal vein the largest amount of the labeled retinol was taken up by the liver within 90 min after injection, although the labeled material was detected in all organs examined [4]. The radioactivity of the retinol in the liver did not change until 6 days after the injection. These results were consistent with previous reports that main storage site of vitamin A in mammals is the liver [5,6].

The hepatic lobule consists of parenchymal cell (PCs) and non-parenchymal cells associated with the sinusoids: endothelial cells (ECs), Kupffer cells, pit cells, dendritic cells, and stellate (SCs) [7]. Sinusoidal endothelial cells (SECs) express lymphocyte costimulatory molecules [8] and form the greater part of the extremely thin lining of the sinusoids, which are larger than ordinary capillaries and more irregular in shape. Kupffer cells are tissue macrophages and components of the diffuse mononuclear phagocyte system. They are usually situated on the endothelium with cellular processes extending between the underlying ECs. The greater part of their irregular cell surface is exposed to the blood in the lumen of the sinusoid. Pit cells are natural killer cells. Dendritic cells, located in the portal triad in human [9], and in periportal and central areas in rat [10] that capture and process antigens, migrate to lymphoid organs and secrete cytokines to initiate immune responses [11], The hepatic stellate cells (HSCs) [5,6,7,12,3,13] that lie in the space between SECs and PCs are considered to be derived from mesenchymal origin. Both ECs and SCs are derived from mesenchymal tissue, namely, septum transversum. Kupffer cells are from monocyte-macrophage system. SCs that store vitamin A in their cytoplasm have been found in extrahepatic organs (kidney, intestine, lung, pancreas, and so on) [14,15,6].

To examine the distribution of vitamin A in the liver, radioactivity per cell was determined after cell fractionation [16]. Specific activity of [^{3}H] retinol (per cell) was the highest in the HSC fraction, both 90 min and 6 days after injection. These results strongly support earlier morphological observations [5,6] that the SC is the storage site of vitamin A in the liver, and are not inconsistent with reports on the retinol transfer from PCs to SCs [17,18,19].

Immunoelectronmicroscopic studies suggest that RBP mediates the paracrine transfer of retinol from hepatic PCs to the SCs and thus SCs bind and internalize RBP by receptor-mediated endocytosis [17]. RBP receptor was cloned and characterized [20]. The SCs may have pivotal roles in type 2 diabetes, because RBP was reported to contribute to insulin resistance in obesity and type 2 diabetes [21].

Retinol plays a central role in many essential biological processes such as vision, immunity, reproduction, growth, development, control of cellular proliferation, and differentiation [1]. The main active forms of retinol are retinoic acids (RAs), except for reproduction and vision, where retinol and retina also play important roles.

Two vehicles are described for mammalian blood transport of retinoids. First, the retinyl esters and carotenoids can be incorporated in intact or remnant chylomicrons or very low-density lipoproteins [22]. Second, the main form of retinol blood transport (1 µmol/l) is associated with a specific binding protein (RBP), which is itself complexed with transthyretin (ratio 1 mol/lmol). The constitution of this ternary complex prevents the glomerular filtration of the small RBP-retinol form (21 kDa) and increases the affinity of RBP for retinol [23]. A binding to other plasma proteins, such as albumin or lipicalins, is also described for retinol. Albumin could serve as a transport for RA, which circulates in very small levels in the blood. The transfer of retinol to target cells involves s specific membrane-bound RBP receptor [24]. To date, the debate still remains concerning the molecular mechanisms of the cellular retinol penetration: endocytosis, dissociation of RBP – retinol complex, and intracellular degradation of RBP or extracellular dissociation of RBP-retinol complex and delivery of retinol via transmembrane pore. The uptake of remnant chylomicrons and very low-density lipoproteins (containing retinyl esters and carotenoids), is realized by target tissues using, respectively, the lipoprotein lipase and low-density lipoproteins receptor pathways. Bound to albumin, RA can be transferred into the tissues by passive diffusion, with an efficiency of transfer, which is cell type and tissue specific [1].

To be biologically active retinol must first be oxidized to retinaldehyde and then to RA. A large number of enzymes catalyze the reversible oxidation of retinol to retinaldehyde: the alcohol dehydrogenases (ADH), the retinol dehydrogenase (RDH) of the microsomal fraction, and some members of the cytochrome P450 family. Several enzymes are able to catalyze irreversibly the oxidation of retinaldehyde to RA: the retinal dehydrogenases (RALDH1, 2, 3, and 4) and also members of the cytochrome P450 family [25]. These enzymatic reactions could be antagonized and/or stopped by several toxic molecules, namely ethanol, citral, nitrofen, or bisdiamine, leading to an exogenous alteration of RA production. Specific isomerization reactions are also likely to occur within the cells, since there are at least two RA stereoisomers *in vivo* (all-trans and 9-cis RA) exhibiting distinct biochemical activities. The catabolism of all-trans and 9-cis RA is also an important mechanism for controlling RA levels in cell and tissues and is carried out by three specific members of cytochrome P450s, CYP26A1, B1, and C1 [19]. RA is catabolized to products such as 4-oxo-RA, 4-hydroxy-RA, 18-hydroxy-RA, and 5,18-epoxy-RA, which are finally excreted. These compounds can also undergo glucoronidation [26]. An alternative metabolic pathway was present for intracellular retinol: the formation and storage as retinyl esters. Indeed, retinol may esterify by two enzymes (lecithin retinol acyltransferase and diacylglycerol O-acyltransferase) into mostly long-chain retinyl esters such as retinyl palmitate, state and oleate. These esters are then stored in cytosolic lipid droplets. The mobilization of these retinyl esters and the release of retinol esters are realized by a retinyl ester hydrolase.

Since retinol, retinaldehyde, and RA are lipids, they lack appreciable water solubility and consequently must be bound to protein within cells. Several intracellular-binding proteins for retinol, retinaldehyde, and RA have been identified and extensively characterized. They include cellular retinol-binding proteins type 1 and 2 (CRBP1 and 2) and cellular RA-binding proteins type 1 and 2 (CRABP1 and 2). The CRBP1 is a key protein to regulate the metabolism of retinol by orientating to storage, export of retinol, or conversion into RA [27]. Both the CRABPs bind RA controlling the intracellular levels of retinoids, acting as cofactors for RA-metabolizing enzymes, and/or participating in the cytoplasmic nuclear transport of RA [28].

The placenta regulates the transport and metabolism of maternal nutrients transferred to the fetus. Abnormalities in these placental functions may have deleterious consequences for fetal development [29]. Since there is no *de novo* fetal synthesis of retinol, the developing mammalian embryo is dependent on the maternal circulation for its vitamin A supply. The presence of measurable hepatic vitamin A stored at birth is indicative of the functionality of placental transport during gestation [30]. A number of studies have investigated the ability of retinoids to pass through the placental barrier in mice or rabbits [31]. It is established that each retinoid (e.g. retinol, 13-cis, all-trans RA, and their glycoronoconjugates) presents a specific rate of transfer. It has been proposed that this peculiarity could account for the variability in teratological effects of comparable amounts of different maternally absorbed retinoids [32].

The different intracellular-binding proteins for retinol, retinaldehyde and RA, are expressed in the mouse [33], rat [34], porcine [35], and human placenta [36]. CRBP1 is detected in the mouse visceral endoderm of the yolk sac, the mouse trophoblastic layer of the placental labyrinth closest to the fetal endothelium, the porcine areolar trophoblasts [35,37], and the human villous trophoblastic cells [36]. Moreover, it was shown that both fetal as well as maternal CRBP2 are required to ensure adequate delivery of vitamin A to the developing fetus when dietary vitamin A is limiting [38]. In addition, Johansson et al [39] precise that retinol metabolism may occur in the CRBP1 positive villous stromal cells and decidual cells of the basal plate in human placenta [39]. For RA transport, cellular RA-binding proteins are also described in placenta [40]. CRABP1 was found in hamster, human, and porcine placenta [35], as well as CRABP2 in human placenta [41]. Throughout mouse placentation, the expression patterns of the CRABP1 and 2 genes partly overlap in the decidual tissue and the vacuolar zones of the deciduas, suggesting a role for these binding proteins in sequestering free RA from maternal blood, thus regulating its availability to the embryo.

Vitamin A is provided to the fetus through a limited and tightly controlled placental transfer [42,43]. The amount of retinol provided to the fetus is usually maintained constant until maternal stores are depleted [30,44,45]. The first step of retinol transfer from maternal blood to embryo implicates the RBP. The exact mechanism of transfer remains discussed but it seems to involve RBP receptor. Indeed, a receptor for RBP has been characterized in the human placenta [46]. It is clearly established that maternal RBP does not cross the placental barrier and does not enter the developing embryo. Similar studies show convincingly that RBP of fetal origin is unable to cross the placenta and enter the maternal circulation. Thus, for retinol bound to RBP in the maternal circulation to be transferred to the fetus, it must be dissociated from maternal RBP after the binding to its receptor at the maternal face of placental barrier. Bound to the CRBPs, the retinol passes through the cytoplasm of the trophoblastic cells and enters the fetal circulation, where a new complex is formed using transthyretin and RBP of fetal origin [47].

If the mammalian placenta is able to regulate the transfer of the retinoids from mother to the fetus, it also expresses several proteins with metabolic activities related to retinoids. In human placenta, a large number of enzymes catalyzing the oxidation of retinol into retinaldehyde are identified; among them are the nonspecific ADH of class I [48] or class III [49]. In the guinea pig, a low-ADH activity is detected in placenta throughout gestation [50], like during late pregnancy in the rat [51] or in the ewe [52]. Specific enzymes like RDH of the microsomal fraction are able to oxidize retinol in retinaldehyde in the human placenta. Among them, the more specific RDH, catalyzing the oxidation of 9-cis but not all-trans retinol, is expressed in human and mouse placenta [52]. Other enzymes with an RDH activity are described in placenta: 17β-hydroxysteroid and 11β-hydroxysteroid dehydrogenases [53,54,55]. Moreover, the human type 1 isoforms of 3β-hydroxysteroid dehydrogenase/isomerase are expressed in the placenta [56], with a potentiality to oxidize the retinol in retinal. An RDH is also found in the yolk sac of rat embryos [34].

Secondarily, retinaldehyde had to be oxidized to RA by retinal dehydrogenase: RALDH1, 2, 3 and 4 [25]. These enzymes were localized in the yolk sac of rat embryos [34]. They were also detected in human choriocarcinoma (JEG-3 cell line) and placental cells. The retinol conversion into all-trans RA was demonstrated using high-performance liquid chromatography (HPLC) experiments [56]. The presence of 9-cis ROH converted to 9-cis RA is also detected in human placenta. Two other mammalian placentas have also been shown to produce RA from retinol: the porcine [57] and the mouse (yolk sac) placenta [34]. This RA generation was experimentally blocked by the presence of ethanol. This point may be a possible linkage between the nutrient supply of retinol to the placenta, the generation of strong developmental morphogene, and placental gene regulation and physiology. During pregnancy, placental cells may be exposed to deleterious maternal conditions, including alcohol abuse. Links have been established between alcohol abuse, fetal malformations, and alterations of retinoid metabolism [58]. The interferences of alcohol on synthesis of functional retinoids from retinol are clearly demonstrated. In this way, the alterations of placental retinoids metabolism by maternal ethanol ingestion may provide a novel and additional explanation for the genesis of fetal alcoholic syndrome and highlight the placental roles in this pathology.

The human term placental tissues (and more precisely, the villous mesenchymal fibroblasts) are able to esterify retinol [59]. Nevertheless the retinyl esters are never detected in human umbilical blood at delivery. It is well accepted that the placenta can be considered as a transitory, primitive functional liver during the first stages of mammalian development. During this period, the placenta stores retinol, waiting for liver maturity and functionality marked by the capacity to secrete RBP. This hypothesis is supported by results concerning the switch in retinoids content of embryonic and placental compartments during the development of the mouse conceptus [60]. During early organogenesis, the retinyl ester content of the placenta is nearly eightfold higher than the embryonic content. At the end of gestation, the embryonic retinyl ester content is nearly fourfold greater than placental one. Abnormalities concerning this switch between placental and embryonic retinyl esters stores are associated with intrauterine growth retardations [61]. Little is known about enzymes implicated in the metabolism (anabolism and catabolism) of placental retinyl esters. The diacylglycerol acyltransferase (DGAT1) showing a nonspecific enzymatic property to esterify the retinol [62] is expressed in the human primordial placenta [63] and perhaps in the amniotic epithelium of amniotic membranes. At the opposite, the lecithin retinol acyltransferase (LRAT) esterifying more specifically the retinol [64] seems to be not expressed in placenta and amniotic membranes. The enzymes involved into the release of retinol from retinyl ester, that is, retinyl ester hydrolase [65] like carboxylesterase, are active in rat placenta [66]. The carboxylesterase-2 isoform is also expressed in human amniotic epithelium [67], and more particularly into microsomal fraction [68]. Moreover, the lipoxygenase is able to oxidize all-trans retinol acetate (one form of retinyl ester) in human term placenta [69].

The maternal and fetal blood levels of the β-carotene (provitamin A) strongly suggest that it may be used as a precursor of retinol in placenta [70]. Note that we also detected the expression of the enzymes β-carotene-15, 15'-dioxygenase (BCDO isoform 2) catalyzing the key step of retinol's cleaving β-carotene into two molecules of retinal [71] in the amniotic part of human term fetal membranes, but not in the placenta. In conclusion, all these data reveal the complex properties of the mammalian placenta in term of retinoids metabolism: the production of active form retinol, the *cis/trans* isomerization and degradation of several RAs, the retinyl ester formation and hydrolysis, and the cleavage of β-carotene into retinal.

Vitamin A deficiency and excess have profound effects on the development of the vertebrate embryo [72,73]. A molecular basis for these phenomena was proposed when it was found that vitamin A active forms, RAs, act through ligand-activated transcription factors and that RA is able to change the expression pattern of homeobox genes clusters [74]. RA is indispensable for patterning the anteroposterior body axis, for morphogenesis and organogenesis [75]. Almost every organ or tissue can be affected by RAs if the embryo is treated with them at a critical time in development [76]. It illustrates the crucial role of RAs in the regulation of distinct developmental events [77]. The biogeneration of RA in the embryo appears to be the first developmental step in the initiation of RA-regulated signaling pathways [78]. Tissue distribution of RA results from the balancing activities of RA-synthesizing enzymes (including retinaldehyde dehydrogenases RALDH1-4), and RA-catabolizing cytochrome P450 hydroxylases (CYP26A1, B1, and C1) [79]. Regulation of retinoid synthesis and catabolism can both be viewed as important ways in which distinct spatiotemporal patterns of active retinoids are maintained in the developing mammalian embryo. Therefore, the function of vitamin A is inseparable from its metabolism.

All of the physiologically important vitamin A metabolites and enzyme systems regulating vitamin A metabolism have been demonstrated in embryos. RA has been detected very early during vertebrate development. Using a transgenic mouse line carrying a β-galactosidase (lacZ) reporter gene under the regulation of three copies of the RARE from the RARβ2 gene, Rossant et al [80] found that prior to implantation sporadic staining was present in the inner cell mass of the blastocyst. RA has also been detected in the preimplantation porcine blastocyst [57]. After implantation egg, cylinder stage or preprimitive streak stage all-trans retinaldehyde (20 fmol/embryo), but not all-trans RA, was identidied in mouse embryos [81].

As previously presented, the ADH family consists of numerous enzymes able to catalyze the reversible oxidation of a wide variety of substrates (ethanol, retinol) to the corresponding aldehydes. Three forms (ADH1, 3 and 4) are highly conserved in vertebrates and mammals. In humans, ADH4 demonstrated higher retinol (ROH) dehydrogenase activity than ADH1, whereas ADH3 had insignificant ROH dehydrogenase activity [82]. The mRNA for cytosolic

ADH4 has been detected by polymerase chain reaction analysis in the egg-cylinder stage mouse embryo [81]. The expression of ADH4 mRNA corresponds well both spatially and temporally with the presence of RA-like activity [83]. However, the enzyme is not absolutely essential for embryogenesis, as homozygous mutant mice null for ADH4 are viable and fertile as are ADH1 null mutant mice [82–84]. The synthesis of RA from ROH may be competitively inhibited by ethanol leading to RA deficiency.

Concerning the other metabolic activities related to the ROH or its precursors during mammalian development, the presence of carotene-15, 15'dioxygenase mRNA has been detected in maternal tissue at the site of embryo implantation during early stages of mouse embryogenesis (7.5 and 8.5 dpc) [85]. It suggests that this enzyme may be acting to provide needed retinoid to the embryo. A weak signal of the carotene-15, 15' dioxygenase mRNA can also be detected in embryonic tissues still 15 dpc, but the functionality of β-carotene cleavage remains still discussed [86]. Vitamin A is mainly stored in the stellate cells of the liver as retinyl esters in lipid droplets but may also be found during embryonic life in lung [87,88]. Fetal CRBP2 is expressed transiently in the mouse yolk sac, lung, and liver during development. Both loss of maternal and loss of fetal CRBP2 contribute to increased neonatal mortality, when dietary vitamin A is reduced to marginal levels. Nevertheless, the role of CRBP2 for retinoids metabolism seems to be limited for the embryonic part. Indeed, the CRBP2 plays a specific role in ensuring adequate transport of vitamin A to the developing fetus, particularly when maternal vitamin A is limited [38]. Similar role can be played by lecithin retinol acyltransferase, during mammalian development [89]. Due to its high expression during mouse development, CRBP1 seemed to be strongly important for the regulation of this retinoids storage. Indeed, CRBP1 (and not CRBP2) is specifically expressed in several tissues including spinal cord, lung, and liver [90,91]. Nevertheless, CRBP1 mutant embryos from mothers fed with a vitamin A-enriched diet are healthy. They do not present any of the congenital abnormalities related to RA deficiency. During development, ROH and retinyl ester levels are decreased in CRBP1 deficient embryos and fetuses by 50% and 80% respectively [27]. The CRBP1 deficiency does not alter the expression patterns of RA-responding genes during development. Therefore, CRBP1 is required in prenatal life to maintain normal amounts of ROH and to ensure its efficient storage as retinyl esters, but seems of secondary importance for RA synthesis, under conditions of maternal vitamin A sufficiency [92].

Folate is necessary for the production and maintenance of new cells [93]. This is especially important during periods of rapid cell division and growth such as infancy and pregnancy. Folate is needed to replicate DNA. Thus folate deficiency hinders DNA synthesis and cell division, affecting most clinically the bone marrow, a site of rapid cell turnover. Because RNA and protein synthesis are not hindered, large red blood cells called megaloblasts are produced, resulting in megaloblastic anemia [94]. Both adults and children need folate to make normal red blood cells and prevent anemia [95]. Folate also helps prevent changes to DNA that may lead to cancer.

In the form of a series of tetrahydrofolate compounds, folate derivatives are substrates in a number of single-carbon-transfer reactions, and also are involved in the synthesis of dtMP (2'-deoxythymidine-5'-phosphate) from dUMP (2'-deoxyuridine-5'-phosphate). It helps convert vitamin B12 to one of its coenzyme forms and helps synthesize the DNA required for all rapidly growing cells. The pathway leading to the formation of tetrahydrofolate (FH_4) begins when folate (F) is reduced to dihydrofolate (FH_2), which is then reduced to tetrahydrofolate (FH_4), dihydrofolate reductase catalyses both steps [96].

Methylene tetrahydrofolate (CH_2FH_4) is formed from tetrahydrofolate by the addition of methylene groups one of three carbon donors: formaldehyde, serine, or glycine. Methyltetrahydrofolate (CH_3-FH_4) can be made from methylene tetrahydrofolate by reduction of the methylene group; formyl tetrahydrofolate (CHO-FH_4, folinic acid results from oxidation of methylene tetrahydrofolate [96].

A number of drugs interfere with the biosynthesis of folic acid and tetrahydrofolate. Among them are the dihydrofolate reductase inhibitors (such as trimethoprim and pyrimethamine), the sulfonamides (competitive inhibitors of para-aminobenzoic acid in the reactions of dihydropteroate synthetase), and the anticancer drug methotrexate (inhibits both folate reductase and dihydrofolate reductase).

Folic acid is very important for all women who may become pregnant. Adequate folate intake during the periconceptional period, the time just before and just after a woman becomes pregnant, helps protect against a number of congenital malformations including neural tube defects [97]. Neural tube defects result in malformations of the spine (spina bifida), skull, and brain (anencephaly). The risk of neural tube defects is significantly reduced, when supplemental folic acid is consumed in addition to a healthy diet prior to and during the first month following conception [98,99]. Women who could become pregnant are advised to eat foods fortified with folic acid or take supplements in addition to eating folate-rich foods to reduce the risk of some serious birth defects. Taking 400 micrograms of synthetic folic acid daily from fortified foods and/or supplements has been suggested. The Recommended Dietary Allowance (RDA) for folate equivalents for pregnant women is 600 micrograms.

Although folic acid does reduce the risk of birth defects, it is only one part of the picture and should not be considered a cure. Even women taking daily folic acid supplements have been known to have children with neural tube defects.

Low concentrations of folate, vitamin B12 or vitamin B6 may increase your level of homocysteine (Hcy), an amino acid normally found in the blood. There is evidence that an elevated homocysteine level is an independent risk factor for heart diseae and stroke [100]. The evidence suggests that high levels of homocysteine may damage coronary arteries or make it easier for blood clotting cells called platelets to clump together and form a clot [101]. However, there is currently no evidence available to suggest that lowering homocysteine with vitamins will reduce of heart disease risk. Clinical intervention trials are needed to determine whether supplementation with folic acid, vitamin B12 or vitamin B6 can lower the risk of developing coronary heart disease.

As of just year, studies have shown that giving folic acid to reduce levels of homocysteine does not result in clinical benefit and suggests that in combination with B12 may even increase some cardiovascular risks [102,103,104].

Some evidence associates low blood levels of folate with a greater risk of cancer [105]. Folate is involved in the synthesis, repair, and functioning of DNA, our genetic map, and a deficiency of folate may result in damage to DNA that may lead to cancer [106]. Several studies have associated diets low in folate with increased risk of breast, pancreatic, and colon cancer [107]. Findings from a study of over 121,000 nurses suggested that long-term folic acid supplementation (for 15 years) was associated with a decreased risk of colon cancer in women 55 to 69 years of age [108].

Folate intake counteracts breast cancer risk associated with alcohol consumption [109] and women who drink alcohol and have a high folate intake are not at increased risk of cancer [110]. Those who have a high (200 micrograms or more per day) level of folate (folic acid) in their diet, are not at increased risk of breast cancer compared to those who abstain from alcohol [111].

However, associations between diet and disease do not indicate a direct cause. Researchers are continuing to investigate whether enhanced folate intake from foods or folic acid supplements may reduce the risk of cancer.

Some evidence links low levels of folate with depression [112]. There is some limited evidence from randomized controlled trials that using folic acid in addition to antidepressant medication may have benefits [113]. However, the evidence is probably too limited at present for this to be a routine treatment recommendation.

In a 3-year trial on 818 people over the age of 50, short-term memory, mental agility and verbal fluency were all found to be better among people who took 800 micrograms of folic acid daily – a high dose - than those who took placebo. The study was reported in The Lancet on 19 January 2007.

Chanarin [114] summarized many studies on folate nutrition and metabolism in pregnancy performed in the 1950s and 1960s. The general conclusion drawn from these studies was that pregnancy was associated with an increased folate demand and in some cases led to overt folate deficiency. The increase in folate requirement during pregnancy is due to the growth of the fetus and uteroplacental organs. However, dietary folate intake does not always meet the increased folate needs in pregnancy. Pregnancy women exhibit rapid plasma clearance of intravenously administered folic acid [114]. Increased folate catabolism [115,116,117,118] and urinary folate excretion [19,20] may also contribute to increased folate needs in pregnancy, but the findings are controversial.

Circulating folate declines in pregnant women who are not supplemented with folic acid [114,119,120-128]. Chanarin [114] reported an average decline in serum of ~ 10 nmol/L (from 20 to 10 nmol/L) during the 40-wk gestation. This decline may represents a physiologic response to pregnancy, but the mechanism still is unknown. The pattern of changes in erythrocyte folate varies, with a decline observed in early pregnancy, followed by a slight increase in midpregnancy [114,100,101]. Possible causes for the declines in blood folate include: increased folate demand for the growth of the fetus and uteroplacental organs [114], dilution of folate due to blood volume expansion [102], increased folate catabolism [118], increased folate clearance and excretion [119,124], decreased folate absorption [114], hormonal influence on folate metabolism as a physiologic response to pregnancy [114], and low folate intake [114]. Although the techniques used in the studies that were conducted in the 1950s and 1960s may be different from those used in recent days, the fundamental conclusions derived from the results are generally reasonable. It is apparent that the first and last causes mentioned above lead to a decrease in folate stores, but it is less apparent whether the observed decline is due to the other factors. For example, Bruinse et al [24] measured plasma volume by a dye dilution method and estimated the total circulating amount of folate during both pregnancy and lactation. They found that serum folate declined up to 42% between 16 and 34 wk of gestation, and this drop was markedly greater than the decline in total circulating folate (28% in the same period), suggesting that the decline in serum folate cannot be explained by hemodilution.

In seemingly similar studies, folate catabolism was reported to increase or remain unchanged in pregnancy. One group reported that excretion of folate catabolites late in pregnancy was higher than in the nonpregnant state [115,117]. These catabolites are cleavage products of the C-9-N-10 bond of folate, including p-acetamidobenzoylglutamate (major urinary catabolite) and p-aminobenzolyglutamate, with the former involving N-acetylation of the latter. The folate-equivalent sum of the catabolites was 349 μg/d (0.9 μmol/d) in the third trimester, an amount double that of the nonpregnant state (0.31 μmol/d), indicating an accelerated folate breakdown. The amounts of catabolites excreted postpartum were similar to the level observed during the first trimester [115,117]. Increased catabolism may be consistent with placental expression of N-acetyltransferase type 1, which catalyzes the N-acetylation of p-aminobenzoylglutamate [104,105]. In contrast, another group did not find an increase in urinary catabolites in the second trimester in women, who received a controlled diet [116]. In the same study, with the use of stable-isotope-labeled folates, they reported no differences in urinary excretion of labeled folates or catabolites between the pregnant and nonpregnant women [118]. The discrepancies between the findings of the 2 groups may be due to differences in the catabolite assay or in the gestational stages analyzed [17]. Why folate catabolism increases late is pregnancy in again unknown [115,117]. Additional studies are needed, particularly studies on how N-acetyltransferase type 1 [104,105] and a ferritin-related folate-catabolizing enzyme that cleaves the C-9-N-10 bond of tetrahydrofolate, possibly regulate intracellular folate concentrations [106].

Results on plasma folate clearance after folic acid administration in pregnancy are consistent. Chanarin et al [107] found that folate clearance after an injection of folic acid was higher in pregnant than nonpregnant women, accelerated as pregnancy progressed, and was greater in pregnant women with megaloblastic anemia than in those without. Landon and Hytten [119] estimated 24h urinary folate serially during pregnancy and postpartum and reported that the mean urinary folate was 32 and 8 nmoles/d, respectively. Fleming [124] also reported that mean folate clearance and urinary folate excretion was higher in pregnancy than in the nonpregnant state. Collectively, administered folic acid is more rapidly incorporated into cells and excreted in urine in pregnant than in nonpregnant women.

Whether a decrease in folate absorption contributes to an increased folate requirement in pregnancy is less certain. Chanarin et al [107] found that the peak serum folate concentration after an oral folic acid dose was significantly lower in pregnant than nonpregnant women, which suggested a decrease in folate absorption. However, Landon and Hytten [108] measured plasma folate after an oral folic acid dose in pregnant women, postpartum women, and adult men and found no difference between the 3 groups, which indicated that folate absorption is not altered in pregnancy. McLean et al [109] reported that oral loading with either folic acid or polyglutamyl folate (yeast) resulted in similar increases in serum folate in pregnant women, which suggested that malabsorption of polyglutamyl folate does not occur. The differences in the quantity of folate administered and the methods used to assess folate absorption may explain the discrepancies between these studies.

Several mechanisms, probably in combination, may explain the decline in blood folate in pregnancy. Whatever the reasons for the decline, it is essential that plasma folate be kept above a critical level (> 7.0 nmol/L) because plasma folate is the main determinant of transplacental folate delivery to the fetus. Adequate plasma folate is likely to be achieved, if prenatal folic acid supplementation or folic acid fortification of foods are practiced. However, in countries without such measures, the risk for gestational folate deficiency remains a public health problem.

Although nutrient transfer via the placenta from the maternal plasma pool must be effective to satisfy the demand for fetal growth, information on placental folate transfer is scarce. Landon et al [110] measured the placental transport of an intravenous dose of [^{3}H] folic acid in women, who were scheduled for pregnancy termination. Tritium uptake was greatest in the fetal liver, and an analysis indicated that a peak of reduced folates in the placenta was detected shortly after the dose was intravenously administered, which suggested that folic acid was rapidly metabolized before or at the time of placental transfer. Baker et al [36] found a strong positive association between maternal plasma, cord plasma, and placental folate concentrations, suggesting that transplacental folate delivery depends on maternal plasma folate concentrations.

In placental perfusion studies, Henderson et al [125] found that 5-methyltetrahydrofolate (the main form of folate found in plasma) is extensively and rapidly bound in the placenta but transferred to the fetus in reduced amounts at a slower pace, and that the transfer is bidirectional and saturable. The placental folate receptor (FR) favors the binding of 5-methyltetrahydrofolate and can transfer folate against a concentration gradient; hence, the fetal perfusate is about 3-fold that of the maternal perfusate, which indicates that folate is concentrated during placental transport. Bisseling et al [126] found that the transfer of 5-methyltetrahydrofolate from the maternal to the fetal perfusate was not saturable in a range well above typical physiologic concentrations.

The placenta is rich in FRs and is one of the tissues (along with the choroids plexus and renal proximal tubules) that expresses the α-isoform of FR (FR-α) in abundance. FR-α is a membrane-bound glycosylphosphatidyl-inositol-linked glycoprotein and the primary form of FR in epithelial cells. The importance of FR-α to placental folate transfer is inferred from the fact that an FR-α knockout mouse in embryo-lethal, whereas the FR-β knockout is not [127]. Placental folate transport may be mediated by FR-α- via a 2-step process [128], which includes the binding of 5-methyltetrahydrofolate to placental FR-α to produce an intravillous concentration 3 times that of maternal plasma and transporting folate to the fetus against a concentration gradient. Maternal folate status should be kept adequate to maintain plasma folate above a certain concentration for placental transfer. High-affinity binding proteins in the maternal circulation, cord blood, and newborns are derived from membrane-associated precursors [129,130].

The activities of dihydrofolate reductase, folylpoly γ-glutamate carboxypeptidase II folate conjugase; [108] methionine synthase [112], MTHFR [113], and serine hydroxymethyltransferase were detected in human placenta, mRNA expression of mitochondrial C_1-tetrahydrofolate synthase [5,10-methylenetetrahydrofolate dehydrogenase; 5,10-methenyltetrahydrofolate cyclohydrolase (reaction8); and 10-formyltetrahydrofolate synthetase (reaction 7)] was detected, although the activity was not measured [131]. Daly et al [113] reported that placenta MTHFR activities were related to C677T MTHFR variants, which suggests a possible association with NTD development. The biochemical and physiologic implications of placental folate metabolism and transport require additional studies and the use of folates labeled with stable isotopes may make such human studies feasible.

Many researchers have evaluated the relations between folate concentrations in maternal, cord, and neonatal blood at or shortly after delivery [132-137]. They reported that blood folate is markedly elevated in fetuses and newborns, which indicates and effective placental folate transport against a concentration gradient. Depsite the elevation of blood folate in cord or newborn blood over maternal blood, total fetal folate stores do not appear to be large, because fetal hepatic folate content is lower than that in adults. Fetal hepatic folate concentrations ranged from 1.5 to 4.0 μg/g [138-140], whereas adult hepatic folate concentrations were > 5.0 μg/g [59,60]. These data suggest that fetal folate acquisition and utilization differ from those of adults. Amniotic fluid folate concentrations range between 3 and 33 nmol/L [141-143], but the metabolic significance of folate in amniotic fluid is unknown.

The ontogeny of folate-dependent enzymes in humans has not been extensively studied due to the obvious diffuculty, with a few exceptions. Gaull et al [144] reported that the activities of methionine synthase in fetal tissues are higher than in adult tissues, whereas those of serine hydroxymethyltransferase were similar. Kalinsky et al [145] reported that the activities of hepatic MTHFR and methionine synthase in preterm infants were higher than those in full-term infants or young children, whereas the activities of hepatic formininotransferase and 5-10-methylenetetrahydrofolate-dehydrogenase were just the opposite. These results suggest dynamic changes in folate-dependent reactions late in fetal life and in neonatal life. In studies conducted in animals, the data indicated that specific activities of some of the folate-dependent enzymes also changed during the perinatal period [146-148]. Furthermore, Xiao et al [149] elucidated the effect of maternal folate status on the regulation of fetal FR in mice. However, it is unclear to what extent the fingings from the animal studies can be extrapolated to human conditions.

Furthermore maternal nutritional status has been shown to contribute significantly to pregnancy outcome [150]. Food intake, processing absorption, metabolism and clearance determine the individual vitamin status. The embryo and foetus are totally dependent on the maternal nutrient status and the maternal-foetal transfer of nutrients. Marginally deficient values or elevated concentrations still within the normal nonpregnant range might have a siginificant impact on early embryonic development as well as on long-term health outcome [151].

Since 1997, a lot of Albanian immigrants have moved into Greece. As ethnic background is of paramount importance in studies of nutritional markers and diseases, this study attempted, for the first time, to compare retinol and folate serum concentrations in a large number of healthy women of two different ethnic groups (Greeks, Albanians) at delivery and in the cord blood of their newborns in relation to their nutritional habits.

MATERIALS AND METHODS

Subjects and Samples

The present study was performed in accordance with the Helsinki Declaration of 1964 (as amended in 1983 and 1989) and approved by the Greek Ethics Committee of Alexandra Maternity Hospital.

Throughout a period of 48 months, serum samples were collected from the cord blood of healthy full-term newborn infants only fulfilling the following criteria: a) null-partum b) singleton live birth; c) eutotic delivery with cephalic presentation; d) gestational age between 36 weeks completed and the end of the 41st week; e) body weight between 2500 and 4000 g and f) Apgar scores of ≥ 9 at the 1st min. From the original 2320 cord blood samples only 1376 fulfilled the above-mentioned criteria and were included in the study. Data concerning mothers of both ethnic groups [Greeks (N=710), Albanians (N=686)], the course of their pregnancy and delivery were obtained from the notes in the records kept by obstetricians and pediatricians, according to the stricted routine practice of the Department of Obstetrics and Gynecology of the "Alexandra" Maternity Hospital of Athens University.

With regards to the Greek pregnant women, no medical and/or obstetrical problem including abortions, have been found. On the contrary, spontaneous abortions and/or malformations followed by abortions were mentioned in 13.8% of the immigrant mothers. The latter information could not be confirmed, because of lack of written Albanian medical records.

As a general trend, the majority of Greek women belong to a moderate or to an upper economic status and deliver their babies in private clinics. Alexandra Maternity Hospital, being a public Institution, receives a rather homogenous population of lower income. Monthly income of the family of the pregnant women could be characterized as high (> 800 euros per month), moderate (500-800 euros per month) and low (< 500 euros per month). Gestational age was determined based on the last menstrual period and the obstetrical findings. No woman smoked, or received micronutrient supplementation at least 3 months before sampling [152,153]. Additionally, a 60 d nutrient intake diary was kept from each woman during the last 2 months of gestation. The amounts of the daily nutrients were calculated according to a coded food list [155].

Immediately after delivery 3.0 ml blood was obtained from mothers and 3.0 ml from umbilical cord in light-protected tubes and centrifuged within 1h. Separated sera were then kept frozen at < -20°C until analysis.

Analytical Procedure

Retinol was measured in deproteinized, hexane-extracted sera using HPLC (Agilent Technologies HP 1100 Series, CA, USA), with an internal standard [10]. Separation was performed with a reversed phase C_{18} column (Bio-Rad Laboratories, Hercules, CA, USA), with 100% methanol mobile phase and detection at 340nm and [155,156,157]. Inter-assay precision was 2.8% and 3.2% respectively. Vitamin A was normalized according to total protein concentrations of the samples. Folate levels were measured by chemiluminescence using the Siemens ADVIA Centaur System (Siemens Medical Solutions, Tarrytown, NY USA). The sensitivity of the assay by this method interassay and intrassay variations were 2.8% and 3.2% respectively [158].

Statistical Analysis

Data were studied by one-way ANOVA. As no variable was simultaneously Gaussian in both groups, differences between groups were tested with the Mann-Whitney-U test. P values < 0.05 were considered statistically significant.

RESULTS

As shown in Table 1, the younger mothers have come from Albania, whereas Greek mothers were almost 1-2 years elder. No statistically significant differences were found between gestational periods, placental weights and birth weights among the studied groups. In contrast, socio-economics status differed greatly between the studied groups. Most of Albanians income per month was chatacterized low (< 600 Euros), whereas most Greeks belonged to a moderate or high (> 800 euros) socio-economic level.

Table 1. Clinical and socio-economics characteristics of Greek and Albanian mothers and their newborns

	Greeks (N=710)	Albanians (N=686)
Age (yrs)	29.7 ± 6.4^a	27 ± 5.9^b
range	(18 – 39)	(14 - 39)
Gestation (weeks)	39.5 ± 1.3^c	38.7 ± 1.4^d
Placenta(g)	480.4 ± 69.2^c	499.3 ± 67^d
Birth weight (g)	3378 ± 386^c	3298 ± 496^d
Sex (M%)	45	52
(F%)	55	48
Socio-economics status (income per month)		
Low (%)	2.0	95.0*
Moderate (%)	82.0	5.0*
High (%)	1.60	-

Values are expressed: mean ± SD;
a/b, c/d NS; * p<0.001.

As presented in Table 2, energy, carbohydrates, total fat, saturated fat and cholesterol intake were significantly increased in the Albanians, as compared with those of Greeks. On the contrary, vitamin A and especially animal protein intake, which is rich of the vitamin [9] mono and polyunsaturated fat and the ratio poly/sat fat were greatly reduced in the immigrant group, whereas folate intake did not differ between Greeks and Albanians.

**Table 2. Estimated 60 d nutrient intakes for the two
studied groups of mothers (Greeks, Albanians)**

Nutrients	Greeks (N = 1125)	Albanian (N = 898)
Energy (Kcal)	2350±150[a]	2900±140[a]
t. Protein (g)	64±14[b]	58±15[b]
Animal prot (g)	50±12[a]	36±10[a]
Veget. Prot (g)	14±9[a]	22±10a
Carbohydrates (g)	280±40[a]	388±44[a]
Total Fat (g)	106±10[a]	124±12[a]
Saturated fat (g)	38± 8[a]	62±10[a]
Monounsaturated (g)	40±12[b]	48±12[b]
Polyunsaturated (g)	28±2.0[a]	14±3.0[a]
Poly / satur (ratio)	0.7±0.1[a]	0.2±0.1[a]
Cholesterol (mg)	380±38[c]	520±40[c]
Vit A μgRE (RNI 800 μg RE[*])	895±98[a]	518±90[a]
Folate μg (RNI 400-600)**	534±95	525±100

Data are presented: mean ± SD (daily values);

**RNI: reference nutrient intake (Garrow J. S., James WP, Ralph A. Human Nutrition and Dietetics 10th Eds Churchill Livingstone 2000 pp 427 – 448).

a/a < 0.001, e/e p<0.05, c/c b/b < 0.01;

*RE, retinol equivalent, 1RE = 1 μg retinol.

As presented in Table 2a, the main source of vitamin A intake with food for Greek mothers comes from animal products, whereas immigrant mothers prefer vegetable food rich of the vitamin. In contrast, Greek mothers preferably eat vegetable food rich of folate and Albania that of animal origin.

As shown in Table 3 retinol level was evaluated statistically significant decreased in Albanian mothers, as compared with that in Greeks. Additionally, subclinical retinol deficiency concentrations were observed in 28% of the Albanians and suboptimal in 52% whereas only in 0.1% of Greeks the vitamin status could be characterized suboptimal.

Retinol levels (Table 4) were determined statistically significant higher in the cord blood of Greek newborns as compared with those of Albanians. Furthermore, the vitamin concentration was suboptimal in 2% of the Greek group only. On the contrary, retinol was determined considerably low in 55% of Albanian newborns and suboptimal in 28%. Interestingly, in 12% of these newborns retinol levels were measured higher compared with those of their mothers in whom the vitamin blood concentrations were found significantly low. Folate levels did not differ among the studied groups.

Table 2a. Nutritional habits (% of the studied population) of Greeks and Albanians

Food consumption	Greeks (N=710)		Albanian(N=686)	
A. Vitamin A rich food[1]		P values		P values
Animal (Oatmeat, liver, chicken, etc		0.02		0.03
Never	2.8		27.8	
≤ 2-3 times/week	12.6		64.2	
≥ 5 times/week	84.6		8.0	
Vegetable (carrots, kate, apricote etc)		0.03		0.04
Never	37		13.0	
≤ 2-3 times/week	56		76.4	
≥ 5 times/weeks	7		10.6	
Folate rich food[1]		0.06		0.04
Animal (Beef liver, etc)				
Never	3.7		18.8	
≤ 2-3 times/week	26.8		76.2	
≥ 5 times/week	69.5		5.0	
Vegetable (spinach, rice, asparagus, beans etc)		0.01		0.02
Never	12.6		3.0	
≤ 2-3 times/week	84.6		58.0	
≥ 5 times/weeks	2.8		39.0	

Only food rich in vitamin A or folate is listed

[1] US Department of Health and Human Services. Advance Data from Vital and Health Statistics. Dietary intake of selected vitamins for the United States population: 1999-2000 Centers for Disease control and Prevention. National Center for Health statistics. Number 339, 2004.

Table 3. Retinol and folate serum concentrations in Greek and Albanian mothers

	Mean ± SD (median)	% retinol (deficient cases)[1]	% retinol (suboptimal cases)[1]	% Folate (suboptimal case)[2]
Greeks (N=710)				
		<0.45 μmol/L[1]	0.45-0.9 μmol/L[1]	<10.5 nmol/L[2]
retinol (μmol/L) (range)	1.3 ± 0.2^a (0.85) (0.6-1.1)	None	0.1	
Folate (nmol/L) Range	18.87 ± 3.8^b (17.8) (2.5 – 24.4)	-	-	2.8
Albanians (N=686)				
		<0.45μmol/L1	0.45-0.9μmol/L1	<10.5 nmol/L2
retinol (μmol/L) (range)	$0.6 \pm 0.1a$ (0.4) (0.2 – 0.8)	28	52	
Folate (nmol/L) Range	$18.1 \pm 4.1b$ (17.0) (2.4 – 23.5)	-	-	2.9

a/a: $p < 0.001$ (retinol), b/b = NS;

[1]McKormick DB and Greene HJ. Vitamins InTietz textbook of clinical chemistry 3rd ed. CA Burtis and ER Ashwood eds 1999. Philadlephia W.B. Saunders Vo pp 999-1028.

[2] Fairbanks VF and Klee GG. Biochemical aspects of hematology

In: Tietz text-book of Clinical Chemistry 2nd ed. Burtis and ER Ashwood Philadelphia, WB Saunders 1999 pp 2046-2049.

As shown in Table 3 retinol level was evaluated statistically significant decreased in Albanian mothers, as compared with that in Greeks. Additionally, subclinical retinol deficiency concentrations were observed in 28% of the Albanians and suboptimal in 52% whereas only in 0.1% of Greeks the vitamin status could be characterized suboptimal.

Retinol levels (Table 4) were determined statistically significant higher in the cord blood of Greek newborns as compared with those of Albanians. Furthermore, the vitamin concentration was suboptimal in 2% of the Greek group only. On the contrary, retinol was determined considerably low in 55% of Albanian newborns and suboptimal in 28%. Interestingly, in 12% of these newborns retinol levels were measured higher compared with those of their mothers in whom the vitamin blood concentrations were found significantly low. Folate levels did not differ among the studied groups.

Table 4. Retinol and folate concentrations in the cord blood of Greeks and Albanians

	Mean ± SD (median)	% retinol (deficient cases)	% retinol (suboptimal cases)	% Folate (suboptimal cases)[2]
Greeks (N=710)		$<0.35\mu mol/L^1$	$0.35-0.70\mu mol/L^1$	$<7.5\ mg/mL^2$
retinol (µmol/L) (range)	0.85 ± 0.1[a] (0.85) (0.6-1.0)		2	
Folate nmol/L Range	26.6 ± 12.0 (24.0)	-	-	0
Albanians (N=686)		$<0.35\mu mol/L1$	$0.35-0.70\mu mol/L1$	$<7.5\ nmol/L2$
retinol (µmol/L) (range)	0.4 ± 0.1a (0.35) (0.6-1.1)	55xx	38	
Folate (nmol/L) Range	24.6 ± 14.7 (23.8)	-	-	1.8

Retinol, a/a p < 0.001;
xx in 12% of cord blood samples retinol levels were evaluated higher as compared to those of their mothers;
[1]McKormick DB and Greene HJ. Vitamins In Tietz textbook of clinical chemistry 3rd ed. CA Burtis and ER Ashwood eds 1999. Philadlephia W.B. Saunders Vo pp 999-1028;
[2]Hick JM, Vitamin B_{12} and Folate, Pediatric reference values 1993, 117:704-6.

DISCUSSION

Individual and population health, in general, is the result of interaction between genetic and a number of environmental factors. The human genetic profile has not changed over the past 10.000 years, whereas major changes have taken place in human food supply and in energy expenditure. Nutrition an environmental factor of major importance is related to a number of factors such as socio-economic standard of living, religion, geographical region, traditions etc. [159]. From this point of view Greek mothers belonged to a unexpected higher socio-economic level than that found in the Albanian immigrant mothers group.

Vitamin A is fundamentally required in physiological processes such as vision, reproduction, cellular differentiation, immune function and growth. During periods of intense proliferative growth and tissue development as in pregnancy, these roles are particularly critical for embryogenesis and fetal development. However, it is assumed that the maternal-fetal transfer of vitamin A must be closely regulated, since either deficiency or excess may be damaging to the fetus [160-163].

Vitamin A occurs in the human diet as retinyl esters in animal products, or as provitamin, β-carotene, which are partly cleared to produce vitamin A in the enterocyte. After intestinal absorption vitamin A is packed into chylomicrons as retinyl esters. The chylomicron remnants are then taken up by hepatocytes, in which the retinyl esters are hydrolyzed into retinol. When vitamin A status is insufficient, the newly formed retinol is bound to retinol binding protein (RBP) and secreted into the blood. The RBP variants are genetically affected [164]. In this study vitamin A intake was found higher in the Greek mothers than that found in the immigrants. This finding may be due to the low economic level of the immigrants since fruits (eg apricots) and animal products rich in the vitamin is costly cost without excluding the immigrants nutritional habits.

Vitamin A metabolism does not seem to be considerably affected during pregnancy. It is transferred from the mother to the embryo across the placenta; vitamin A concentrations in fetal blood are approximatelly half of those in the mother [165].

Concentrations of ~ 1 μmol/L, as found in the sera of the Greek mothers, are frequent and are not considered indicative of a deficient status. The situation is more critical for premature deliveries and may pose a direct threat to the child's health. Indicator of low vitamin A status include a serum retinol level (< 0.7 μmol/L) and poor dietary habits, as determined in the sera of Albanian mothers and in their dietetic diaries [164].

Vitamin A and its active derivatives, the retinoids, are fundamental for the development of mammalian fetus [166-170]. The placenta plays a crucial role in the regulation of transport and metabolism of maternal nutrients transferred to the fetus. Abnormalities in these placental functions may have deleterious consequences on fetal development [171,172]. Maternal vitamin A status, placental function and the duration of gestation are some of the factors, which would be expected to influence the delivery of vitamin A to the fetus [173 – 175]. Gebre-Medhin and Valquist [166] have reported an exponential increase in liver retinol concentrations during the later part of pregnancy in Swedish, but not in Ethiopian fetuses. Presumably, the vitamin A status of the mothers in the latter group was too low to have an impact on the fetal liver store. Similarly Shah et al [167] reported that low income group women, as the Albanian group of this study, had lower plasma vitamin A levels compared with the high income group women in each of the trimester. Moreover, in a longitudinal study, Sivakumer et al [176] have demonstrated that food rich of vitamin A and only long term maternal supplementations was effective in raising cord level and hence fetal status.

It is well recognized that the placenta could be considered as a transitory, primitive functional liver during the first stages of development. The capacity of the human placenta at term to esterify retinol may have activity during early embryonic and fetal development. The retinyl ester content of embryo is nearly 4-fold greater than that of placenta. The timing of this crossover correlates with the apparent onset of retinol storage of the embryonic liver [164]. The placentae, which were found normal in both groups of this study, could be considered as an efficient buffer to control retinol exchange between mother and fetus by: a) releasing retinol to the fetus when maternal intake is deficient, as we found in a group of the immigrant mothers with very low serum retinol levels and, b) protecting the embryo from a potential excess of maternal retinol, thus preventing the fetus from retinoid teratogenicity [168,170].

Retinol plasma concentration was measured normal in the Greek mothers as their vitamin A intake. On the contrary, the vitamin levels in the Albanians were found half of that in Greeks. The mean retinol levels in the cord blood of the Greek newborns reflected its adequate intake by their mothers. On the contrary, the reduced vitamin intake by the immigrant mothers resulted in either deficient or suboptimal vitamin concentrations in their newborns. Almost similarly, low concentrations of retinol were observed in the immigrant Albanian mothers, as those determined by Shah et al [167], in the blood of mothers with low income. As already mentioned, the placenta appearance, both in Greeks and Albanians, was normal and their weights did not differ among the groups of study (Table 1). The above suggest that the observed low vitamin A levels in the immigrant mothers and in the cord blood of their newborns could be due to their inadequate nutritional intake of the vitamin during pregnancy in relation to their low socio-economic status as Braesco and Pascal reported [164] or even due to their nutritional habits.

A subclinical mother vitamin A deficiency may produce no effect on the fetal circulating retinol, but may affect the placental handling of retinol and carotenoids to ensure an adequate retinol supply to the fetus. Besides, vitamin A concentration in fetal circulation is significantly lower than in maternal circulation [171,172], as found in our study too. Additionally, when maternal retinol levels are extremely low, as determined in a great number of Albanian mothers, the trans-placental flow may favor the fetus and, in this situation, fetal circulating retinol levels are maintained to ensure only tissue demands in preference to liver storage, [166,177]. In agreement with this hypothesis, the same authors observed lower liver retinol concentration in fetuses of poorly nourished, compared to well nourished. Under conditions of maternal/fetus vitamin A deficiency the requirement of the fetus would take precedence and the concentration of cord blood approximates and in some cases exceeds that of mothers [162] as we found in a great part of the Albanian neonates (Table 4), whose mother retinol levels were measured extremely low.

In practice, vitamin recommendations vary greatly according to the endemicity and socioeconomic conditions of the country. In developed countries, there is no endemicity of low vitamin A status [166] and consequently there is no need for vitamin A supplementation. Such a measure could be even harmful, because of the potential risk of teratogenesis from high doses of vitamin A. From the other side, it is possible that a significant part of the low-income female population in some of the developed countries, who do not usually undergo prenatal examinations, suffers from undiagnosed low vitamin A status [164]. From all the above reasons, prenatal "follow up" could be the best public health measure to prevent vitamin deficiencies in both mothers and their neonates.

Furtheromore, the effect of folate status on pregnancy outcomes has long been recognized [114]. Since Wills [178] successfully treated megaloblastic anemia in pregnancy with a yeast extract (Marmite) in 1931, researchers have studied the prevalence and treatment of pregnancy-related folate deficiency and megaloblastic anemia [114]. Studies conducted in the 1950 and 1960s led to the fact that supplementation with folic acid reduced the prevalence of folate deficiency in pregnancy, and prenatal folic supplementation in the second and third trimesters became a common public health measure. In 1970, the US Food and Nutrition Board [179] recommended folic acid supplementation (200-400 μg/d) for pregnant women, and this became a common practice in developed countries and substantially reduced pregnancy-induced severe folate deficiency, which can lead to megaloblastic anemia. Prenatal folic acid, along with iron, supplementation reduced the prevalence of 2 of the most common pregnancy-related deficiencies. In this study, both Greek and Albanian mothers folate intake were found normal as recommended above [179] but the sources were not similar and may be related to the different socio-economics status of our participants.

The second major achievement with the use of folic acid occurred in the 1990s. For many years, researchers suspected an association between maternal folate status and fetal malformations, particularly neural tube defects (NTDs) [93,94]. However, this relation was not confirmed until the early 1990s, when periconceptional folic acid supplementation was found to reduce both the recurrence [95] and occurrence [96] of NTDs. This periconceptional folic acid supplementation no longer aims to treat or prevent pregnancy-induced severe folate deficiency, but only to correct abnormal folate metabolism or a subtle folate inadequacy that is possibly present in a certain segment of the population. These discoveries led to mandate folic acid food fortification in several countries [180-183]. These distinctively various uses of folic acid-prenatal folic acid supplementation, periconceptional folic acid supplementation, and folic fortification of staple foods-may well be ranked among the most significant public health measures for the prevention of pregnancy-related disorders. From this point of view no malformation and particularly NTDs were found among the newborns of the present study.

Chanarin et al [184] measured folate content in individually prepared meals collected from pregnant women and found that mean folate intake was 676 μg/d, which significantly correlated with erythrocyte folate concentrations. However, this value is condisered extremely high. Moscovitch and Cooper [185] measured the folate content of meals consumed by women, who were in the second trimester of pregnancy and who prepared duplicate diets and their mean folate intake was found 242 μg/d. The large difference between the 2 groups of those studies may be due to variety in food selection and folate assay methods. Since these reports, more than 30 y ago, there have been no reports on direct folate analyses of self-selected diets, consumed by pregnant women. Instead, investigators have estimated dietary intakes by dietary recalls or food-frequency questionnaires and calculated the values for folate intake from food tables [186-192]. In these reports, the mean folate intakes of pregnant women varied widely form 85 to 668 μg/d.

Studies were conducted in the 1960s to determine the quantity of folic acid required, in addition to regular dietary intake, to maintain adequate folate status in pregnancy [114,194-196]. Willoughby and Jewell [193] measured the dose-response effect of prenatal folic (50-530 μg/d) on serum folate concentrations in the postpartum period and found that serum folate increased linearly with the amount of folic acid supplemented, which was given from ~3 mo of gestation to delivery. To keep postpartum serum folate > 7.0 nmol/L, they concluded that the minimum dose of folic acid needed during late pregnancy, in addition to a dietary folate intake of 50 μg/d, was close to 300μg/d. Hansen and Rybo [194] conducted a similar study by monitoring blood folate concentrations in late pregnancy. Plasma folate increased linearly, when folic acid was given at 200-500 μg/d. They suggested that an oral dose of 200 μg folic acid/d is close to the minimum requirement to maintain normal blood folate concentrations, although dietary folate intake was not reported in that study. Greek mothers were supplemented with folic acid (100 μg/d) during the 2th and 3d trimester of their pregnancy. In contrast, we cannot verify that the same happened in the immigrant group, because of language difficulties and lack of strict follow up during their pregnancy.

In addition to the blood folate assay, various biochemical (ie, formiminoglutamic acid analysis after a histidine load or deoxyuridine-suppression test) and hematologic (ie, neutrophil lobe count, mean corpuscular volume, or bone marrow test) tests were used to diagnose deficiency, assess the degree of folate deficiency, or measure responses to folic acid therapy in pregnancy [132,184,193,197-201]. In the 1990s, the plasma tHcy assay was added as a tool to assess folate adequacy. Of these tests, assays of folate and total homocysteine (tHcy) concentrations are the most extensively used; the other tests noted are used less, because they lack sensitivity and specificity. The normal folate levels measured in the sera of the groups of this study in relation to the absence of malformations or NTD in the newborns as well as the absence of mothers' hematological problems lead us to the decision not to evaluate Hcy plasma levels in the studied groups.

Before prenatal folic acid supplementation effectively reduced the prevalence of folate deficiency in developed countries, many cases of folate deficiency or megaloblastic anemia in pregnancy were reported [132,195-201]. However, folate deficiency was prevalent worldwide in the 1970s. For example, > 30% of women with pregnancy-related anemia in Venezuela were folate deficient [202], and a prevalence of folate deficiency of >10% was reported in pregnant women in Australia and the United States [203,204]. The presence of folate deficiency with or without megaloblastic anemia is still a public health problem of pregnant women in developing countries [205,206]. A short interpregnancy interval associated with inadequate folate status was found to lead to unfavorable pregnancy outcome [187,207 – 208].

Birth weight is probably the most important pregnancy outcome, because fetal growth restriction (FGR; birth weigh <10th percentile of a given population) is highly related to high mortality and morbidity [209]. Many researchers examined the relations between birth weight and the rates of FGR, low-birth weight (<2500 g), or very-low-birth weight (< 1500g) and maternal folate status [205-209], folate intake or folic acids supplementation [185,186,210-214], or megaloblastic anemia in pregnancy [111]. Conclusions as to whether maternal folate nutrition and metabolism affect fetal growth could not be made, because of the lack of consistency between the studies and the insufficient statistical power, due to small sample sizes. It is essential to understand that potential deficiencies in nutrients other than folate acting as confounding variables make it difficult to draw a solid conclusion, and this issue applies to interpreting data on the association between folate status and other pregnancy outcomes. Additionally, in 1992, Burke et al [212] first noted the possible relation between elevated tHcy and FGR. In a large Norwegian cohort, Vollset et al [213] later reported that the total growth risk of (FGR) infants was significantly increased in women, who were in the higher quartiles of tHcy that those in the lower quartiles, and others reported similar findings [214,215]. In this study none FGR newborn was found in both ethnic groups.

Retinol and folate serum levels were found normal in Greek mothers and in most of their newborns, probably due to their higher standard of living and their mediterranean diet. On the contrary, in the 1/3 of the Albanian mothers, retinol levels were evaluated significantly low and in 1/2 suboptimal. As a consequence, in more than 1/2 of their newborns retinoids were measured very low and in 1/3 suboptimal. With regards to folate, the vitamin was determined normal in most of the two ethnic groups both in mothers and their infants. As a general recommendation, programmes for the elevation of the immigrant socio-economic level along with strict follow up of the immigrant pregnant women should be planned in Greece.

ACKNOWLEDGMENT

The authors are highly indepted to Mrs Anna Stamatis and Mrs Maria Kalogerakou for their wonderful assistance in preparing this manuscript.

REFERENCES

[1]   Chawla A, Repa JJ, Evans RM and Mangelsdorf DJ (2001): Nuclear receptors and lipid physiology: Opening the X-files. *Science 294*, 1866-1870.

[2]   Blomhoff R (1994): *Vitamin A in Health and Disease*. Marcel Dekker Inc., New York.

[3]   Senoo H, Wake K, Wold HL, Higashi N, Imai K, Moskaug JO, Kojima N, Miura M, Sato T, Sato M, Roos N, Berg T. et al (2004): Decreased capacity for vitamin A storage in hepatic stellate cells in arctic animals. *Comp. Hepatol.* 3 (Suppl. 1), S18.

[4]   Senoo H, Hata R, Nagai Y and Wake K (1984): Stellate cells (vitamin A-storing cells) are the primary site of collagen synthesis in non-paranchymal cells in the liver. *Biomed. Res. 5*, 451-458.

[5]   Wake K (1971): Sternzellen in the liver: Perisinusoidal cells with special reference to storage of vitamin *A. Am J Anat. 132*, 429-462.

[6]   Wake K (1980): Perisinusoidal stellate cells (fat-storing cells, interstitial cells, lipocytes), their related structure in the around the liver sinusoids, and vitamin A-storing cells in extrahepatic organs. *Int. Rev. Cytol. 66*, 303-353.

[7]   Bloom E and Fawcett DW (1994): *A Textbook of Histology*. 12th ed. Pp. 652-668. Chapman & Hall, New York.

[8]   Kojiama N, Sato M, Suzuki A, Sato T, Sotah S, Kato T, and Senoo H (2001): Enhanced expression of B7-1, B7-2, and intercellular adhesion molecule 1 in sinusoidal endothelial cells by warm ischemia/reperfusion injury in rat liver. *Hepatology 34*, 751-757.

[9]   Prickett TCR, McKenzie JL, and Hart DNJ (1988): Characterization of interstitial dendrtitic cells in human liver. *Transplantation 46*, 754-761.

[10] Steiniger B, Klempnauer J and Wonigeit K (1984): Phenotype and histological distribution of interstitial dendritic cells in the rat pancreas, liver, heart and kidney. *Transplantation 38*, 169-175.

[11] Senoo H, Imai K, Wake K, Wold HL, Moskaug JO, Kojima N, Matano Y, Miura M, Sato M, Ross N, Langvatn R, Norum KR et al (1999): Vitamin A-storing system in mammals and birds in Arctic area: A study in the Svalbard archipelago. *Cells Hepatic Sinusoid 7*, 34-35.

[12] Sato M, Suzuki S, and Senoo H (2003): Hepatic stellate cells: Uniwque characteristics in cell biology and phenotype. *Cell Struct. Funct. 28*, 105-112.

[13] Senoo H, Sato M, and Imai K (1997): Hepatic stellate cells – From the viewpoint or retinoid handling and function of the extracellular matrix. *Acta Anat. Nippon 72*, 79-94.

[14] Matano Y, Miura M, Kojima N, Sato M, Imai K, and Senoo H (1999): Hepatic stellate cells and extrahepatic stellate cells (extrahepatic vitamin A-storing cells). *Cells Hepatic Sinusoid 7*, 26-27.

[15] Nagy NE, Holven KB, Roos N, Senoo H, Kojima N, Norum KR and Blomhoff R (1997): Storage of vitamin A in extrahepatic stellate cells in normal rats. *J. Lipid Res, 38*, 645-658.

[16] Senoo H, Hata R, Wake K and Nagai Y (1991): Isolation and serum free culture of stellate cells. *Cells Hepatic Sinusoid 3*, 259-262.

[17] Malaba L, Smeland S, Senoo H, Norum KR, Berg T, Blomhoff R and Kindberg GM (1996): Retinol-binding protein and asialo-orosomucoid are taken up by different pathoways in liver cells. *J Biol Chem 270*, 25686-15692.

[18] Senoo H, Stang E, Nilsson A, Kindberg GM, Berg T, Ross N, Norum KR and Blomhoff R (1990): Internalization of retinol-binding protein in parenchymal and stellate cells of rat liver. *J Lipid Res 31*, 1229-1239.

[19] Senoo H, Smaland S, Malaba L, Bjerkness T, Stang E, Roos N, Bert T, Norum KR, and Blomhoff R (1993): Transfer of retinol- binding protein from HepG2 human hepatoma cells to cocultured rat stellate cells. *Proc Natl Acad Sci USA 90*, 3616-3620.

[20] Smeland S, Bjerknes T, Malaba L, Eskild W, Norum KR and Blomhoff R (1995): Tissue distribution of the receptor for plasma retinol-binding protein. *Biochem J 305*, 419=424.

[21] Yang Q, Graham TE, Mody N, Preitner F, Peroni OD, Zabolotny JM, Kotani K, Quadro L and Kahn BB (2005): Serum retinol binding protein 4 contributes to insulin resistance in obesity and type 2 diabetes. *Nature 436*, 356-362.

[22] Debier C and Larondelle Y (2005): Vitamins A and E: Metabolism, roles and transfer to offspring. *Br J Nutr 93*, 153-174.

[23] Bellovino D, Apreda M, Gragnoli S, Massimi M, and Gaetani S (2003): Vitamin A transport: In vitro models for the study of RBP secretion. *Mol Aspects Med 24*, 411-420.

[24] Sivaprasadarao A, Sundraram M and Findlay JB (1998): Interactions of retinol-binding protein with transthyretin and its receptor. *Methods Mol Biol 89*, 155-163.

[25] Liden M and Eriksson U (2006). Understanding retinol metabolism-structure and function of retinol dehydrogenases. *J Biol Chem 281 (19)*, 13001-13004.

[26] Marill J, Idres N, Capron CC, Nguyen E and Chabot GG (2003): Retinoic acid metabolism and mechanism of action: A review. *Curr Drug Metab 4*, 1-10.

[27] Ghyselinck NB, Bavik C, Sapin V, Mark M, Bonnier D, Hindelang C, Dierich A, Nilsson CB, Hakansson H, Sauvant P, Azais-Braesco V, Frasson M et al. (1999):

Cellular retinol-binding protein I is essential for vitamin A homeostasis, *EMBO J 18*, 4903-4914.

[28] Napoli JL (1999): Interactions of retinoid binding proteins and enzymes in retinoid metabolism. *Biochim Biophys Acta 1440*, 139-162.

[29] Rossant J and Cross JC (2001): Placental development: Lessons from mouse mutants. *Nat. Rev Genet 2*, 538-548.

[30] Ross AC, and Gardner EM (1994). The function of vitamin A in cellular growth and differentiation and its roles during pregnancy and lactation. *Adv. Exp. Med. Biol 352*, 187-200.

[31] Sass JO, Tzimas G, Elmazar MM and Nau H (1999): Metabolism of retinaldehyde isomers in pregnant rats: 13-Cis- and all-trans-retinaldehyde, but not 9-cis-retinaldehyde, yield very similar patterns of retinoid metabolites. *Drug Metab Dispos. 27*, 317-321.

[32] Nau H, Elmazar MM, Ruhl R, Thiel R and Sass JO (1996): All-trans-retinoyl-beta-glucuronide is a potent teratogen in the mouse because of extensive metabolism to all-trans-retinoic acid. *Teratology 54*, 150-156.

[33] Sapin V, Ward SJ, Bronner S, Chambon P and Dolle P (1997): Differential expression of transcripts encoding retinoid binding proteins and retinoic acid receptors during placentation of the mouse. *Dev Dyn 208*, 199-210.

[34] Bavik C, Ward SJ and Ong DE (1997): Identification of a mechanism to localize generation of retinoic acid in rat embryos. *Mech Dev 69*, 155-167.

[35] Johansson S, Dencker L and Dantzer V (2001): Immunohistochemical localization of retinoid binding proteins at the meterno-fetal interface of the porcine epitheliochorial placenta. *Biol Reprod 64*, 60-68.

[36] Blanchon L, Sauvant P, Bavik C, Gallot D, Charbonne F, Alexandre-Gouabau MC, Lemery D, Jacquetin B, Dastugue B, Ward S and Sapin V (2002): Human choriocarcinoma cell line JEG-3 produces and secretes active retinoids from retinol. *Mol Hum Reprod 8*, 485-493.

[37] Johansson S, Gustafson AL, Donovan M, Romert A, Eriksson U and Dencker L (1997): Retinoid binding proteins in mouse yolk sac and chorio-allantoic placentas. *Anat Embryol (Berl.)195*, 483-490.

[38] Xueping E, Zhang L, Lu J, Tso P, Blaner WS, Levin MS and Li E (2002): Increased neonatal mortality in mice lacking cellular retino-binding protein II. *J Biol Chem 277*, 36617-36623.

[39] Johansson S, Gustafson AL, Donovan M, Eriksson U and Dencker L (1999): Retinoid binding proteins-expression patterns in the human placenta. *Placenta 20*, 459-465.

[40] Levin MS, Li E, Ong DE, and Gordon JI (1987): Comparison of the tissue-specific expression and developmental regulation of two closely linked rodent genes encoding cytosolic retinol-binding proteins. *J Biol Chem 262*, 7118-7124.

[41] Astrom A, Pettersson U and Voorhees JJ (1992): Structure of the human cellular retinoic acid-binding protein II gene. Early transcriptional regulation by retinoic acid. *J Biol Chem 267*, 25251-25255.

[42] Bates CJ (1983): Vitamin A in pregnancy and lactation. *Proc Nutr Soc 42*, 65-79.

[43]   Moore T (1971): Vitamin A transfer from mother to offspring in mice and rats. *Int. J Vitam Nutr Res 41*, 301-306.

[44]   Ismadi SD and Olson JA (1982): Dynamics of the fetal distribution and transfer of vitamin A between rat fetuses and their mother. *Int J Vitam Nutr Res 52*, 112-119.

[45]   Pasatiempo AM and Ross AC (1990): Effects of food or nutrient restriction on milk vitamin A transfer and neonatal vitamin A transfer and neonatal vitamin A stores in the rat. *Br J Nutr 63*, 351-362.

[46]   Sivaprasadarao A and Findlay JB (1994): Structure-function studies on human retinol-binding protein using site-directed mutagenesis *Biochem J 300*, 437-442.

[47]   Quadro L, Hamberger L. Gottesman ME, Colantuoni V, Ramakrishnan R and Blaner WS (2004): Transplacental delivery of retinoid: The role of retinol-binding protein and lipoprotein retinyl ester. *Am J Physiol Endocrinol Metab 286*, 844-851.

[48]   Estonius M, Svensson S and Hoog JO (1996): Alcohol dehydrogenase in human tissues: Localisation of transcripts coding for five classes of the enzyme. *FEBS Lett 397*, 338-342.

[49]   Sharma CP, Fox EA, Holomquist B, Jornvall H and Vallee BL (1989): cDNA sequence of human class III alcohol dehydrogenase. *Biochem Biophys Res Commun 164*, 631-637.

[50]   Card SE, Tomplins SF, and Brien JF (1989): Ontogeny of the activity of alcohol dehydrogenase and aldehyde dehydrogenases in the liver and placenta of the guinea pig. *Biochem Pharmacol 38*, 2535-2541.

[51]   Zorzano A and Herrera E (1989): Disposition of ethanol and acetaldehyde in late pregnant rats and their fetuses. *Pediatr Res 25*, 102-106.

[52]   Gamble MV, Shang E, Zott RP, Mertz JR, Wolgemuth DJ, and Blaner WS (1999): Biochemical properties, tissue expression and gene structure of a short chain dehydrogenase/reductase able to catalyze cis-retinol oxidation. *J Lipid Res 40*, 2279-2292.

[53]   Brown WM, Metger LE, Barlow JP, Hunsaker LA, Deck LM, Royer RE and Vander Jagt DL (2003): 17-Beta-Hydroxysteroid dehyydrogenase type 1: Computation design of active site inhibitors targeted to the Rossmann fold. *Chem Biol Interact 143-144*, 481-491.

[54]   Lin SX, Shi R, Qiu W, Azzi A, Zhu DW, Dabbagh HA and Zhou M (2006): Structural basis of the multispecificity demonstrated by 17beta-hydrozysteroid dehydrogenase types 1 and 5. *Mol. Cell Endocrinol 248*, 38-46.

[55]   Persson B, Krook M and Jornvall H (1991): Characteristics of short-chain alcohol dehydrogenases and related enzymes. *Eur J Biochem 200*, 537-543.

[56]   Thomas JL, Duax WL, Addlagatta A, Kacsoh, B, Brant SE and Norris WB (2004): Structure/function aspects of human 3 beta-hydroxysteroid dehydrogenase. *Mol Cell Endocrinol 215*, 73-82.

[57]   Parrow V, Horton C, Maden M, Laurie S, and Notarianni E (1998): Retionoids are endogenous to the procine blastcyst and secreted by trophecroderm cells at functionally-active levels. *Int J Dev Biol 42*, 629-632.

[58] Leo MA and Lieber CS (1999): Alcohol, vitamin A, and beta-carotene: Adverse interactions, including hepatotoxicity and carcinogenicity. *Am J Clin Nutr* 69, 1071-1085.

[59] Sapin V, Chaib S, Blanchon L, Alexandre-Gouabau MC, Lemery D, Charbonne F, Gallot D, Jacquetin, B, Dastugue B, and Azais-Braesco V (2000): Esterification of vitamin A by the human placenta involves villous mesenchymal fibroblasts. *Pediatr Res 48*, 565-572.

[60] Satre MA, Ugen KE and Kochhar DM (1992): Developmental changes in endogenous retinoids during pregnancy and embryogenesis in the mouse. *Biol Reprod 46*, 802-810.

[61] Sapin V, Gallot D, Marceau G, Dastugue B and Lemery D (2004): Implications trophoblastiques des retinoides: Aspects fondamentaux et hypothese physiopathologiqque. *Reprod Hum Horm 17*, 155-158.

[62] Orland MD, Anwar K, Cromley D, Chu CH, Chen L, Bilheimer JT, Hussain MM and Cheng D (2005): Acyl coenzyme A depender retinol esterification by acyl coenzyme A: Diacylglycerol acyltransferase 1. *Biochim Biophys Acta 1737*, 76-82.

[63] Gimes G, and Toth M (1993): Low concentration of Triton X-100 inhibits diacylglycerol acyltransferase without measurable effect on phosphatidate phosphohydrolase in the human primordial placenta. *Acta Physiol Hung 81*, 101-108.

[64] O'Byrne SM, Wongsiriroj N, Libien J, Vogel S, Goldberg IJ, Baehr W, Palczewski K, and Blaner WS (2005): Retinoid absorption and storage is impaired in mice lacking lecithin: retinol acyltransferase (LRAT). *J Biol Chem 280*, 35647-35657.

[65] Linke T, Dawson H and Harrison EH (2005): Isolation and characterization of a microsomal acid retinyl ester hlydrolase. *J Biol Chem 280*, 23287-23294.

[66] Lassiter TL, Barone S, IR, Moser VC, and Padilla S (1999): Gestatrional exposure to chlorpyrifos: Dose response profiles for cholinesterase and carboxylesterase activity. *Toxicol Sci 52*, 92-100.

[67] Zhang W, Xu G, and McLeod HL (2002): Comprehensive evaluation of carboxylesterase-2 expression n normal human tissues using tissue array analysis. *Appl Immunohistoche Mol Morphol 10*, 374-380.

[68] Yan B, Matoney L and Yang D (1999): Human carboxylesterase in term placentae: Enzymatic characterization, molecular cloning and evidence for the existence of multiple forms. *Placenta 20*, 599-607.

[69] Datta K and Kulkarni AP (1996): Co-oxidation of all-trans retinol acetate by human term placental lipoxygenase and soybean lipoxygenase. *Peprod Toxicol 10*, 105-112.

[70] Dimenstein R, Trugo NM, Donangelo CM, Trugo LC and Anastacio AS (1996): Effect of subadequate maternal vitamin-A status on placental transfer of retinol and beta-carotene to the human fetus. *Biol Neonate 69*, 230-234.

[71] Kiefer C, Hessel S, Lampert JM, Vogt K, Lederer MO, Breithaupt, DE and von Lintig J (2001): Identification and characterization of a mammalian enzyme catalyzing the asymmetric oxidative cleavage of provitamin A. *J Biol Chem 276*, 14110-14116.

[72] Lammer EJ, Chen DT, Hoar RM, Agnish ND, Benke PJ, Braun JT, Curry CJ, Fernhoff PM, Grix AW Ir, Lott IT, Macash RG, Nada GR et al. (1985): Retinoic acid embryopathy. *N. Engl J Med 313*,837-841.

[73] Wilson JG, Roth CB, and Warkany J (1953): An analysis of the syndrome of malformations induced by maternal vitamin A deficiency. Effects of restoration of vitamin A at various times during gestation. *Am J Anat 92*, 189-217.

[74] Conlon RA (1995): Retinoic acid and pattern formation in vertebrates. *Trends Genet 11*, 314-319.

[75] Mark M and Chambon P (2003): Functions of RARs and RXRs in vivo: Genetic dissection of the retinoid signalling pathway. *Pure Appl Chem 75*, 1709-1732.

[76] Shenefelt RE (1972): Morphogenesis of malformation in hamsters caused by retinoic acid: Relation to dose and stage at treatment. *Teratology 5*, 103-118.

[77] Ross SA, McCeffery PJ, Drager UC and De Luca LM (2000): Retinoids in embryonal development. *Physiol Rev 80*, 1021-1054.

[78] Zile MH (2001): Function of vitamin A in vertebrate embryonic development. *J Nutr 131*, 705-708.

[79] Mark M, Ghyselinck NB and Chambon P. (2004): Retinoic acid signalling in the development of branchial arches. *Curr Opin Genet Dev 14*, 591-598.

[80] Rossant J, Zirngibl R, Cado D, Shago M and Giguere V (1991): Expression of a retinoic acid response element-hsplacZ transgene defines specific domains of transcriptional activity during mouse embryogenesis. *Genes Dev 5*, 1333-1344.

[81] Ulven SM, Gundersen TE, Weedon MS, Landaas VO, Sakhi AK, Fromm SH, Geronimo BA, Moskaug JO, and Blomhoff R (2000): Identification of endogenous retinoids, enzymes, binding proteins and receptors during early postimplantation development in mouse: Important role of retinal dehydrogenase type 2 in synthesis of all-trans retinoic acid. *Dev Biol 220*, 379-391.

[82] Deltour L, Foglio NH and Duester G (1999a): Impaired retinol utilization in Adh4 alcohol dehydrogenase mutant mice. *Dev Genet 25*, 1-10.

[83] Ang HL, Dletour L, Hayamizu TF, Zgombic-Knight M, and Duester G (1996): Retinoic acid synthesis in mouse embryos during gastrulation and craniofactial development linked to class IV alcohol dehydrogenase gene expression. *J Biol Chem 271*, 9526-9534.

[84] Deltour L, Foglio MH and Duester G (1999b): Metabolic deficiencies in alcohol dehydrogenase Adh1, Adh3 and Adh4 null mutant mice. Overlapping roles of Adh1 and Adh4 in ethanol clearance and metabolism of retinol to retinoic acid. *J Biol Chem 274*, 16796-16801.

[85] Paik J, During A, Harrison EH, Mendelsohn CL, Lai K and Blaner NS (2001): Expression and characterization of a murine enzyme able to cleave beta-carotene. The formation of retinoids. *J Biol Chem 276(34)*, 32160-32168.

[86] Redmond TM, Gentleman S, Duncan T, Yu S, Wiggert B, Gantt E and Cunningham FX Jr (2001): Identification, expression and substrate specificity of a mammalian beta-carotene 15, 15'-dioxygenase. *J Biol Chem 276*, 6560-6565.

[87] Chytil F (1996): Retinoids in lung development. *FASEB J 10*, 986-992.

[88] Zachman RD, and Grummer MA (1998): The interaction of ethanol and vitamin A as a potential mechanism for the pathogenesis of Fetal Alcohol syndrome. *Alcohol Clin Exp Res 22*, 1544-1556.

[89] Liu L and Gudas LJ (2005): Disruption of the lecithin: retinol acyltransferase gene makes mice more susceptible to vitamin A deficiency, *J Biol Chem 280*, 40226-40234.

[90] Dolle P, Ruberte E, Leroy P, Morriss-Kay G and Chambon P (1990): Retinoic acid receptors and cellular retinoid binding proteins I. A systematic study of their differential pattern of transcription during mouse organogenesis. *Development 110*, 1133-1151.

[91] Gustafson AL, Dencker L and Eriksson U (1993): Non-overlapping expression of CRBPI and CRABP I during pattern formation of limbs and craniofacial structures in the early mouse embryo. *Development 117*, 451-460.

[92] Matt N, Schmidt CK, Dupe V, Dennefeld C, Nau H, Chambon P, Mark M and Ghyselinck NB (2005). Contribution of cellular retinol-binding protein type 1 to retinol metabolism during mouse development. *Dev. Dyn 233*, 167-176.

[93] Hibbard ED, Smithells RW. (1965): Folic acid metabolism and human embryopathy. *Lancet i*: 1254.

[94] Smithells RW, Sheppard S, Schorah CJ.(1976): Vitamin deficiencies and neural tube defects. *Arch Dis Childh 51*: 944-50.

[95] MRC Vitamin Study Research Group. Prevention of neural tube defects: results of the Medical Research Council Vitamin Study. *Lancet 1991*; 338:131-7.

[96] Czeizel AE, Dudas I. (1992): Prevention of the first occurrence of neural-tube defects by periconceptional vitamin supplementation. *N Engl J Med 327*:1832-5.

[97] Wagner C. (1995): Biochemical role of folate in cellular metabolism. In: Bailey LB, ed. *Folate in health and disease*. New York, NY: Marcel Dekker, 23-42.

[98] Selhub J, Jacques PF, Wilson PWF, Rush D, Rosenberg IH. (1993): Vitamin status and intake as primary determinants of homocysteinemia in an elderly population. *JAMA 270*: 2693-8.

[99] Green R, Jacobsen DW. (1995): Clinical Implications of hyperhomocysteinemia. In: Bailey LB, ed. *Folate in health and disease*. New York, NY: Marcel Dekker, 75-122.

[100] Bates CJ, Fuller NJ, Prentice AM (1986): Folate status during pregnancy and lactation in a West African rural community. *Hum Nutr: Clin Nutr 40C*: 3-13.

[101] Qvist I, Abdulla M, Jagerstad M, Svensson S. (1986): Iron, zinc and folate status during pregnancy and two months after delivery. *Acta Obstet Gynecol Scand 65*: 15-22.

[102] Bruinse HW, van den Berg H. (1995): Changes of some vitamin levels during and after normal pregnancy. *Eur J Obstet Gynecol Reprod Biol 61*:31-7.

[103] Cikot RJLM, Steegers-Theunissen RPM, Thomas CMG, de Boo TM, Merkus HMWM, Steegers EAP.(2001): Longitudinal vitamin and homcysteine levels in normal pregnancy. *Br J Nutr 85*: 49-58.

[104] Smelt VA, Upton A, Adjaye J, et al. (2000): Expression of arylamine N-acetyltransferase in preterm placentas and in human primplantation embryos. *Hum Mol Genet 9*: 1101-7.

[105] Upton A, Smelt V, Mushtag A. et al. (2000): Placental arylamine N-acetyltransferase type 1: potentiala caontributory source of urinary folate catabolite p-aminobenzoylglutamate during pregnancy. *Biochim Biophys Acta 1542*: 143-8.

[106] Suh JR, Oppenheim EW, Girgis S, Stover PJ. (2000): Purification and properties of a folate-catabolizing enzyme. *J Biol Chem 275*: 35646-55.

[107] Chanarin I, MacGibbon BM, O'Sullivan WJ, Mollin DL. (1959): Folic acid deficiency in pregnancy. The pathogenesis of megaloblastic amaemia of pregnancy. *Lancet ii*: 634-9.

[108] Landon MJ, Hytten FE. (1972): Plasma folate levels following an oral load of folic acid during pregnancy. *J Obstet Gynaecol Br Comm 79*: 577-83.

[109] McLean FW, Heine MW, Held B, Streiff RR. (1970): Folic acid absorption in pregnancy: comparison of the pteroylpolyglytamate and pteroylmonoglutamate. *Blood 36*: 628-31.

[110] Landon MJ, Eyre DH, Hytten FE. (1975): Transfer of folate to the fetus. *Br J Obstet Gynaevil 82*:12-9.

[111] Baker H, Frank O, Deangelis B, Feingold S, Kaminetzky HA. (1981): Role of placenta in maternal-fetal vitamin transfer in humans. *Am J Obstet Gynecol 141*: 792-6.

[112] Utley CS, Marcell PD, Allen RH, Antony AC, Kolhouse JF. (1985): Isolation and characterizatio of methionine synthetase from human placenta. *J Biol Chem 260*: 13656-65.

[113] Daly SF, Molloy AM, Mills JL, et al. (1999): The influence of 5,10 methylenetetrahydrofolate reductase genotypes on enzyme activity in placental tissue. *Br J Obstet Gynaecol 106*: 1214-8.

[114] Chanarin I. (1969): *The megaloblastic anaemias*. Longon United Kingdom: Blackwell 786-829.

[115] McPartin J, Halligan A, Scott JM, Darling M, Weir DG. (1993): Accelerated folate breakdown in pregnancy. *Lancet 341*: 148-9.

[116] Caudill MA, Gregory IF III, Hutson AD, Bailey LB. (1998): Folate catabolism in pregnant and non-pregnant women with controlled folate intakes. *J Nutr 128*: 204-8.

[117] Higgins JR, Quinlivan EP, McPartlin J, Scott JM, Weir DG, Darling MRN (2000): The relationship between increased folate catabolism and the increased requirement for folate in pregnancy. *Br J Obstet Gynaecol 107*: 1149-54.

[118] Gregory JF III, Caudill MA, Opalko J, Bailey LB. (2001): Kinetics of folate turnover in pregnant women (second trimester) and nonpregnancy controls during folic acid supplementation: stable-isotopic labelling of plasma folate, urinary and folate catabolites shows subtle effects of pregnancy on turnover of folate pools. 131: 1928-37.

[119] Landon MJ, Hytten FE. (1971): The excretion of folate in pregnancy: *J Obstet Gynaecol Br Comm 78*: 769-75.

[120] Ball EW, Giles C. (1964): Folic acid and vitamin B12 levels in pregnancy and their relation to megaloblastic anaemic. *J Clin Path 17*: 165-74.

[121] Marti JD, Davis RE (1964): Serum folic acid activity and vaginal bleeding in early pregnancy. *J Obstet Gyn Br Comm 71*: 400-3.

[122] Ek J, Magnus EM. (1981): Plasma and red blood cell folate during normal pregnancies. *Acta Obstet Gynecol Scand 60*: 247-51.

[123] Bruise HW, van den Berg H, Haspels AA. (1985): Maternal serum folacin levels during and after normal pregnancy. *Eur J Obstet Gynecol Reprod Biol 20*: 153-8.

[124] Fleming AF. (1972): Urinary excretion of folate in pregnancy. *J Obstet Gynaecol Br Comm 79*: 916-20.

[125] Henderson Gl, Perez T, Schenker S, Mackins J, Antony AC. (1995): Maternal-to-fetal transfer of 5-methyltetrahydrofolate by the perfused human placental cotyledon: evidence for a concentrative role by placental folate receptors in fetal folate delivery. *J Lab Clin Med 126*:184-203.

[126] Bisseling TM, Steegers EAP, van den Heuvel JJM, et al (2004): Placental folate transport and binding are not impaired in pregnancies complicated by fetal growth restriction. *Placenta 25*: 588-93.

[127] Piedrahita JA, Oetama B, Bennet GD, et al (1999): Mice lacking the folic acid-binding protein Folbpl are defective in early embryonic development. *Nat Genet 23*: 288-32.

[128] Antony AC. ((1996): Folate receptors, *Annu Rev Nutr 16*:501-21.

[129] da Costa M, Rothenberg SP. (1974): Appearance of a folate binder in leukocytes and serum of women who are pregnant or taking oral contraceptives. *J Lab Clin Med 83*: 207-14.

[130] Gross S, Kamen B, Fanaroff A, Caston D. (1980): Folate compartments during gestational maturation. *J Pediatr 96*:842-4.

[131] Prasannan P, Pike S, Peng K, Shane B, Appling DR. (2003): Human mitochondrial C1-tetrahydrofolate synthase. Gene structure, tissue distribution of the mRNA, and immunolocalization in Chinese hamster overy calls. *J Biol Chem 31*:43178-87.

[132] Giles C. (1966): An account of 335 cases of megaloblastic anaemia of pregnancy and the puerperium. *J Clin Pathol 19*: 1-11.

[133] Ladon MJ, Oxley A. (1971): Relation between maternal and infant blood folate activities. *Arch Dis Childh 46*:810-4.

[134] Baker H, Frank O, Thomson AD, et al (1975): Vitamin profile of 174 mothers and newborn at parturition. *Am J Clin Nutr 28*:56-65.

[135] Ek J. (1980): Plasma and red cell folate values in newborn infants and their mothers in relation to gestational age. *J Pediatr 97*: 288-92.

[136] Molloy AM, Mills JL, Mc Partlin J, Kirke PN, Scott JM, Daly S. (2002): Maternal and fetal plasma homocysteine concentrations at birth: the influence of folate, vitamin B12 and the 5,10-methylenetetrahydrofolate reductase 677C→T variant. *Am J Obstet Gynecol 186*:499-503.

[137] Guerra-Shinohara EM, Paiva AA, Rondo PHC, Yamasaki K, Terzi CA, D'Almeida V. (2002): Relationship between total homocysteine and folate levels in pregnant women and their newborn babies according to maternal serum levels of vitamin B12. *BJOG 109*:784-91.

[138] Iyengar L, Apte SV. (1972): Nutrient stores in human foetal livers. *Br J Nutr 27*: 313-7.

[139] Vaz Pinto A, Torras V, Sandoval JFF, Dillmann E, Ramiarez Mateos C, Cordova MS. (1975): Folic acid and vitamin B12 determination in fetal liver. *Am J Clin Nutr 28*:1085-6.

[140] Loria A, Vaz-Pinto A, Arroyo P, Ramirez-Mateos C, Sanchez-Meda L. (1977): Nutritional anemia. VI. Fetal hepatic storage of metabolites in the second half of pregnancy. *J Pediatr 91*:569-73.

[141] Gardiki-Kouidou P, Seller MJ. (1988): Amniotic fluid folate, vitamin B12 and transcoblamins in neural tube defects. *Clin Genet 33*: 441-8.

[142] Weekes EW, Tamur T, Davis RO, et al (1992): Nutrient levels in amniotic fluid from women with normal and neural tube defect pregnancies. *Biol Neonate 61*:226-31.

[143] Tamura T, Weekes EW, Birch R, et al (1994): Relationship between amniotic fluid and maternal blood nutrient levels. *J Perinatal Med 22*:227-34.

[144] Gaull GE, von Berg W, Raiha NCR, Sturman JA (1973): Developent of methyltransferase activities of human fetal tissues. *Pediatr Res 7*:527-33.

[145] Kalnitsky A, Rosenblatt D, Zlotkin S. (1982): Differences in liver folate enzyme patterns in premature and full term infants. *Pediatr Res 16*:628-31.

[146] Ordonez LA, Villarroel OA. (1976): Increased brain activity of methylene reductase during early development. *J Neurochem 27*:305-7.

[147] Snell K. (1980): Liver enzyme of serine metabolism during neonatal development of the rat. *Biochem J 190*: 451-5.

[148] Thompson HR, Jones GM, Narkewicz MR. (2001): Ontogeny of hepatic enlism in rabbits. *Am J Physiol 280*:G873-8.

[149] Xiao S, Hansen DK, Horsley ETM et al (2005): Maternal folate deficiency results in selective upregulation of folate receptors and heterogeneous nuclear ribonucleoprotein-E1 associated with multiple sublte aberration in fetal tissues. *Birth Defects Res A Clin Mol Teratol 73*:6-28.

[150] Baker M, Erdberg R, Pasher J, Soburka M, (1984): Study of folic acid and vitamin B12 in blood and urine during normal pregnancy. *Proc Sur Exp Biol Med 94*:511-6.

[151] Selhub J (1984): Folate binding protein mechanism for placenta and intestinal uptake. *Adv Exp Med Biol 152*: 141-5.

[152] Stryker WS, Kaplan LA, Stein EA, Stampfer MJ, Sober A, Willen WC. (1988): The relation of diet, cigarette smoking and alcohol consumption in plasma β-carotene and α-tocopherols levels. *Am J Epidemiol 127*: 283-96.

[153] Vogel S, Contois JH, Tucker KL, Wilson PWF, Schaefer EJ, Lamin-Keefe CJ. (1997): Plasma retinol and plasma lipoprotein tocopherol and carotenoids concentrations in healthy elderly participants of the Framingham Heart Study. *Am J Clin Nutr*, 66:950-8.

[154] Paul AA, Southgate DA and Russel J. *The composition of the food*. London HMSO 1980.

[155] Lachili B, Faure H, Smail A, Zema N, Belnatreche C, Rousel AM. (1999): Plasma vitamin A, E and β-Carotene levels in adult Post-Partum Algerian Women. *Int J Vitam Nutr Res 69*: 239-242.

[156] Nierenberg DW and Lester DC. (1985): Determination of vitamins A and E in serum and plasma using a simplified clarification method and high-performance liquid chromatography. *J Chromatography*, 345: 275-285.

[157] Arnaoud J, Fortis I, Blachier S, Kia D and Favier A (1991): Simultaneous determination of retinol, α-tocopherol and β-carotene in serum by high-performance liquid chromatography. *J Chromatography* 572, 103-116.

[158] Ferre-Masferrer M, Fuentes-Ardeteu X, Goma-Llongueras M, Aluna-Trullas A, Aranendi-Ranes MG, Castano-Vidriales JL et al. (2001): Regional reference values fos some quantities measured with the ADVIA Centraur analyser. A model of co-operation between the in vitro diagnostic industry and clinical laboratories. *Clin Chem Lab Med* 39:166-9.

[159] Simopoulos AP. Childs B. (1990): Genetic variation and nutrition. *World Rev Nutr Diet*, 63:1-300.

[160] El. Sohemy, A. Baylin, A. Ascherio, E. Kabagambe, D. Spiegelman, H. Campos. (2001): Population-based study of α and γ-tocopherol in plasma and adipose tissue as biomarkers of intake in Costa Rican adults. *Am J Clin Nutr* 74:356-63.

[161] Ascherio A, Stampfer MJ, Coldditz G.A., Rimm EB, Litin J, Willet WC. (1992): Correlations of carotenoids and tocopherols among American men and women. *J Nutr*, 122:1792-1801.

[162] Dimenstein R, Trugo NMF, Donangelo CM, Trugo LD, Anastacio AS. (1996): Effect of subadequate maternal vitamin A status on placental transfer of Retinol and β-carotene to the human fetus. *Biol Neonate*, 69: 230-234.

[163] Ghebremeskel K, Burns L, Burden TJ, Harbige L, Costeloe K, Powell JJ, Grawford MA. (1994): Vitamin A and related essential nutrients in cord blood relationship with anthropometric measurements at birth. *Early Hum Dev* 39: 177-188.

[164] Azais – Braesco V and Pascal G. (2000): Vitamin A in pregnancy: requirements and safety limits. *AJCN*: 71 (5) 1325S-1345.

[165] Sklan D, Shalit J, Lasebnic N, Spirer Z, Weisman Y. (1985): Retinol transport proteins and concentrations in human amniotic fluid, placenta, fetal and maternal sera. *Br J Nutr*, 54:577-83).

[166] Gebre-Medhin M, A Valiquist. (1984): Vitamin A nutrition in the human fetus. A comparison of Sweden and Ethiopia. *Acta Paediatr Scand*, 73: 333-40.

[167] Shah RS, Rajalakshmi R, Bhatt RV, Hazza M, Patel BC, Swamy NB. (1987) Liver stores of vitamin A in human fetuses in relation to gestational age, fetal size and maternal nutritional status *Br J Nutr*, 58:181-189.

[168] Sapin V, S Chaib, L Blachon, MC Gonabau, D. Lemery, F. Charbone et al. (2000): Esterification of Vitamin A by human placenta involve Villous Mesenchymal Fibroblasts. *Ped Res* 48; 565-575.

[169] Chambon P. (1994): The retinoid signalling pathway: molecular and genetic analyses. *Semin Cell Biol*, 5: 115-125.

[170] Morris - Kay GM, Ward SJ. (1999): Retinoids and embryonic development. *Int Rev Cytol* 188: 73-133.

[171] Ross AC, Gardner EM. (1994): The function of vitamin A in cellular growth and differentiation and its roles during pregnancy and lactation. *Adv Exp Med Biol* 352: 187-200.

[172] Miller RK, Faber W, Asai M, D'Gregorio RP, Ng WW, Shah Y, Neth-Jessee I. (1993): The role of the human placenta in embryonic nutrition: impact of environmental and social factors. *Ann NY Acad Sci* 678:92-107.

[173] Gross GC, Werb Z, Fisher SJ. (1994): Implantation and the placenta: Key pieces of the development puzzle. *Science*, 266: 1508-1518.

[174] Greeoh-Kraft J, Nau H, Lammer E, Olney J. (1987): Embryonic retinoid concentration after maternal intake of Isotretinoin. *N Engl J Med* 321: 262-264.

[175] Jaques PF, Sulsky SI, Sadowski JA, Phillips JCC, Rush D, Willett WC. (1993): Comparison of micronutrient intake measured by a dietary questionnaire and biochemical indicators of micronutrient status. *Am J Clin Nutr* 57: 182-9.

[176] Sivakumer B, Panth M, Shatrugna V, Raman L. (1995): Vitamin A requirements assessed by plasma response to supplementation during pregnancy. *Internat J Vit Nutr Res* 49: 134-136.

[177] Srinivasan SR, Berenson CS. Serum lipoprotein in children and methods for study, In: *Lewis LA-ed Lipoprotein methodology and human studies* CBC Vol III, Boca Raton FL, CRC Press 1983: 185-204.

[178] Wills L. (1931): Treatment of "pernicious anaemia of pregnancy" and "tropical anaemia" with special reference to yeast extract as a curative agent. *Br. Med J 1*:1059-64.

[179] Food and Nutrition Board, National Research Council. Maternal nutrition and the course of pregnancy. Washington, DC: National Academy of Sciences, 1970.

[180] Food and Drug Administration. Food standards:amendment of standards of identify for enriched grain product to require addition of folic acid. *Fed Regist* 1996; 61:8781-97.

[181] Ray JG (2004): Folic acid food fortification in Canada. *Nutr Rev 62*:S35-9.

[182] Chen LT, Rivera MA (2004): The Costa Rican experience reduction of neural tube defects following food fortification programs. *Nutr Rev 62*:S40-3.

[183] Hertrampf E, Cortes F. (2004): Folic acid fortification of wheat flour: Chile. *Nutr Rev 62*:S44-8.

[184] Chanarin I, Rothman D, Perry J, Stratfull D (1968): Normal dietary folate, iron and protein intake, with particular reference to pregnanty. *Br Med J 2*:394-7.

[185] Moscovitch LF, Cooper BA. (1973): Folate content of diets in pregnancy: comparison of diets collected at home and diets prepared from dietary records. *Am J Clin Nutr 26*:707-14.

[186] Lowenstein L, Cantlie G, Ramos O, Brunton L. (1966): The incidence and prevention of folate deficiency in a pregnant clinic population. *Can Med Ass J 95*:797-806.

[187] Martinez OB. (1980): Red cell folate values of a group of non pregnant mothers. *Can J Public Health 71*:163-9.

[188] Bates CJ, Prentice AM, Paul AA. (1994): Seasonal variations in vitamins A, C, riboflavin and folate intakes and status of pregnant and lactating women in a rural Gambian community: some possible implications, *Eur J Clin Nutr 48*:660-8.

[189] Scholl TO, Hediger ML, Schall JI, Khoo C-S, Fischer RL. (1996): Dietary and serum folate: their influence on the outcome of pregnancy. *Am J Clin Nutr 63*:520-5.

[190] Boushey CJ, Edmonds JWm Welshimer KJ. (2001): Estimates of the effects of folic-acid fortification and folic-acid bioavailability for women. *Nutriotion 17*: 873-9.

[191] Siega-Riz AM, Savitz DA, Zeisel SH, Thorp JM, Herring A. (2004): Second trimester folate status and preterm birth. *Am J Obstet Gynecol 191*: 1851-7.

[192] Stark KD, Pawlosky RJ, Beblo S et al. (2005): Status of plasma folate after folic acid fortification of the food supply in pregnant African American women and the influences of diet, smoking, and alcohol consumption. *Am J Clin Nutr 81*:669-77.

[193] Willoughby MLN, Jewell FJ. (1966): Investigation of folic acid requirements in pregnancy. *Br Med J 2*: 1568-71.

[194] Hansen H, Rybo G. (1967): Folic acid dosage in prophylactic treatment during pregnancy. *Acta Obstet Gynecol Scand 46 (suppl)*: 107-12.

[195] Chanarin I, Rothman D, Ardeman S, Berry V. (1965): Some observations on the changes preceding the development of megaloblastic anaemia in pregnancy with particular reference to the neutrophil leucocytes. *Br J Haematol 11*:557-62.

[196] Hibbard BM, Hibbard ED. (1971): Neutrophil hypersegmentation and defective folate metabolism in pregnancy. *J Obstet Gynaecol Br Comm 78*: 776-80.

[197] Chanarin I, Rothman D. (1971): Further observations on the relation between iron and folate status in pregnancy. *Br Med J 2*:81-4.

[198] Luhby AL, Cooperman JM, Teller DN. (1959): Histidine metabolic loading test to distinguish folic acid deficiency from vit. B12 in megaloblastic anemias. *Proc Exp Biol Med 101*: 350-2.

[199] Metz J. (1984): The deoxyuridine suppression test. *CRC Crit Rev Clin Lab Sci 20*:205-41.

[200] Gatenby PBB, Lillie EW (1960): Clinical analysis of 100 cases of severe megaloblastic anaemia of pregnancy. *Br Med J 2*:1111-4.

[201] Ainley NJ. (1961): Megaloblastic anaemia of pregnancy and the puerperium. *J Obstet Gynaecol Br Comm 68*: 245-60.

[202] Diez-Ewald M, Molina RA (1972): Iron and folic acid deficiency during pregnancy in western Venezuela. *Am J Trop Med Hyg 21*:587-91.

[203] Fleming AF, Martin JD, Stenhouse NS (1974): Pregnancy anaemia, iron and folate deficiency in Western Australia. *Med J Aust 2*: 479-84.

[204] Wouters MGAJ, Thomas CMG, Boers GHJ, et al (1993): Hyperhomocysteinemia: a risk factor in women with unexplained recurrent early pregnancy loss. *Fertil Steril 60*:820-5.

[205] Fleming AF, Ghatoura GBS, Harrison KA, Briggs ND, Dunn DT (1986): The prevention of anaemia in pregnancy in primigravidae in the guinea savanna of Nigeria. *Ann Trop Med Parasitol. 80*:211-33.

[206] Fleming AF (1989): The aetiology of severe anaemia in pregnancy in Ndola, Zambia. *Ann Trop Med Parasitol 83*:37-49.

[207] Smitz LJM, Essed GGM (2001): Short interpregnancy intervals and unfavourable pregnancy outcome: role of folate depletion. *Lancet 358*:2074-7.

[208] Doyle W, Srivastava A, Crawford MA, Bhatti R, Brooke Z, Costeloe KL. (2001): Inter-pregnancy folate and iron status of women in an inner-city population. *Br J Nutr 86*:81-7.

[209] Wilcox AJ (2001): On the importance-and the unimportance- of birth-weight, *Int J Epidemiol 30*:1233-41.

[210] Shaw GM, Liberman RF, Todoroff K, Wasserman CR (1977): Low birth weight, preterm delivery, and periconceptional vitamin use. *J Pediatr 130*:1013-4.

[211] Michell EA, Robinson E, Clark PM, et al. (2004): Maternal nkutritional risk factors for small for gestational age babies in a developed country: acase-control study. *Arch Dis Child Fetal Neonat 89*:F431-5.

[212] Burke G, Robinson K, Refsum H, Stuart B, Drumm J, Graham I. (1992): Intrauterine growth retardation , perinatal death, and maternal homocysteine levels. *N Engl J Med 326*:69-70.

[213] Vollset SE, Refsum H, Irgens LM, et al (2000): Plasma total homocysteine, pregnancy complications, and adverse pregnancy outcomes: the HOrdaland Homocysteine Study. *Am J Clin Nutr 71*:96208.

[214] El-Khairy L, Vollset SE, Refsum H, Ueland PM (2003): Plasma total cysteine, pregnancy complications, and adverse pregnancy outcomes: the Hordaland Homocysteine Study. *Am J Clin Nutr 77*:467-72.

[215] Murphy MM, Scott JM, Arija V, Molly AM, Fernandez-Ballart JD (2004): Maternal homocysteine before conception and throughout pregnancy predicts fetal homocysteine and birth weight. *Clin Chem 50*:1406-12.

In: Micronutrients and Health Research
Editor: Takumi Yoshida, pp. 107-146

ISBN: 978-1-60456-056-5
© 2008 Nova Science Publishers, Inc.

Chapter III

CURRENT STATUS OF MICRONUTRIENT SUPPLEMENTATION IN PREGNANCY

Olivera Kontic-Vucinic and Milan Terzic

Institute of Ob/Gyn., School of Medicine, University of Belgrade, 11000 Belgrade, Serbia.

ABSTRACT

Well-balanced and adequate maternal nutrition prior conception and during pregnancy affects the course and outcome of pregnancy, and enables achievement of a: 1) healthy pregnancy, 2) uncomplicated delivery of a full-term and well-developed baby, 3) lower risk of maternal postpartum complications, and 4) sufficient source for lactation. Adequate maternal nutrition also improves future maternal health in general and reproductive health in particular. As it is now widely recognized that the risk of various chronic diseases in adulthood might have their origins in intrauterine life, the new goal of the contemporary approach in pregnancy nutrition is to establish the nutritional foundations for a healthy adults during intrauterine life.

Pregnancy represents a special maternal demand for high-quality nutrients, as it is regarded as a metabolic stress that is increasing according to the course of the gestation. Although it is not completely clear how nutritional status of the mother influences her own health as well as fetal growth/development, nutrition imbalance could be harmful to the pregnant woman, influencing both the outcome of pregnancy and the composition of breast milk.

In well-nourished women these increased needs are best met by biological and metabolic adaptation to pregnancy. Increasing demands should be achieved by appropriate dietary intake, which contains all nutrition requirements. In cases of imbalanced dietary intake, preexisting deficiencies of micronutrients, previous adverse pregnancy outcomes, and in all cases of high-risk pregnancies micronutrient supplementation is especially important. However, until now there is insufficient evidence to define whether there is a need for routine antepartum supplementation or should nutritional intervention be restrained to deficient populations and high-risk pregnancies. As the data on the effectiveness of supplementation in preventing or treating pregnancy-related disorders and perinatal complications are contradictory, future well designed randomized control trials would try to solve this dilemma.

Micronutrient supplementation supporters have a standpoint that the potential benefits of routine supplementation overweigh any potential adverse reaction that can be attributed. In the other hand, the daily requirements are easily met in all individuals having a balanced diet. Although deficiency states are rare, several pharmaceutical companies produce over-the-counter vitamin – plus- mineral nutritional supplements, despite the lack of clear evidence to support their supplemental consumption.

Currently, micronutrient supplementation should be chosen on an individual basis. In the near future, the goal would be to estimate micronutrient status prior to conception or in the early pregnancy, in order to define patients who must receive appropriate micronutrient supplementation.

INTRODUCTION

A successful pregnancy implies several goals, the most important of which are: maintaining maternal health and well-being during pregnancy and delivery, giving birth to a healthy full-term well-developed neonate as the result of the previous, lowering the risk of maternal postpartum complications, providing a good basis for adequate breastfeeding, and creating conditions for future maternal health, including reproductive health (Ramakrishnan U et al, 1999; Allen LH, 2003).

Pregnancy creates a specific metabolic demand for high-quality nutrients. Adequate maternal nutrition before conception and during pregnancy influences the course and outcome of pregnancy. Although the pausity of evidence regarding the increased nutrient needs in pregnancy does exist, the effect of the mother's nutritional status on her health, fetal growth and development is not completely understood (Black RE, 2001). There is a rising interest in women's diet preconceptionally, during pregnancy and during the breastfeeding period, in order to reduce potential fetal, neonatal, and maternal risks. Pregnancy induces a metabolic stress for the mother, which changes and increases according to the progression of the gestation (Baker H et al, 2002). It is possible that these increased requirements in well-nourished women are met by biological adaptation to pregnancy which is reflected on maternal metabolism; daily requirements are easily met by women who have a balanced diet (Harding JE, 2001). Subsequently, deficiency states in women in reproductive years in developed countries are rare. Although micronutrient malnutrition is primarily related to inadequate dietary intake, nutrition is also highly dependant on the economic status, social and cultural environment, and personal habits of the mother. This becomes even more important for the underprivileged groups and population in developing countries.

Evidence-based recommendations indicate that a well-balanced diet during pregnancy generally provides for the recommended daily allowance (RDA) of all nutrients, except for elemental iron. A personal interview and counseling on the daily dietary intake should be an integral part of both preconceptional and antenatal care. Consequently, prenatal supplements are not necessary for every pregnant patient, and should be chosen on an individual basis and only in cases of proven deficiency (Hösli I et al, 2007). Nevertheless, prenatal supplementation has been widely accepted as a routine clinical approach. There are several reasons for such practice. Firstly, nutritional deficiencies during pregnancy might be difficult to diagnose, and supplementation makes good sense in an attempt to provide broad coverage. Also, subclinical deficiencies are likely to exist in multiparous patients, and if the period between consecutive deliveries is less than two years. The same goes for different underprivileged and high-risk groups. Furthermore, we should not underestimate the placebo effect of supplementation, because many women feel more comfortable knowing that they receive all that is necessary for a successful pregnancy outcome. Finally, and most importantly, the potential benefits of routine supplementation seem to overweigh any potential adverse effect. Considering increasing demands, it could be unsafe for the mother and outcome of her pregnancy to be solely dependent upon her dietary intake. It is therefore important to provide adequate reserves. The effect of incorrect nutrition may depend on its timing during gestation, severity, or both.

It is now widely accepted that the risk of a number of chronic diseases in adulthood may have their origins in intrauterine life (hypertension, coronary heart disease, and non insulin-dependent diabetes mellitus). The incidence of those diseases is increasing both in developed and developing world. Barker first suggested that fetal nutrition has lifelong effects on metabolism, with a far-reaching impact on risk of chronic disease in adulthood (Barker DJP, 1998). Biomedical research using animal models has been widely employed to gain a deeper understanding of the underlying mechanisms involved (Oliver MH et al, 2007). There is good experimental evidence that nutrition can be an important and probably central programming stimulus for susceptibility to adult disease (Harding JE, 2001). The fetus carries its own genetic potential for development, which can only be fully realized in interrelation with other necessary cofactors - one of the most important is supply of nutrients. It has been shown that maternal nutrition around time of conception has important effects on the duration of gestation, intrauterine growth, as well as postnatal growth and health. The pattern of fetal growth restriction confers a high risk of adult chronic disease. It is hypothesized that this is the result of programming events in fetal life, leading both to altered birth size and permanent changes in structure and function, which constitute a predisposition to disease in adult life. Recent epidemiological evidence has shown increased rates of cardiovascular mortality and associated risk factors in those born small.

It is estimated that every year 62 million women in developing countries experience pregnancy-related illnesses, labor, delivery, and postpartum complications and chronic conditions that result from pregnancy (Koblinsky MA et al, 1992). Nutrition has been confirmed to be a part of underlying causes for various disorders, with micronutrients playing an important role. Furthermore, micronutrient malnutrition is common in pregnancy, particularly in low-income countries. Reported deficiences include iron, iodine, zinc, vitamin A, vitamin B complex, with multiple micronutrient deficiences more common than single ones (Ramakrishnan U et al, 1999).

Nutrition has long been hypothesized to have a role in etiology of one of the most investigated pregnancy-related disorders in the last decade - preeclampsia. Preeclampsia is a disease influencing both maternal and fetal health/wellbeing, confirmed to be a leading cause of maternal morbidity, as well as perinatal morbidity and mortality. Worldwide, preeclampsia will affect more than four million women, and cause about 60,000 deaths each year (WHO, 2005). It is now well understood that, while preeclampsia is clinically evident late in pregnancy, the causal exposure and many of the pathophysiologic changes are present months earlier.

The pathogenesis of preeclampsia comprises endothelial dysfunction, defect trophoblast invasion, consequent placental hypoperfusion, as well as immune maladaptation and inflammation (Roberts JM & Redman CWG, 1993). The most probable link, connecting these events in pathological circle, is oxidative stress, characterized by excessive production of reactive oxygen species (ROS), coupled with inadequate or overwhelmed antioxidant defense mechanisms. A ROS is an atom or molecule with one unpaired electron in its outer orbit that is capable of existing independently for a short period of time. ROS is generated continuously through leakage from the electron transport chain in the process of cellular respiration within the mitochondria. ROS is essential factor for cell replication, differentiation and growth, especially during pregnancy. There is also evidence that ROS plays a role in remodeling of uterine tissues, implantation of the embryo and placentation (Aurousseau B et al, 2006). Oxidative metabolism leads to generation of ROS, which has the potential to cause further oxidative reactions, especially to cell membranes or nucleic acids (Evans P & Halliwell B, 2001). The potential to cause damage is limited by antioxidant mechanisms (Shenkin A, 2006). Antioxidants achieve their defensive role through inhibition of peroxidation reactions, thus protecting enzymes and proteins, as well as cells from destruction.

In women with established preeclampsia there is evidence of oxidative stress - oxidative stress markers are present both in the placenta and maternal circulation of affected women. While markers of lipid peroxidation are increased, concentrations of both water and lipid soluble antioxidants are decreased in plasma and placenta, providing the further support for the causative concept of increased oxidative stress (Mikhail MS et al, 1994; Staff AC et al, 1999). Moreover, oxidative stress is also involved in serious, even life-threating complications affecting preterm neonates, such as respiratory distress syndrome (RDS), chronic lung disease, intraventricular haemorrhage (IVH), retinopathy of prematurity, and necrotizing enterocolitis (Hubel CA et al, 1996; Mikhail MS et al, 1994; Saugstad OD, 2001). These data provide the basis for possible prophylaxis with antioxidants, in attempt to prevent oxidative stress, and consequently reduce the risk of both preeclampsia in pregnant women and perinatal complications in their infants (Evans P & Halliwell B, 2001; Schenkin A, 2006).

There is pausity of data on periconceptional nutrition and preeclampsia risk. As mentioned above, preeclampsia is the late clinical manifestation of an earlier causal exposure. Periconceptional exposures may be particularly important, as they may affect implantation and/or decidual vascular remodeling - a physiologic process known to be abnormal in preeclampsia. Implantation is characterized by vascular remodeling, heightened inflammation, oxidative stress, and rapid cell division – all of which can be affected by nutritional status. Inadequate nutrient intake has the potential to compromise the inflammatory response, antioxidant defense mechanism, and DNA and protein synthesis. All of these could lead to abnormal implantation and reduced placental perfusion, causing the preeclampsia (Jauniaux E et al, 2000). It is biologically plausible that periconceptional multivitamin use protects against preeclampsia, but research will be needed to improve that and to elucidate the specific mechanisms and the most relevant nutrients (Roberts JM et al,

2003). This was the rationale for extensive investigation of the supplementation antioxidant therapy aimed at preventing or overcoming preeclampsia.

Fetal growth is a complex process dependant on several nutritional and non-nutritional interreacting factors. The extend and consequences of such interactions are still not completely understood. Approximately 20 million children, or 15.5 percent of all births, are born worldwide every year weighing less than 2500gr. The majority of them (more than 95 percent) are born in developing countries (United Nations Children's Fund, 2004). The etiology of low birth weight (LBW) is preterm delivery and/or a slow intra-utero growth with delivery at term. Preterm delivery, the leading underlying cause of mortality among infants with nonlethal congenital anomalies, is also a major factor determining the rate of LBW infants. Two-thirds of LBW infants in the developed world are born preterm. The remaining one-third of infants is born at term, but is growth-restricted in utero. On the other hand, most infants weighting <2500gr in the developing world are growth restricted. A low birth weight (<2500gr) increases the risk of neonatal complications, and presents a major predictor of neonatal and infant mortality (Ramakrishnan U et al, 1999; United Nations Children's Fund and WHO, 2004; Gillman MW, 2005). Compared to normal-weight infants, LBW infants have a dramatically increased mortality rate (Osrin D & de L.Costello AM, 2000). Accordingly, nutritional intervention for the purpose of increasing the size of infants should be a priority in developing nations. Intrauterine growth restriction (IUGR) also carries a risk of perinatal mortality that is 6-10 times higher than the risk for infants with normal growth (Scholl TO & Johnson WG, 2000). Additionally, as mentioned above, infants who are small/disproportionate at birth have an increased risk of developing various diseases in adult life (Barker DJP, 1998). Consequently, the new goal is to set the nutritional foundations for a healthy adult life, while the individual is still in utero.

IUGR and preeclampsia are pregnancy-specific disorders that have in common abnormal placental implantation (Roberts JM & Hubel CA, 1999). Unlike preeclampsia presented by maternal manifestations of the disease and often accompanied by subnormal fetal growth, IUGR has no notable clinical impact on the mother's health, but always involves impairment of fetal growth. Nevertheless, it was reported recently that women who have had an IUGR baby also have an increased risk for ischemic heart disease in later life - this elevated risk is independent of preeclampsia and other potentially confounding factors (Smith GC et al, 2001). Furthermore, before and after pregnancy, non preeclamptic women with growth-restricted babies are more likely to experience elevated blood pressure (Lawlor DA et al, 2002).

Preterm premature rupture of the membranes (PPROM), the main known cause of preterm delivery, remains critically important clinical and public health problem, complicating approximately 10-20% of all pregnancies. The pathophysiology of PPROM is very complex, and the role of ROS is considered to be important. The generation of ROS, as potentially damaging molecules, may impair the physical integrity (elasticity, strength) of amniotic epithelium and collagen in the amnion and chorion, thus resulting in PPROM. Also, the role of microorganisms in PPROM is well known. ROS plays a crucial function in destruction of microorganisms by phagocytic cells (Woods JR et al, 2001). During microbial elimination and phagocytosis ROS is released by monocytes, neutrophils, and macrophages.

The leakage of ROS from these cells is capable of damaging collagen and amniotic epithelium in the amniotic membrane.

Apart from playing a central part in metabolism and maintaining a tissue function, some micronutrients have antioxidant properties. During pregnancy these antioxidant micronutrients prevent an imbalance between production and scavenging of ROS, which might be detrimental to the mother and her fetus (Aurousseau B et al, 2006).

Smoking is a leading risk factor for PPROM, as it is associated with oxidative stress. Tobacco smoke contains a mixture of smoke-borne ROS and aromatic hydrocarbons. Those substances induce systemic oxidative damage to different tissues. Low concentrations of several micronutrients, especially the antioxidants vitamin C and beta-carotene, are also associated with smoking. Moreover, smoking is associated with reduced dietary intake of vitamin C and carotenoid-containing foods. Smoking most likely does not deliver ROS directly to the amnion and chorion. Instead, smoking generates its damage to tissues by consuming antioxidants, leaving amniotic membranes vulnerable to ROS (Woods JR et al, 2001; Northrop-Clewes CA & Thurnham DI, 2007). Second trimester bleeding is also recognized as a risk factor for PPROM. The release of free iron from hemolyzed red blood cells can catalyze the conversion from H_2O_2 to hydrohyl ion, thereby exposing tissues, including fetal membranes, to risk of oxidative damage.

Much research has been done into the possible role of micronutrients throughout pregnancy (Kontic-Vucinic O et al, 2006a). How much do we really know? Is there a place for routine supplementation in antenatal care, or should we limit our interventions just to deficient population, and high risk pregnancies? Some, but not all nutrients have been studied extensively. Very little is known about the significance of interactions among several micronutrients for pregnancy outcomes. On the other hand, data on the effectiveness of supplementation in preventing or treating pregnancy-related disorders and perinatal complications are often contradictory and future well-designed randomized control trials are needed to solve this dilemma.

With these considerations in mind, this chapter reviews the available scientific information related to women's reproductive health, in particular to pregnancy and lactation.

Vitamin A

The main physiologic functions of vitamin A involve maintenance of epithelial tissues and night vision, and a role in various basic physiologic processes, including reproduction, immunity and growth. Vitamin A is essential during the entire life of an individual, but its role is critical during life periods characterized by rapid proliferation and differentiation of cells (i.e., gestation and early childhood). Experimental studies confirmed its essential role in embryonic development (Ghyselinck NB et al, 1997). Vitamin A deficiency affects millions of women and children worldwide. Insufficient supply during pregnancy results in low vitamin A status at birth and in early infancy. Those children have a depressed immune function and higher morbidity and mortality due to infectious diseases and respiratory disability (Spears K et al, 2004). Increased mother-to-child transmission of HIV-1 is also associated with vitamin A deficiency (Semba RD, 1997).

Potential teratogenicity of excessive ingestion of vitamin A during early pregnancy was also a concern, particularly regarding high-dose supplementation in population with normal vitamin A status (Werler MM et al, 1990). Vitamin A supplementation should be carefully initiated in each inidivual case and based on the estimation of the mother's vitamin A status and the availability of vitamin A-rich food in her diet (Azais-Braesco V & Pascal G, 2000). Consequently, in developed countries where there is no endemic hypovitaminosis A, there is no need for vitamin A supplementation of pregnant women or women of reproductive age. However, this is not applicable to a significant proportion of the low-income population or underprivileged groups in some developed countries who were found to suffer from undiagnosed low vitamin A status (Stephens D et al, 1996; Saunders C et al, 2004).

In regions with endemic vitamin A deficiency, the situation is completely different. Supplementation in those areas is the most efficient way of correcting deficiency, with important, sometimes life-saving benefits, outweighting all potential risks (Wedner SH et al, 2004). Apart from night blindness, pregnant vitamin A deficient women are more likely to have symptoms of genitourinary and gastrointestinal infections, and preeclampsia/eclampsia (Christian P et al, 1998), and to be at increased risk of death (Christian P et al, 2000a). Maternal vitamin A or beta-carotene supplementation might improve womens' reproductive health, particularly during late pregnancy, at the time of birth, as well as six months postpartaly (Christian P et al, 2000b). It has been found that weekly supplementation of women of reproductive age with normal dietary levels of vitamin A or beta-carotene could reduce pregnancy-related deaths by 40 and 49%, respectively. (West KP Jr et al, 1999). Reduce of infant mortality was not proved (Christian P et al, 2004). Weekly vitamin A and beta-carotene supplementation did not have any influence on pregnancy and postpartum complications occurrence at <29 weeks, but vitamin A supplementation exerts benefits in the third trimester of the pregnancy, influencing predominantly the duration of labor and symptoms of nausea, faintness and night blindness. Beta-carotene supplementation also reduced symptoms of postpartum fever.

Vitamin D

Vitamin D is an important micronutrient for maintaining calcium homeostasis and, consequently, normal bone metabolism. Deficiency leads to two well defined phenomena: rickets in infants and osteomalacia in adults. The discovery that most tissues and cells in the body have a vitamin D receptor, provided new aspects of the function of this vitamin. Apart from well known skelethal regulatory role, it is also possible that vitamin D has a high potential for antiproliferative and immunomodulatory activity. It gives the bases for potential role of this vitamin in decreasing the risk of many chronic diseases, including cancers, autoimmune disorders, infectious and cardiovascular diseases. It has been estimated that 1 billion people worldwide have some degree of vitamin D deficiency (Holick MF, 2007).

During pregnancy, significant changes in maternal vitamin D and calcium metabolism occur in an atempt to provide the additional calcium required for fetal bone mineralization. Vitamin D deficiency is more common in pregnant women who are poorly exposed to sunlight (for environmental, cultural, or medical reasons) or have a low dietary intake of vitamin D. Thus, maternal vitamin D deficiency is more likely to occur in winter, in regions where certain food products are not routinely fortified with vitamin D, among ethnic or religious groups whose members cover most of their skin, and among individuals with heavily pigmented skin (Specker B, 2004).

Adequat maternal vitamin D status is important for both the mother and the growing fetus. Deficiency during pregnancy is associated with lower maternal weight gain. Maternal deficiency could cause biochemical evidence of disturbed skelethal homeostasis in the infant. In extreme circumstances, deficiency results in reduced bone mineralization, rickets and fractures, as well as growth retardation. Additionaly, such newborns may have low vitamin D stores and continue to receive insufficient vitamin D intake if they are exclusively breastfed without supplementation for a long period. If those neonates have dark skin and/or receive little sun exposure, the risk further increases (Gartner LM & Greer FR, 2003). Importantly, it was recently suggested that current dietary recommendations for adults may not be sufficient to maintain circulating 25(OH)D levels at or above the required level, especially for pregnant and lactating women (Hollis BW, 2005). However, there is still not enough evidence to evaluate the requirements and effects of vitamin D supplementation during pregnancy. Further studies are required to determine the optimal vitamin D intakes for women during pregnancy and lactation, including the above mentioned groups with increased needs (Hollis BW, 2005).

Vitamin E

Vitamin E is confirmed to be a membrane antioxidant. As a potent nonenzymatic antioxidant in lipid membranes, it promotes protective effect by inhibiting damage of cellular and intracellular structures caused by oxidative stress and production of lipid peroxides. Cell membrane polyunsaturated free fatty acids posses available hydrogen atoms and are targets for ROS. Vitamin E donates hydrogen atoms to ROS and prevents disruption of the polyunsaturated free fatty acid double bonds. Vitamin E, in turn, blocks the progression of lipid peroxidation by becoming a tocopheryl free radical. Having those antioxidative properties, vitamin E is also assumed to exert a protective activity against oxidative stress related disorders (Traber MG, 1999).

Maternal blood levels of vitamin E rise throughout pregnancy and in the third trimester reach a level that is 60% higher than in the pregestational period. It is important to emphasize that abnormal pregnancies are characterized by lower maternal concentrations of vitamin E than healthy pregnant women of the same gestational age (von Mandach U et al, 1994). It is not clearly understood what regulates placental transfer of vitamin E. After oral intake, maternal plasma vitamin E concentrations increase, and are higher than umbilical cord levels, correlating with concentration of this vitamin in the chorioamnion. The newborns have significantly lower levels of vitamin E than their mothers. The fetus and premature neonate are deficient in vitamin E, and therefore at risk for lipid peroxidation-induced hemolysis (Pressman EK et al, 2003; Sanchez-Vera I et al, 2004).

Free radicals and causative oxidative stress are associated with several pregnancy-related disorders, including preeclampsia, diabetic embryopathy, preterm premature rupture of the membranes, and intrauterine growth restriction. This was the pathophysiological background for a potential benefit of early antioxidant supplementation therapy in the prevention of such disorders, in particularly preeclampsia (Rodrigo R et al, 2005).

First observational and randomized controlled trials have shown that antioxidant prophylactics in high-risk women lowered the prevalence of preeclampsia (Kharb S, 2000; Poston L et al, 2004; Chappell LC et al, 1999). Moreover, vitamin supplementation was associated with better endothelial function and less placental dysfunction. However, a Cochrane review (Rumbold A & Crowther CA, 2005c; Rumbold A et al, 2005d) and more recent studies concluded that data are too insufficient to suggest that vitamin E supplementation, either alone (Beazley D et al, 2005) or in combination with other supplements (Gulmezoglu AM et al, 1997), is beneficial in reducing the risk of pre-eclampsia, and other pregnancy complications associated with oxidative stress.

Nevertheless, as mentioned above, since the chorion and amnion contain polyunsaturated free fatty acids, vitamin E may protect them from lipid peroxidation. Additionaly, it was established through measurements of maternal plasma concentrations of vitamin E that plasma concentrations of this vitamin at 16th and at 28th week were positively related to increased fetal growth, a decreased risk of small-for-gestational-age births, and an increased risk of large-for-gestational-age births. The concentration of alpha-tocopherol at week 28 was positively related to the use of prenatal multivitamins and dietary intake of vitamin E. Early and late circulating concentrations of alpha-tocopherol were positively associated with fetal growth (Scholl TO et al, 2006). Despite these encouraging findings, the data are still too few to claim that vitamin E supplementation is beneficial for pregnancy (Rumbold A & Crowther CA, 2005c) .

It was mentioned that premature infants might be especially low in vitamin E due to their inability to accumulate sufficient fat during the third trimester of pregnancy. Several complications associated with preterm infants, such as hemolytic anemia, bronchopulmonary dysplasia, and retinopathy, were thought to be related to vitamin E status (Gonzales-Reyes S et al, 2003; Liu PM et al, 2005). Cochrane data base review assessed the effects of vitamin E supplementation on morbidity and mortality in preterm infants. It was concluded that vitamin E supplementation in preterm infants reduces the risk of intracranial hemorrhage, but increases the risk of sepsis. In very low birth weight infants it increases the risk of sepsis, and reduces the risk of severe retinopathy and blindness. Overall, a Cochrane review failed to support routine use of vitamin E supplementation in preterm infants (Brion LP et al, 2005).

Vitamin C

Apart from the best known physiological role in the prevention of scurvy, vitamin C (ascorbic acid) has many functions in complex physiological processes, including acting as an antioxidant and a potent 'free-radical fighter', regenerating other antioxidants, such as vitamins A, E and some B vitamins, and serving as a key immune system nutrient. Vitamin C scavenges free radicals in the aqueous phase. Ascorbic acid functions as a reducing agent by delivering a hydrogen atom with its single electron to ROS with a single unpaired electron in its outer ring. ROS, now with paired electrons in its outer ring, is stabilized. In turn, ascorbic acid becomes a weak ROS, called dehydroascorbic acid, and is eliminated in the urine.

Pregnant and lactating women warrant special attention with respect to vitamin C requirements (Bsoul SA & Terezhalmy GT, 2004). Plasma levels of vitamin C normally decline about 10-15% during pregnancy. Therefore, supplementation of vitamin C seems reasonable. It is even more justified for pregnant smokers, lactating women and their babies, considering the fact that smoking is a source of oxidant stress (Proskocil BJ et al, 2005). Maternal plasma vitamin C levels after oral ingestion correlate with concentration of this vitamin in amniotic fluid. Vitamin C is found to be the highest in amniotic fluid, somewhat lower in fetal plasma, and the lowest in maternal plasma. (Pressman EK et al, 2003). Human milk ascorbic acid concentration can be doubled or tripled by increasing intake in women with low baseline content (Daneel-Otterbech S et al, 2005).

Ascorbic acid deficiency during pregnancy has been associated with increased risk of infections, premature rupture of the membranes (PROM), prematurity and hypertensive disorders in pregnancy. Regarding fetal membranes, ascorbic acid serves to strengthen and stabilize collagen by direct stimulation of collagen synthesis through activation of multiple genes. Additionaly, vitamin C may use products of lipid peroxidation to regulate collagen synthesis (Woods et al, 2001). It was observed that women who had a preconceptional low total vitamin C intake had twice the risk of preterm delivery due to premature rupture of membranes. The risk is even greater for the women with low vitamin C intake, both preconceptionally and during the second trimester (Siega-Riz AM et al, 2003). Additionally, low maternal blood and leukocyte levels of vitamin C are associated with increased risk for PROM (Casanueva E et al, 1995). Prelabor ruptured membranes had a reduced collagen and ascorbic acid concentrations. Tissue ascorbic acid status may be an important mediator of these events (Stuart EL et al, 2005). Accordingly, it was postulated that maintaining adequate vitamin C status could decrease the incidence of PROM.

The evidence regarding the role of vitamin C is conflicting. Although some studies have shown that daily supplementation with 100mg vitamin C after 20 week of gestation effectively lessens the incidence of PROM (Casanueva E et al, 2005), supplementation of women at risk of preterm labour failed to prove that gestation could be prolonged with supplementation. Moreover, increase in spontaneous preterm labour was noted in the supplemented patients (Rumbold AR et al, 2005a).

So far, there has been no sufficient evidence to recommend vitamin C supplementation, either alone or in combination with other supplements, in order to reduce the risk of stillbirth, perinatal death, growth restriction and hypertensive disorders in pregnancy. The potential role of vitamin C and other antioxidants in the prevention of impaired glucose tolerance in pregnancy is still uncertain.

Vitamin C and E

Extensive research has been conducted over the past ten years in different pregnant patient groups in an attempt to prove the presumed beneficial influence of antioxidants, predominantly related to the combined use of vitamins C and E on preeclampsia. Almost all studies used the same regiment, as vitamin C in dose of 1000 mg per day results in plasma saturation, and vitamin E, in dose of 400 IU per day has been shown to prevent low-density lipoprotein oxidation, with limited evidence that higher doses are more effective.

The obtained results were conflicting. Although first observational studies were encouriging, further differently designed trials did not support the previous beneficial findings (Chappell LC et al, 1999; Poston L et al, 2004; Beazley D et al, 2005; Rumbold AR et al, 2005b; Polyzos NP et al, 2007). Nevertheless, these findings directed further studies either to earlier initiation of the therapy, or to different combination of antioxidants (Gulmezoglu AM et al, 1997).

Cosidering the fact that previous studies were not powered to detect differencies in preeclampsia, it became clear that multicenter randomized placebo-controlled trials were needed to provide answers to many crucial questions regarding the issue whether antioxidants are benefitial in high-risk women (Poston L et al, 2006); in nulliparous women (Fraser WD et al, 2005; Roberts JM, 2006); in women considering to be at increased risk for preeclampsia, including women with diabetes (Holmes VA et al, 2004); and in those who had preeclampsia during a previous pregnancy (Fraser WD et al, 2005; Poston L et al, 2006; Spinnato JA, 2006). Recently, several such studies were published with compatible, although disappointing results. Routine daily supplementation in healthy nulliparous women showed no reduction in the risk of preeclampsia, and the risk of serious perinatal outcomes in their infants, including the risk of intrauterine growth restriction (Rumbold AR et al, 2006). Moreover, it became clear that vitamin supplemented patients were more likely to develop hypertensive disorders in pregnancy. In the case of low dietary intakes of antioxidants, these results, such as they were, could not be extrapolated. Women with low antioxidant status in the first trimester pregnancy benefit from antioxidant supplementation regarding better maternal (preeclampsia, abortion, hypertension) and perinatal (preterm deliveries, IUGR) outcome, compared to women supplemented with iron and folate alone (Rumiris D et al, 2006).

In patients with identified risk of preeclampsia, concomitant supplementation with vitamin C and vitamin E does not prevent pre-eclampsia, but does increase the rate of babies born with low birthweight. Striking, unexpected result regarding the earlier onset of preeclampsia, first noted in healthy nulliparous women, was also observed in vitamin supplemented high-risk patients (Poston L et al, 2006). Within the above mentioned trials, very interesting results were obtained regarding the secondary outcomes, such as preterm birth, IUGR, and LBW. There is an adverse association between supplementation with antioxidants and low birthweight, and an umbilical artery cord pH of less than 7.0, which could be attributable to the earlier onset of pre-eclampsia in supplemented groups. Overall, more low birthweight babies were born to women who took antioxidants, but small size for gestational age did not differ between supplemented and nonsupplemented patients; growth restriction was not increased in women who took antioxidants. The question then arose how safe it is to use multivitamins that contain vitamins C and E during pregnancy. Although neither antioxidant is contraindicated in pregnancy, evidence on their safety is limited. A speculated reason for increased rate of LBW in supplemented patients could be the detrimental effect of supraphysiological doses of vitamins C and E on placental function and possible direct effect on fetal growth. Cochrane reviews of vitamin E (Rumbold A et al,

2005c), and vitamin C (Rumbold A et al, 2005a) supplementation in pregnancy emphasise the need to establish the safety of their use in high doses in pregnant women. According to contemporary data, the use of these antioxidants in high doses is not justified in pregnancy.

Although preeclamptic studies showed that maternal supplementation was not associated with any overall benefits with respect to the primary infant outcomes, intrauterine growth restriction, rate of preterm birth, it was associated with a reduced risk of the respiratory distress syndrome and the use of surfactant. It is possible that maternal supplementation with antioxidant vitamins may increase the antioxidant status of at-risk infants and thus reduce the risk of diseases associated with oxidative stress (Rumbold AR et al, 2006).

Despite the disappointing findings of the mentioned studies, the results should not be extrapolated to other antioxidants, other regiments, different timing of intervention, or different patient groups. Above all, this should not detract from the potential importance of oxidative stress in preeclampsia. For example, antioxidant supplementation in pregnant women with proved low antioxidant status in early pregnancy was associated with better perinatal outcome (preterm deliveries and IUGR) (Rumiris D et al, 2006). Currently, there are some ongoing trials whose results are expected with great enthusiasm. It was well established that the rates of preeclampsia in women with type 1 diabetes are two to four times higher than in normal pregnancy. Diabetes is associated with antioxidant depletion and increased free radical production. Also, an increasing body of evidence suggests that oxidative stress and endothelial cell activation may be relevant to disease pathogenesis in pre-eclampsia. An ongoing study, The Diabetes and Pre-eclampsia Intervention Trial - DAPIT, aims to establish if pregnant women with type 1 diabetes supplemented with vitamins C and E have lower rates of preeclampsia and endothelial activation compared with placebo treatment (Holmes VA et al, 2004). Another very important ongoing trial, Combined Antioxidant and Preeclampsia Prediction Studies (CAPPS), has a hypothesis that antioxidant therapy initiated prior to 16 weeks of gestation will reduce the frequency of serious maternal and infant complications associated with pregnancy-related hypertension (Roberts JM, 2006).

PROM is also extensively investigated. The vitamin C to E ratio may be of central importance in protecting against the damaging effects of reactive oxygen species, considered to be important for etiopathogenesis of PROM. An interaction between vitamin C and vitamin E was suggested, with vitamin C possibly exerting a 'redox' recycling effect on oxidised vitamin E within lipoproteins and membranes (Hamilton IMJ et al, 2000). Supplementation of vitamin C and E was suggested for prevention against ROS-induced PPROM (Plessinger MA et al, 2000). In the absence of ascorbic acid, alpha-tocopheryl radicals are not recycled to alpha-tocopherol-OH, but instead accumulate as evidence of ongoing lipid peroxidation (Woods JR et al, 2001). It was assumed that enhanced dietary consumption or supplementation with vitamins C and E during pregnancy may reduce risks of PPROM (Woods JR et al, 2001), but the effects of this intervention are uncertain.

It is obvious that many questions still remain unanswered regarding the influence of vitamins C and E on pregnancy outcomes, including the issue of the optimal dose of vitamins C and E.

Folic Acid

Widespread cell division is a centrale feature of embryonic/fetal development, and folate is critically important for that process. Once absorbed, folate acts as a cofactor for many essential cellular reactions. Folate-containing coenzymes are responsible for the synthesis of DNA and methionin. DNA methylation is essential in mammalian development and represents one of several mechanisms that regulate genome programming and imprinting during embryogenesis (McKay JA et al, 2004). Additionaly, folate coenzymes are required for the synthesis of methionine from homocysteine and, consequently, deficiency results in decreased synthesis of methionin and increased levels of homocysteine.

Humans are entirely dependent on dietary source/supplements for their folate supply. Additionally, folate requirements are high in pregnancy. This fact increases the prevalence as well as the risk of deficiency, which can be consequence of low dietary folate intake or increased metabolic requirement caused by specific genetic defect(s). Behavioral factors, such as nicotin and alcohol abuse, as well as oral contraceptives, are also associated with poor folate status. Inadequate folate may lead to alterations in DNA synthesis and chromosomal aberrations. Folic acid deficiency, through interference with DNA synthesis, leads to impaired mitosis, altered protein syntesis and gives rise to abnormal cell division. Rapidly dividing cells are the most susceptibile to irregularities in DNA production. During pregnancy, folate-dependent processes include an increase in red cell mass, enlargement of the uterus and mammary gland, and growth of the placenta and the fetus. Even marginal folate nutriture can impair cellular growth and replication in the fetus or placenta. One of the most important consequences of inadequate folate status during pregnancy is an increased risk of neural tube defects (NTD) in the offspring. The discovery that folic acid in early pregnancy reduces the risk of neural tube defects is one of important public health advances of recent years. The benefit of folic acid supplementation during the periconceptional period in reducing the risk of neural tube defects in offspring has been demonstrated both in experimental and observational studies. The risk of NTD in the United States, after fortification of specific foods with folic acid, was reduced by between 60% and 100% in women who consumed folic acid supplementation in addition to a varied diet during the periconceptional period (about one month prior and throughout the first trimester of pregnancy) (Centers for Disease Control and Prevention, 2004). Folic acid fortification of cereal products has almost halved the risk of neural tube defects among babies born in Canada. The decrease was greatest in areas in which the baseline rate was high (De Wals P et al, 2007).

Surprisingly, despite the proven benefits and effectiveness of folic acid supplementation, a significant proportion of women of reproductive age, and as many as 50% of pregnant women did not follow the recommendation. More aggressive food fortification program is considered by many as the only option which is likely to succeed (Scholl TO & Johnson WG, 2000; Botto LD et al, 2005; De Wals P et al, 2007).

Folate intake may need to be sustained after complete closure of the neural tube to decrease the risk of other undesirable pregnancy outcomes. The correlation between adequate folate status and reduced risk of pregnancy complications, apart from NTD (other birth defects, preterm delivery, low birth weight, restricted fetal growth, spontaneous abortions, preeclampsia and placental abruption) is less clear, with studies showing an effect (Scholl TO & Johnson WG, 2000; Siega-Riz AM et al, 2004) or no effect (Charles DHM et al, 2005). It was recently observed that periconceptional intake of folic acid seemed to reduce the risk of isolated cleft lip with or without cleft palate by about a third. It was also suggested that other nutritional factors correlating in diet with folates may have a role in preventing this anomaly (Wilcox AJ et al, 2007). Early data showed that low folate intake was associated with significant increase in risk of infant low birth weight and preterm delivery (Scholl TO et al, 1996; Malinow MR et al, 1998). Unlike observational studies, randomized trials of folic acid supplementation have shown less uniform benefit (Czeizel AE et al, 1994). Nevertheless, some women, especially from economically unprivileged groups, may benefit from receiving additional folic acid during, as well as before pregnancy (Scholl TO & Johnosn WG, 2000). General suggestion of these observational and supplemental trials is that poor dietary folate intake and low circulating concentrations of folate are associated with an increased risk of adverse birth outcomes. It is possible that a more abundant supply of folate to mother and fetus could support growth and gestation, leading to improved infant birth weight and increased gestation duration (Scholl TO & Johnosn WG, 2000).

A Cochrane review of folate supplementation in pregnancy found insufficient evidence to conclusively demonstrate that folate supplementation reduces the above mentioned poor pregnancy outcomes, other than suggestion of a lowering the risk for low birth weight (Mahomed K, 2000b). Also, data regarding the alleged cause-and-effect relationship between an increased twining rate and folic acid supplementation are still controversial (Czeizel AE & Vargha P, 2004; Kàllen B, 2004).

It should be mentioned that human milk has a relatively high content of folate, which is unaffected to a large extent by maternal intake. Consequently, the infant is relatively well protected from maternal deficiency, unlike the mother who remains exposed to greater risk of depletion during lactation (Allen LH, 2003).

Hyperhomocysteinemia, a marker for folate deficiency or metabolic abnormality, has been associated with serious pregnancy complications, such as habitual spontaneus abortion, pregnancy-induced hypertension, preeclampsia, and placental abruption (Dekker GA et al, 1995; Leeda M et al, 1998). All of the above present risk factors for limited intrauterine growth and preterm delivery. There are still no data from well-controlled studies to determine whether supplementation with folic acid and B vitamins reduces the risk associated with maternal hyperhomocysteinemia (Scholl TO & Johnosn WG, 2000). Although supports for these findings are not consistent, it seems reasonable to maintain folic acid supplementation throughout pregnancy (Bailey LB & Berry RJ, 2005; Holmes VA et al, 2005).

Vitamin B1 (Thiamine)

Thiamine pyrophosphate is an essential coenzyme for a few very important enzymes involved in decarboxylation of carbohydrate metabolism and energy production.

Thiamin deficiency may result from inadequate thiamin intake, increased requirement, excessive loss, dietary anti-thiamin factors, or a combination of the above. Insufficient intake is common amongst populations on high carbohydrate-based diets, particularly in underdeveloped countries and low-income populations. Increased requirements for thiamin occur during pregnancy, lactation and in patients with hyperemesis.

As pregnancy increases energy expenditure, a proportional increase in thiamine requirement appears. The concentration of thiamin in human milk falls rapidly and substantially in vitamin-depleted mothers, which can result in infantile beriberi within a few weeks after birth (Allen LH, 2003). It was estimated that during pregnancy approximately 50% of women develop a biochemical thiamin deficiency, which in turn might cause alteration in glucose tolerance and intrauterine growth, and an increased risk of viscerocranial malformations (Baker H et al, 2002; Krapels IP et al, 2004). In addition, deficiency might impair brain development, as thiamine dependent enzymes play an important role in cellular energy metabolism necessary for lipid and nucleotide synthesis in the developing brain. Thiamin supplementation increases intrauterine fetal growth in women treated for gestational diabetes mellitus, whereas conventional treatment of this condition, without thiamine, increases the risk of low birth weight. So, thiamine supplementation appears to be an effective, preventive measure in women with gestational diabetes mellitus (Bakker SJ et al, 2000).

Vitamin B2 (Riboflavin)

Riboflavin, acting as a part of flavoprotein enzyme complex, is involved in carbohydrate metabolism and energy production by catalyzation of important oxidation reactions. Consequently, riboflavin requirement is dependant on caloric expenditure and the carbohydrate content of the diet.

The additional energy requirement during pregnancy increases the demand for riboflavin. Considering the fact that riboflavin is an essential constituent of muscle tissue, riboflavin intake during pregnancy is related to birth weight: growing fetal tissue demand increased amounts of this vitamin during pregnancy (Bates CJ et al, 1994). During both the pre- and postnatal periods, riboflavin has an important co-enzyme role in energy utilization, and can be considered as an indirect antioxidant. Moreover, it was suggested that women at risk of preeclampsia were 4.7 times more likely to develop the disorder if they were riboflavin deficient, compaired to those with adequate riboflavin nutritional status. It is possible that decreased intracellular levels of flavin coenzymes could affect preeclampsia associated mitochondrial function, oxidative stress and blood vessel dilatation (Wacker J et al, 2000). Low riboflavin concentration at birth could be indicative of an insufficient antioxidative protection of the neonate. Moreover, human milk riboflavin concentration is very sensitive to maternal intake and status and responds to maternal supplementation (Allen LH, 2003). Breast milk riboflavin levels may have a significant influence on the nutritional status and health of the breast-feeding babies, especially in certain clinical conditions such as phototherapy for hyperbilirubinemia.

Vitamin B6 (Pyridoxine)

Functions of vitamin B6 are primarily evident in the metabolism of proteins, fat, and carbohydrates. Its active form pyridoxal phosphate acts as a coenzyme for more than 100 essential chemical reactions in the human body. The need for vitamin B6 is closely linked with protein requirements and protein intake. Pyridoxine plays a major role in the development of the central nervous system, synthesis of neurotransmitters in the brain and nerve cells, and is an essential cofactor in the muscle tissues.

Severe deficiency of vitamin B6 is uncommon, except in strict vegetarians, who might need to increase their vitamin B6 intake. During pregnancy, the enchanced demand for protein and the enhanced conversion of tryptophan to niacin increases the requirement for vitamin B6. Animal studies have shown that maternal vitamin B6 deficiency might have harmful effects on the fetus, but the relationship between vitamin B6 status and pregnancy outcomes has not been well studied in humans. Maternal blood levels decline during pregnancy and are at their lowest between the 4th and 8th month of gestation. The demand for vitamin B6 is increased in pregnancies compromised by preeclampsia, HELLP syndrome, and placental insufficiency (Herrmann W et al, 2004).

Vitamin B6 has been used to treat pregnancy-related nausea. According to a Cochrane review, vitamin B6 appears to be more effective than other substances in reducing the severity of nausea in early pregnancy (Jewell D & Young G, 2003).

Niacin

Niacinamide, a functional form of niacin, exerts its function as a part of two essential coenzyme systems (NAD and NADP) that catalyze oxidation-reduction reactions for glycolysis, fatty acid metabolism, and oxidative phosphorylation. As many as 200 enzymes require NAD and NADP to accept or donate electrons for redox reaction, and over 40 biochemical reactions depend on one of these coenzyme systems. Niacin deficiency may result from inadequate dietary intake of niacin and/or tryptophan. As pregnancy increases energy expenditure, a proportional increase is required for niacin. During the first trimester, a strikingly high proportion of niacin deficiency among healthy, vitamin supplemented women was observed. This deficiency worsened later on, throughout pregnancy (Baker et al, 2002).

Vitamin B12 (Cyanocobalamin)

Vitamin B12 is the only vitamin that contains an essential mineral element, cobalt. The two basic coenzyme functions of this vitamin are conversions of homocysteine to methionine, and methyl malonyl CoA to succinyl CoA. As both reactions are important for different metabolic processes, deficiency can cause defective DNA synthesis, reduced cell multiplication, and metabolic disorders. Vitamin B12 deficiency usually occurs as a consequence of pernicious anemia and malabsorption of dietary vitamin B12. Vegetarian diet is likely to be low in vitamin B12, and therefore presents a risk factor for deficiency.

Requirements for vitamin B12 are increased during pregnancy and lactation. Deficiency has been reported in some infants born to mothers who were strict vegetarians (Weiss R et al, 2004). Also, maternal smoking negatively influences hematological parameters and cobalamin function in the infants (Bjorke-Monsen AL et al, 2004).

During pregnancy decreased vitamin B12 blood levels have been associated with an increased risk of neural tube defects. Increased intake of folate and vitamin B12 neutralizes the negative effects of the mutated alleles on homocystein metabolism (Zetterberg H, 2004). Accordingly, addition of vitamin B 12 to folic acid might be beneficial in the prevention of NTD (Groenen PM et al, 2004a). It is also possible that periconceptional supplementation with folate and vitamin B12 decreased the incidence of miscarriage in women planning a pregnancy (Zetterberg H, 2004). Maternal vitamin B12 defficiency was also linked with increased risk for nonsyndromic orofacial clefts in the offspring (van Rooij et al, 2003). There is limited evidence to connect vitamin B12 deficiency with prematurity, low birth weight and even intra-uterine death (Allen LH, 1994).

As it goes with other B vitamins, except for folate, low maternal intake or low stores during lactation reduce the concentration of this vitamin in human milk, and consequently reduces the infants' stores. The prevalence of some B vitamin deficiencies, especially deficiencies of riboflavin and vitamin B12, are probably underestimated. So, providing adequate amounts of B vitamins to infants and young children seems reasonable (Allen LH, 2003).

Biotin

Biotin acts as a coenzyme in carbohydrate and fatty acid metabolism, citrulline and purine synthesis, and in amino acid catabolism. Requirements for biotin increase during pregnancy due to the synthesis of essential carboxylases in rapidly dividing cells of the developing fetus, whereas maternal biotin status declines. A marked proportion of marginal biotin deficiency was noted even during healthy pregnancy (Mock DM et al, 2002). Although the observed deficiencies were subclinical, and although only experimental studies established a link between biotin deficiency and birth defects, it seems reasonable to ensure adequate biotin intake throughout pregnancy (Mock DM et al, 2002).

Pantothenic Acid (vitamin B5)

Pantothenic acid is a constituent of coenzyme A, a vital coenzyme in numerous chemical reactions and a constituent of acyl-carrier protein. These two systems are responsible for transferring acetyl and acyl groups during glucose and fatty acid oxidation, and for the synthesis of fatty acid, cholesterol, porphyrin, neurotransmitters (acetylcholine) and hormones (melatonin). Effects of pantothenic acid defficiency come from animal studies, since this condition is rare in humans. It is possible that pantothenic acid requirement is increased during pregnancy, as maternal blood levels decrease during gestation, and remain low during puerperium. Pregnant and lactating women might need to consume more pantothenic acid in order to maintain non-pregnant blood levels (Song WO et al, 1985).

Vitamin K

Vitamin K is essential for blood clotting. Although rare, deficiency states may be fatal for infants. Vitamin K content in human milk is relatively low compared to baby formulas. Neonates exclusively breast-fed, or those born to mothers taking anticonvulsants, are at increased risk of vitamin K deficiency. The American Academy of Pediatrics recommended that an injection of vitamin K1 is to be administered to all newborns (Thorp JA et al, 1995).

MINERALS AND TRACE ELEMENTS

Calcium

Calcium, the most abundant mineral in the human body, is the main structural element of the skeleton. More than 99% of the total body calcium is stored in bones and teeth, where it functions to support their structure. The remaining 1% is found throughout the body. Calcium has extremely important biochemical and physiological roles. Homeostatic control mechanisms exist to maintain a relatively constant blood level of calcium, so these vital body processes can function efficiently. In cases of insufficient dietary intake or rapid loss of calcium from the body, calcium is withdrawn from bones. Conditions that increase calcium requirements, such as pregnancy and lactation, present the challenge to these homeostatic systems. Since the skeleton provides a large reserve of calcium for maintaining normal blood levels, deficiencies are rarely due to low dietary intake.

During pregnancy, high calcium requirements occur, with the accretion rate reaching its maximum in the third trimester. Calcium absorption and urinary excretion are higher during pregnancy, and are back to normal after delivery. Most of the additional calcium is required for adequate mineralization of the fetal skeleton. Although no data demonstrates that pregnancy causes a permanent negative effect on bone density, it is possible that in some cases pregnancy could be a risk factor for maternal osteomalacia (Di Gregorio S et al, 2000). Moreover, some longitudinal studies suggest that skeletal response to pregnancy may lead to an increase in the biological activity of the skeleton and thus may not be entirely independent of maternal calcium intake, especially in women with low calcium intake (Zeni SN et al, 2003). Potential negative consequences of deficiency in calcium intake during pregnancy are hypertensive disorders, adverse influence on bone metabolism and fetal growth.

Data from developing countries suggest an inverse relationship between calcium intake and the incidence of pregnancy induced hypertension (PIH). These observations lead to the assumption that in population of low calcium intake the incidence of preeclampsia can be decreased by calcium supplementation (Belizan JM et al, 1988). Moreover, results of numerous clinical trials and several meta-analyses have suggested that calcium supplementation reduce the incidence of preeclampsia (Carroli G et al, 1994; Bucher HC et al, 1996).

However, data on the effectiveness of prophylactic calcium in preventing or treating PIH are contradictory (Ritchie LD & King JC, 2000). Reviews of previously cited reports revealed important differences in the study design that limit acceptance of these trials. Meta-analysis of randomized placebo-controlled studies showed that calcium supplementation reduced the incidence of high blood pressure and preeclampsia in women at high risk of PIH, as well as in pregnant women with low dietary calcium intake. Accordingly, calcium supplementation could be a promising nutritional intervention for those groups of pregnant women, although a final confirmation is not established yet. Cochrain review confirmed that reduction of preeclampsia incidence with calcium supplementation was the most evident in the group with the low baseline calcium intake (Attalah AN et al, 2002). However, in healthy nulliparous women, in low risk pregnant women, as well as in those with adequate calcium intake, the beneficial effects of calcium supplementation are not found to be significant for prevention of preeclampsia, PIH, or adverse perinatal outcomes (Levine RJ et al, 1997).

In this context it is important to stress that the average calcium dietary intakes in the United States are currently beneath the adequate intake recommendation, especially in females (Harville EW et al, 2004). Supplements may be a good nutritive alternative. For the general female population, achieving current recommendation for calcium during pregnancy may be preventable for PIH, but the question of adequate doses for different risk groups still remains open.

It is possible that deficiency during pregnancy may reduce neonatal bone density and affect neonatal size. Also, there are some evidences that maternal calcium supplementation could permanently program lipid metabolism during intrauterine life, thus influencing cardiovascular risk factors during adult life (Morley R et al, 2004). Another potential benefit of maternal mid-gestational calcium supplementation may be lowering blood pressure in the offspring, and prevention of hypertension in the next generation (Gillman MW et al, 2004).

Sodium

Sodium and water retention are normal findings in pregnancy. Sodium intake has long been a target for dietary intervention in preeclampsia. A Cochrane review indicated that manipulating sodium intake does not affect the rate of preeclampsia (Duley L & Henderson-Smart D, 2002). As preeclampsia is characterized by intravascular depletion, dietary sodium restriction could have an adverse effect on uteroplacental perfusion (Norwitz ER et al, 1999). Sodium restriction or supplementation has no place in the management of hypertensive disorders in pregnancy.

Iodine

Iodine is a critically important micronutrient in the human diet. It is an essential constituent of thyroid hormones, which play a vital role in the regulation of metabolic processes, such as growth and energy expenditure. Approximately 3/4 of the body's iodine is stored in the thyroid gland. Iodine deficiency is an important health problem worldwide. According to the WHO, iodine deficiency disorders (IDD) affect 740 million people in the world, and nearly 50 million people suffer from some degrees of IDD-related brain damage. The spectrum of IDD includes mental retardation, hypothyroidism, goiter, reproductive dysfunction, and different growth and development abnormalities. Nearly two-thirds of the population of Western and Central Europe live in regions of mild-to-severe iodine deficiency (Delange F, 2002; Zimmermann M & Delange F, 2003). In addition, there is an increased risk for people whose diets exclude iodized salt, fish and seaweed. Iodine deficiency during pregnancy is the commonest worldwide cause of preventable intelectual impairment, as well as damage to the development of the fetus and the newborn. In areas where iodine deficiency is severe, IQ scores in children are decreased by 10 to 15 points, psychomotor deficits are more common, hearing may be impaired, and there is markedly increased prevalence of attention deficit hyperactivity disorders (ADHD). Baby's birth size is decreased and infant mortality is increased in iodine deficiency regions (Das SC et al, 2006).

Iodine requirements are increased in pregnant and lactating women. More iodine is required to ensure maternal thyroid hormone production at the level almost double than in non-pregnant state. During pregnancy, the fetus derives very little thyroid hormone from the mother, and consequently has to obtain the necessary iodine from the mother in order to synthesize its own supply. The fetus is entirely dependant on thyroxine (T4) transferred from the mother during the first and second trimester, and on iodine transfer for fetal thyroid hormone synthesis during the last trimester. Any compromise in the placental transfer of T4 or iodine to the fetus directly influences normal central nervous system development. Iodine deficiency may adversely affect all stages of development, but it is most damaging to the developing brain. In early pregancy the fetus is particularly vulnerable to damage from decreased circulating maternal levels of T4, be it from environmental iodine deficiency or thyroid disease. Thus, if supplementation begins only at the first prenatal care visit, this critical period may be missed (Morreale de Escobar G et al, 2004). Iodine deficiency during pregnancy has been associated with an increased incidence of miscarriage, stillbirth, and long-term neuropsychological deficits in infants (Ohara N et al, 2004).

One of the most devastating consequences of maternal iodine deficiency is congenital hypothyroidism (cretinism) associated with irreversible mental retardation. Even mild or sublinical maternal hypothyroidisms during pregnancy may have subtle effects on neuropsychological development of the offspring (Vermiglio F et al, 2004). Iodine deficiency in lactating women may result in insufficient iodine to the infant.

Iodine intake in the U.S. decreased significantly over the past 20 years. Almost 7% of pregnant women and 14.5% of women of childbearing age have insufficient iodine intake (Hollowell JG et al, 1998). In Europe, median iodine intakes are approximately half of the recommended levels for women of child-bearing age. Moreover, although data suggest that most women in Europe are iodine-deficient during pregnancy, only 13-50% received iodine-containing supplements (Zimmermann M & Delange F, 2003). Because iodine-containing supplements have a beneficial impact on the iodine and thyroid status of both mother and newborn, this should be considered and recommended for pregnant women and for those women planning a pregnancy, if they are not adequately covered by iodized salt (Glinoer D, 2004).

Iron

Iron is an essential constituent of numerous proteins and enzymes required for various important vital functions, such as growth, reproduction, and immune function. The main role of iron is oxygen transport. Iron is essential to life, because of its unique ability to serve as both an electron donor and acceptor. Iron intestinal absorption is regulated by its level in the body, form of iron (heme or non-heme), and by dietary factors such as vitamin A, copper, zinc, calcium and ascorbic acid.

Iron deficiency is the most common nutritional disorder, affecting millions in both developed and developing countries. Most of the symptoms result from the associated anemia. The WHO estimated that the global incidence of anemia amongst pregnant women is about 50%. Moreover, anemia contributes to 20% of the maternal deaths in Africa and 23% in Asia (World Health Organization, 1996).

An additional amount of iron throughtout pregnancy is required to increase red cell mass, expand the plasma volume and to support the growth of the feto-placental unit. Due to these physiological changes, and increased iron utilization, pregnant women must double their iron intake. Since iron requirement is high, it is difficult to meet that demand through dietary intake alone. That gives the basis for routine iron supplementation during pregnancy (Ramakrishnan U, 2004).

Severe anemia in pregnant women is correlated with adverse pregnancy outcomes, such as low birth weight, premature birth and maternal mortality. As anemia and iron-deficient anemia (despite being a major contributory factor) are not synonymous, it remains unclear whether iron deficiency anemia is a causal factor in poor pregnancy outcome. Maternal iron deficiency anemia affects also lactation, maternal infections, emotions and cognition (Beard JL et al, 2005).

When detected early in pregnancy, iron-deficient anemia (IDA) is associated with a more than double increase in the risk of preterm delivery. There are at least three potential mechanisms explaining how maternal IDA might lead to preterm delivery: hypoxia, oxidative stress, and infection (Allen LH, 2001). Maternal anemia diagnosed before mid-pregnancy is also associated with a substantially increased risk of preterm delivery. Early iron supplementation is associated with some decrease in the risk of low birth weight or preterm low birth weight, but not in preterm delivery (Cogswell ME et al, 2003). Although relatively common, maternal anemia during the third trimester is usually not associated with increased risk of adverse pregnancy outcomes, unless it is followed by an episode of postpartum hemorrhage which sometimes could be fatal. It is difficult to establish causal associations between iron deficiency anemia during third trimester with low birth weight and compromised neonatal status in human population. Data from appropriate animal models indicated that inadequate intake of iron from diet during pregnancy can lead to compromised hematologic status of the neonate without indications of growth retardation or impaired neurologic function at birth (Golub MS et al, 2006).

On the other hand, high levels of hemoglobin, hematocrit and ferritin are associated with an increased risk of fetal growth restriction, preterm delivery and preeclampsia (Lao TT et al, 2000). Also, iron and different markers of iron status, such as increased free iron, increased ferritin, and decreased transferrin levels, have been reported as abnormal in preeclampsia (Hubel CA et al, 1996). But, as inflammatory responses are increased in preeclampsia, markers relating to iron homeostasis need to be interpreted carefully (Roberts JM et al, 2003).

In addition, iron supplementation and increased iron stores have recently been linked to maternal complications (such as gestational diabetes) and increased oxidative stress during pregnancy. Consequently, whereas iron supplementation may improve pregnancy outcome in iron deficient mothers, it is possible that prophylactic supplementation may increase the risk of adverse outcomes when mother is not iron deficient (Scholl TO, 2005). Recently, it has been found that routine iron supplementation in nonanemic women is not rational, and moreover may even be harmful. That is, iron supplementations could predispose pregnant women who are not anemic to high blood preasure and small babies (Ziaei S et al, 2007). It may be reasonable to identify an upper limit for iron-replete pregnant women beyond which prophylactic supplementation is not indicated (Scholl TO, 2005).

The most recent Cochrane database found insufficient data to evaluate routine antenatal supplementation with iron or combination of iron and folic acid on clinically important maternal and infant outcomes (Pena-Rosas JP & Viteri FE, 2006).

Magnesium

Magnesium is predominantly located in bone, and involved in more than 300 essential metabolic reactions. Among other properties, magnesium has an indirect antithrombotic effect upon thrombocytes and the endothelial functions, microvascular leakage and vasospasm through its function similar to calcium channel blockers. Magnesium deficiency is rare in healthy adults on balanced diet. Nevertheless, about 20% of the population, particularly women, consume less than two-thirds of the RDA for magnesium.

Pregnant women also have inadequate dietary intake of magnesium, and supplementation may be necessary to meet higher demand for this nutrient during pregnancy and lactation. Magnesium intake in the first trimester possitively corelates with birth weight, while the second and third trimester supplementation had no effect on the pregnancy outcome (Sibai BM et al, 1989).

Magnesium deficiency during pregnancy can induce maternal, fetal and even long-lasting consequences. Animal studies show that magnesium deficiency may produce, among other, detrimental effects on fetal growth/development. Chronic maternal magnesium deficiency or magnesium depletion could contribute to premature delivery. Magnesium deficiency might be associated with preeclampsia and preterm delivery, and possibly with low birth weight and other adverse fetal outcomes (Almonte RA et al, 1999). Regarding fetal malformations, it was suggested that a low preconceptional intake of magnesium, among other nutrients, is associated with a 2- to 5-fold increased risk of spina bifida (Groenen PM et al, 2004b).

While some maternal magnesium supplementation trials found association with fewer maternal hospitalizations, preterm births, growth restriction, admissions to the neonatal intensive care unit, and a significant influence on the maternal morbidity both before and after delivery (Sibai BM et al, 1989; Makrides M & Crowther MA, 2000; Pathak P & Kapil U, 2004), other were not able to prove significant differences regarding pregnancy outcomes in terms of preterm labor and delivery (Arikan GM et al, 1999).

High dose intravenous magnesium sulfate has been widely accepted as a therapy of choice for preventing eclamptic seizures. Since convulsions are the result of cerebral vasospasm, the vasodilatatory effect of magnesium seems to be the major prophylactic mechanism. Furthermore, magnesium sulphate therapy for eclampsia reduce maternal mortality rate. It was speculated that magnesium might be deficient in women with preeclampsia, as reduced maternal magnesium concentrations in serum, intracellularly and in erythrocyte membranes were found in some (Kisters K et al, 2000) but not all studies (Seydoux J et al, 1992). Still, there is not enough high quality evidence to confirm beneficial effect of dietary magnesium supplementation during pregnancy (Pathak P & Kapil U, 2004; Roberts JM et al, 2003).

Copper

Copper is an essential component of numerous cuproenzymes that are present in energy production, free radical destruction, connective tissue, melanin and norepinephrine synthesis, as well as in iron utilization.

Pregnancy is characterized by progressively increased copper retention in all the three trimesters (Anetor JI, 2003). The fetus is fully dependent on the maternal copper supply, and copper deficiency during embryonic and fetal development might lead to gross structural and biochemical abnormalities, including neural tube defects (Pathak P & Kapil U, 2004; Czeizel AE, 1995). The most common clinical signs of copper deficiency appear in low-birth weight infants and young children and include anemia (unresponsive to iron therapy), neutropenia, osteoporosis, and other abnormalities of bone development. The suggested importance of copper deficiencies in preeclampsia relates to the fact that this trace element is present in ceruloplasmin and superoxide dismutase. Copper, as a transition metal, can catalyze the formation of free radicals. Finally, there is also an association between low plasma ascorbate and copper levels with preeclampsia (Gandley RE et al, 2005). It is still not clearly documented what is the importance of copper deficiency in human placental development.

Zinc

Zinc is an essential component of over 100 metalloenzymes involved in different physiological events, including growth and development, cell division, reproduction, and immunity. Importantly, it also plays a vital role in the expression of certain genes.

Zinc deficiency is recognized as an important public health issue, especially in developing countries. Severe zinc deficiency can cause growth retardation, hypogonadism, and impaired immunity. Even mild zinc deficiency could contribute to impaired physical and neuropsychological development, and increased susceptibility to life-threatening infections in children (Hambidge M, 2000). Identified groups with an increased risk for zinc deficiency are infants, children, pregnant and lactating women (especially teenagers), strict vegetarians, and those with debilitating and certain chronic diseases or infections.

It was estimated that more than 50% of pregnant women worldwide have zinc deficiency. Currently, the cause remains unclear: it is possible that pregnancy leads to zinc deficiency due to increased fetal needs, or the women are zinc deficient when they become pregnant (Pathak P & Kapil U, 2004). Still, there is much to define about the zinc status of pregnant women and its relation to the zinc levels in the newborn. Throughtout pregnancy, there is a decrease in circulating zinc, possibly due to increased transfer of zinc from the mother to the fetus (Anetor JI et al, 2003). Little is known about zinc absorption in late pregnancy, and from the daily diet (Hambridge KM et al, 2006; Harvey LJ et al, 2007). Even with adequate supplementation zinc levels decrease by 20-35% below prepregnancy levels. Plasma zinc concentrations decline more precipitously when iron is supplemented orally as a result of competition for absorption by these two ions.

In the absence of the valid indicator of zinc deficiency in pregnancy, observational data regarding association between the deficiency and adverse fetal outcomes are conflicting. Evidences exist about relationship between lowered zinc concentrations during pregnancy and low birth weight, suggesting a threshold for serum zinc concentration below which adverse pregnancy outcome may significantly increase (Pathak P & Kapil U, 2004). Although some previous reports associated poor maternal zinc status with low birth weight, congenital abnormalities, premature delivery, prolonged labor and other delivery complications, and a negative correlation with fetal distress, maternal infection and pregnancy induced hypertension, more recent studies failed to confirm this connection (Osendarp SJ et al, 2000; Black RE, 2001; Hafeez A et al, 2005). However, a positive effect of zinc supplementation on fetal bone growth and development of fetal heart rate was confirmed (Merialdi M et al, 2004a; Merialdi M et al, 2004b). Low levels of zinc were also associated with gestational hyperglycemia (Bo S et al, 2005). Attempts to modify the frequency of PIH/preeclampsia with zinc supplementation have not been successful (Osendarp SJ et al, 2000; Black RE, 2001). The suggested importance of the deficiencies of zinc in preeclampsia could relate to the fact that it is present in superoxide dismutase, and metallothionein. On the other hand, leukocyte concentrations of zinc are increased in women with preeclampsia (Mahomed K et al, 2000a).

Overall, studies of human pregnancy and zinc supplementation, including those from developing countries, have failed to document a consistent beneficial effect on fetal growth, duration of gestation, and early neonatal survival (Ruz M, 2006; Akman I et al, 2006; Shah D & Sachdev HP, 2006). There is insufficient evidence to evaluate fully the effect of zinc supplementation during pregnancy (Mahomed K, 2000c). Also, there is no evidence that zinc has any beneficial effects on pregnancy outcome in HIV-infected women (Fawzi WW et al, 2005).

Chromium

Chromium is an essential microelement which participates in glucose metabolism. Specifically, it assists in binding insulin to its cell membrane receptors. Therefore, chromium deficiency results in glucose intolerance. It has been hypothesized that deffiency could contribute to the development of Type 2 diabetes. Although it is possible that pregnancy may result in chromium depletion, a few studies evaluating effects of chromium supplementation on gestational diabetes yielded conflicting results (Gunton JE et al, 2001).

Molybdenum

Molybdenum is an essential component of three oxidation-reduction enzymes involved in purine, copper, and sulfur metabolism. Dietary molybdenum deficiency has never been observed in healthy people. No data are available for determining the daily requirement for molybdenum during pregnancy (Kontic-Vucinic O et al, 2006 b).

Manganese

Manganese is necessary for normal carbohydrate, lipid and protein metabolism. In mitochondria, it is an essential component of superoxide dismutase. Manganese is required for the formation of healthy bone and cartilage, as well as for wound healing. In the human placenta, manganese assists in the oxidation of diamines (Nielsen FH, 1999). Increased demands during pregnancy lead to increased blood levels. Environmental factors and personal habbits, such as smoking, may influence blood manganese levels. Because manganese is widely available in food, a deficiency syndrome has not been reported in humans, although negative balance has been observed in some pregnant women.

Selenium

Selenium is an essential micronutrient for the functioning of enzymes known as selenoproteins. These enzymes, the best known of which are antioxidants glutathione peroxidase and superoxide dismutase, are involved in the body's antioxidant defense system and thyroid hormone metabolism. Accordingly, insufficient selenium intake results in decreased activity of glutathione peroxidases, and leads to increased susceptibility to physiological stresses.

It has been found that depletion in plasma selenium occurs during pregnancy. In healthy pregnant women umbilical cord selenium serum concentration increases and maternal-umbilical selenium difference declines, according to the progression of gestation, probably as a consequence of fetal accretion of selenium (Makhoul IR et al, 2004). Average decrease in selenium concentrations in the third trimester is approximately 30%, reaching the lowest levels just before delivery. Plasma gluthatione peroxidase activities started to decrease after the 20th week of pregnancy, while the same trend was observed in red blood cell gluthatione peroxidase activity after the 30th week of gestation. These results suggest that the requirement for selenium significantly increases in pregnant women with low or even moderate blood selenium concentrations (Rayman MP, 1997).

Selenium apparently plays an important role in human fertility, predominantly female infertility. It appears that selenium deficiency results in significantly higher risk of spontaneous abortions. Selenium is involved in the protection of the embryo from oxidative damage (Kingsley PD et al, 1998), and thought to be one of the factors responsible for neural tube defect (Cengiz B et al, 2004). The potential role of selenium deficiency in abnormal placentation was also investigated (Rayman MP et al, 2003). Selenium deficiency has been implicated in accelerated disease progression and poorer survival among HIV pregnancies (Kupka R et al, 2004).

Diseases in pregnancy can further deteriorate selenium status. There is evidence of significant inverse association of selenium serum levels with preeclampsia and gestational diabetes (Bo S et al, 2005; Rayman MP et al, 2003), while selenium excess could be associated with pathologic pregnancies, including preeclampsia (Mahomed K et al, 2000a).

Preterm infants had significantly lower serum selenium concentrations than full term infants and serum selenium concentrations in malformed infants tend to be lower than those in normal infants. Selenium deficiency may have adverse effects on premature infants (Makhoul IR et al, 2004). Low selenium levels in blood of women at preterm delivery were also related to retinopathy of prematurity and respiratory distress syndrome in preterm infants (Dobrzynski W et al, 1998).

It is important to stress that selenium requirement during lactation is increased and selenium content and gluthatione peroxidase activity of human milk are directly influenced by maternal selenium supply.

MULTIVITAMINS

There is important evidence about the role of selected nutrient interactions and multivitamin-mineral supplements in improving pregnancy outcomes (Ramakrishnan U et al, 1999). Maternal micronutrient deficiences may contribute to different adverse pregnancy outcomes. Apart from the fact that iron and folate supplementation to pregnant women are routine practice, the prenatal dietary intake of other micronutrients is frequently considered to be insufficient to meet increased requirements during pregnancy (Allen LH, 2005). This is especially thrue for developing countries, where multivitamin supplementation was found to increase birthweight (Osrin D et al, 2005). Multivitamins may led to better birth outcomes in at least two ways: possible reduction of the risk of intrauterine infections by improving maternal nutritional status and immunity during pregnancy; and increase of hemoglobin levels, and consequently decrease of adverse pregnancy outcome. Having in mind these benefits and the low cost of the supplements, the use of multivitamins should be encouraged for all pregnant women in developing countries (Fawzi WW et al, 2007). Even authors from developed countries suggest that multivitamin use before and during pregnancy can diminish diet-related deficiencies of certain micronutrients and potentially prevent preterm birth (Vahratian A et al, 2004).

Most of the randomized trials regarding micronutrient supplementation in pregnancy were conducted in developing countries. The obtained results considering birthweight and other pregnancy outcomes are conflicting. Trials conducted in Nepal (Christian P et al, 2003) and Mexico (Ramakrishnan U et al, 2003) involving pregnant presumably human immunodeficiency virus (HIV) negative women showed no significant effects on pregnancy outcomes. Moreover, the obtained data suggest that micronutrient supplementation may even increase the risk of perinatal death. The possible explanation for the finding is that higher birth weight, at least among short and chronically undernourished South Asian women, could lead to difficulty in labor, probably because of cephalopelvic disproportion, with associated perinatal mortality (Christian P et al, 2005). Others noticed reduced incidence of low birth weight, but no effect on preterm birth (Osrin D et al, 2005).

Unlike the above mentioned studies, which used RDA doses of micronutrients, a study conducted in Tanzania evaluated the use of multiple RDA on comparable population of pregnant women (Fawzi WW et al, 2007). HIV-negative Tanzanian women who received prenatal supplementation with vitamin B complex and vitamins C and E, have a reduced incidence of low birth weight and small-for-gestational-age births, but without significant influence on prematurity or fetal death. Multivitamins also reduced the risk of birth size that was small for gestational age, and resulted in significant although modest improvements in hemoglobin levels and CD4+ cell counts among mothers 6 weeks after delivery. These benefits, including the reduction of the risk for fetal death, were even more significant among HIV-positive women previously evaluated (Fawzi WW et al, 1998; Fawzi WW et al, 2004). Another trial, conducted in Guinea-Bissau, confirmed the beneficial use of supplements containing twice the RDA (Kaestel P et al, 2005). The possible explanation is that RDA for pregnant women may be different in developing countries, given that the RDA is the level recommended for healthy women in North America. This level of supplementation may be inadequate to meet the requirements of pregnant women in many developing countries, because of undernutrition and parasitic infections which additionally compromise pregnancies in these countries.

Multivitamins contain a number of micronutrients that have been hypothetisized to be relevant for preeclampsia prevention (Roberts JM et al, 2003). There is evidence that periconceptional multivitamin use could be important for the course and outcome of pregnancy. Confirmation came from the study completed and published last year (Bodnar LM et al, 2006). It was observed that regular use of multivitamins in the periconceptional period was associated with a 45% reduction in preeclampsia risk. Protective effect of multivitamins may be limited to women who enter pregnancy with a body index of less than 25. Among lean women periconceptional multivitamins use makes a significant difference in the indicence of preeclampsia. Unfortunately, multivitamins make no difference for overweight women. Although these findings need to be confirmed by other investigations, they mark a modifiable risk factor for preeclampsia for which there is a relatively inexpensive and safe intervention available. Further investigation is needed to establish which nutrients may be most relevant for the prevention of preeclampsia.

The lack of protective effects of multivitamins on overweight women remains an intriguing finding. Apart from being a well recognized health problem in developed countries, obesity is also a contributory risk factor for several pregnancy-related disorders. Body mass index must be considered as an important modification factor in pregnancy related nutritional studies (Werler MM et al, 1996). This may be related to heightened inflammation, oxidative stress, and endothelial dysfunction characteristic of both preeclampsia and the overweight pregnant state, and alterations in maternal-fetal disposition of some trace elements and antioxidant enzyme status (Ramsay JE et al, 2002; Al-Saleh E et al, 2006). It is possible that typical multivitamins, which contain low nutrient doses, may not be adequate to overcome these disturbances. This issue need to be investigated further.

In developing countries, prepregnancy and pregnancy undernutrition are important predictors of reduced birth weight. In those resource-poor settings, both macronutrients and micronutrients dietary intake may be deficient (Allen LH, 2005). Even in developed countries mothers who gave birth to LBW were reported to have low baseline intake of most of the micronutrients. Compared with iron and folic acid supplementation, the administration of multimicronutrients to undernourished pregnant women may reduce the incidence of low birth weight and early neonatal morbidity (Gupta P et al, 2007). Antenatal micronutrient supplementation may be one of the strategies for increasing birth size (Friis H et al, 2004).

Cochrane database review evaluated micronutrient supplementation during pregnancy and its effects on the pregnancy outcome. Statistically significant reduction in the number of low birthweight and small-for-gestational-age babies and maternal anemia were found with a multiple-micronutrient supplementation, when compared with supplementation with two or less micronutrients or no supplementation or a placebo. But, analyses revealed no added benefit of multiple-micronutrient supplements compared with iron-folic acid supplementation alone. There was also insuffitient evidence to identify adverse affects and to say that excess multiple-micronutrient supplementation during pregnancy is harmful to the mother or the fetus (Haider BA & Bhutta ZA, 2006).

REFERENCES

Akman, I; Arioglu, P; Koroglu, OA; Sakalli, M; Ozek, E; Topuzoglu, A; Eren, S; Bereket, A. Maternal zinc and cord blood zinc, insulin-like growth factor-1, and insulin-like growth factor binding protein-3 levels in small-for-gestational-age newborns. *Clin Exp Obstet Gynecol* 2006;33:239-240.

Allen, LH. Vitamin B-12 metabolism and status during pregnancy, lactation and infancy. In: Allen LH, King J, Lonnerdal B (Eds). *Nutrient regulation during pregnancy, lactation and infant growth.* New York: Plenum Press; 1994; 173-186.

Allen, LH. Biological mechanisms that might underlie iron's effects on fetal growth and preterm birth. *J Nutr* 2001;131: 581S-589S.

Allen, LH. B vitamins: proposed fortification levels for complementary foods for young children. *J Nutr* 2003;133:3000S-3007S.

Allen, LH. Multiple micronutrients in pregnancy and lactation: and overview. *Am J Clin Nutr* 2005;81:1206S-1212S.

Almonte, RA; Heath, DL; Whitehall, J; Russell, MJ; Pathole, S; Vink, R. Gestational magnesium deficiency is deleterious to fetal outcome. *Biol Neonate* 1999;76:26-32.

Al-Saleh, E; Nandakumaran,M; Al-Harmi, J; Sadan, T; Al-Enezi, H. Maternal-fetal status of copper, iron, molybdenum, selenium, and zinc in obese pregnant women in late gestation. *Biol Trace Elem Res* 2006;113:113-123.

Anetor, JI; Adelaja, O; Adekunie, AO. Serum micronutrient levels, nucleic acid metabolism and antioxidant defence in pregnant Nigerians: implications for fetal and maternal health. *Afr J Med Sci* 2003;32:257-262.

Arikan, GM; Panzitt, T; Gucer, F; Scholz, HS; Reinisch, S; Haas, J; Weiss, PA. Course of maternal magnesium levels in low risk gestations and in preterm labor and delivery. *Fetal Diagn Ther* 1999;14:332-336.

Atallah, AN; Hofmeyr, GJ; Duley, L. Calcium supplementation during pregnancy for preventing hypertensive disorders and related problems. *Cochrane Database Syst Rev* 2002;4:CD001059.

Aurousseau, B; Gruffat, D; Durand, D. Gestation linked radical oxigen species fluxes and vitamins and trace mineral deficiencies in the ruminant. *Reprod Nutr Dev* 2006;46:601-620.

Azais-Braesco, V; Pascal, G. Vitamin A in pregnancy: requirements and safety limits. *Am J Clin Nutr* 2000;71:1325S-1333S.

Bailey, LB; Berry, RJ. Folic acid supplementation and the occurrence of congenital heart defects, orofacial clefts, multiple births, and miscarriage. *Am J Clin Nutr* 2005;81:1213S-1217S.

Baker, H; De Angelis, B; Holland, B; Gittens-Williams, L; Barrett, TJr. Vitamin profile of 563 gravidas during trimesters of pregnancy. *J Am Coll Nutr* 2002;21:33-37.

Bakker, SJ; ter Maaten, JC; Gans, RO. Thiamine supplementation to prevent induction of low birth weight by conventional therapy for gestational diabetes mellitus. *Med Hypothese* 2000;55:88-90.

Barker, DJP. *Mothers, Babies and Disease in Later Life*, 2nd ed. London, Harcourt Brace, 1998.

Bates, CJ; Prentice, AM; Paul, AA. Seasonal variations in vitamins A, C, riboflavin and folate intakes and status of pregnant and lactating women in a rural Gambian community: some possible implications. *Eur J Clin Nutr* 1994;48:660-668.

Beard, JL; Hendricks, MK; Perez, EM; Murray-Kolb, LE, Ber, A; Vernon-Feagans, L; Irlam, J; Isaacs, W; Sive, A; Tomlinson, M. Maternal iron deficiency anemia affects postpartum emotions and cognition. *J Nutr* 2005;135: 267-272.

Beazley, D; Ahokas, R; Livingston, J; Griggs, M; Sibai, BM. Vitamin C and E supplementation in women at high risk for preeclampsia: a double-blind, placebo-controlled trial. *Am J Obstet Gynecol* 2005;192:520-521.

Belizan, JM; Villar, J; Repke, J. The relationship between calcium intake and pregnancy-induced hypertension: Up-to-date evidence. *Am J Obstet Gynecol* 1988;158:898-902.

Bjorke-Monsen, AL; Vollset, SE; Refsum, H; Markestad, T; Ueland, PM. Hematological parameters and cobalamin status in infants born to smoking mothers. *Biol Neonate* 2004;85:249-255.

Black, RE. Micronutrients in pregnancy. *Br J Nutr* 2001;85:193S-197S.

Bo, S; Lezo, A; Menato, G; Gallo, ML; Bardelli, C; Signorile, A; Berutti, C; Massobrio, M; Pagano, GF. Gestational hyperglycemia, zinc, selenium, and antioxidant vitamins. *Nutrition* 2005;21:186-191.

Bodnar, LM; Tang, G; Ness, RB; et al. Periconceptional multivitamine use reduces the risk of preeclampsia. *Am J Epidemiol* 2006;164:470-477.

Botto, LD; Lisi, A; Robert-Gnansia, E; et al. International retrospective cohort study of neural tube defects in relation to folic acid recommendations: are the recommendations working? *BMJ* 2005;330:571.

Brion, LP; Bell, EF; Raghuveer, TS. Vitamin E supplementation for prevention of morbidity and mortality in preterm infants (Cochrane Review). The Cochrane Library, Issue 2, 2005.

Bsoul, SA; Terezhalmy, GT. Vitamin C in health and disease. *J Contemp Dent Pract* 2004;5:1-13.

Bucher, HC; Cook, RJ; Guyatt, GH; Lang, JD; Cook, DJ; Hatala, R; Hunt, DL. Effect of calcium supplementation on pregnancy-induced hypertension and preeclampsia: a meta-analysis of randomized controlled trials. *JAMA* 1996;275:1113-1117.

Carroli, G; Duley, L; Belizan, JM; Villar, J. Calcium supplementation during pregnancy: a systematic review of randomised controlled trials. *Br J Obstet Gynaecol* 1994;101:753-758.

Casanueva, E; Avila-Rosas, H; Polo, E; et al. Vitamin C status, cervico-vaginal infection and premature rupture of amniotic membranes. *Arch Med Res* 1995;26:5149-5152.

Casanueva, E; Ripoll, C; Tolentino, M; Morales, RM; Pfeffer, F; Vilchis, P; Vadillo-Ortega, F. Vitamin C supplementation to prevent premature rupture of the chorioamniotic membranes: a randomized trial. *Am J Clin Nutr* 2005;81:859-863.

Cengiz, B; Soylemez, F; Ozturk, E; Cavdar, AO. Serum zinc, selenium, copper and lead levels in women with second-trimester induced abortion resulting from neural tube defects: a preliminary study. *Biol Trace Elem Res* 2004;97:225-235.

Centers for Disease Control and Prevention. Spina bifida and anencephaly before and after folic acid mandate – United States, 1995-1996 and 1999-2000. *Morb Mortal Wkly Rep* 2004;53:362-365.

Chappell, LC; Seed, PT; Briley, AL; Kelly, FJ; Lee, R; Hunt, BJ; Parmar, K; Bewley, SJ; Shennan, AH; Steer, PJ; Poston, L. Effect of antioxidants on occurrence of preeclampsia in women at increased risk: a randomised trial. *Lancet* 1999;354:810-816.

Charles, DHM; Ness, AR; Campbell, D; Davey Smith, G; Whitley, E; Hall, MH. Folic acid supplementations in pregnancy and birthoutcome: re-analysis of a large randomised controlled trial and update of Cochrane review. *Paediatr Perinat Epidemiol* 2005;19:112-124.

Christian, P; West, KPJr; Khatry, SK; Katz, J; Shrestha, SR; Pradhan, EK; LeClerq, SC; Pokhrel, RP. Night blindness of pregnancy in rural Nepal: Nutritional and health risks. *Int J Epidemiol* 1998;27:231-237.

Christian, P; West, KPJr; Khatry, SK; Kimbrough-Pradhan, E; LeClerq, SC; Katz, J; Shrestha, SR; Dali, SM; Sommer, A. Night blindness during pregnancy and subsequent mortality among women in Nepal: Effects of vitamin A and beta-carotene supplementation. *Am J Epidemiol* 2000a; 152:542-547.

Christian, P; West, KP Jr; Khatry, SK; Katz, J; LeClerq, SC; Kimbrough-Pradhan, E; Dali, SM; Shrestha, SR. Vitamin A or beta-carotene supplementation reduces symptoms of illness in pregnant and lactating Nepali women. *Journal of Nutrition* 2000b;130:2675-2682.

Christian, P; Khatry, SK; Katz, J; et al. Effects of alternative maternal micronutrient supplements on low birth weight in rural Nepal: double blind randomised community trial. *BMJ* 2003;326:571.

Christian, P; West, KP Jr; Katz, J; Kimbrough-Pradhan, E; LeClerq, SC; Khatry, SK; Shrestha, SR. Cigarette smoking during pregnancy in rural Nepal. Risk factors and effects of beta-carotene and vitamin A supplementation. *Eur J Clin Nutr* 2004;58:204-211.

Christian, P; Osrin, D; Manandhar, DS; et al. Antenatal micronutrient supplements in Nepal. *Lancet* 2005;366:711-712.

Cogswell, ME; Parvanta, I; Ickes, L; Yip, R; Brittenham, GM. Iron supplementation during pregnancy, anemia, and birth wight: a randomized controlled trial. *Am J Clin Nutr* 2003;78:773-781.

Czeizel, AE; Dudas, I; Metneki, J. Pregnancy outcomes in a randomised controlled trial of periconceptional multivitamin supplementation. *Arch Gynecol Obstet* 1994;255:131-139.

Czeizel AE. Nutritional supplementation and prevention of congenital abnormalities. *Curr Opin Obstet Gynecol* 1995;2:88-94.

Czeizel, AE; Vargha, P. Pericinceptional folic acid/multivitamin supplementation and twin pregnancy. *Am J Obstet Gynecol* 2004;191:790-794.

Daneel-Otterbech, S; Davidsson, L; Hurrell, R. Ascorbic acid supplementation and regular consumption of fresh orange juice increase the ascorbic content of human milk: studies in European and African lactating women. *Am J Clin Nutr* 2005;81:1088-1093.

Das, SC; Mohammed, AZ; Al-Hassan, S; Otokwula, AA; Isichei, UP. Effect of environmental iodine deficiency (EID) on foetal growth in Nigeria. *Indian J Med Res* 2006;124:535-544.

De Wals, P; Tairou, F; Van Allen, MI; Uh, S-H; Lowry, RB; Sibbald, B; Evans, JA; et al. Reduction in neural-tube defects after folic acid fortification in Canada. *N Engl J Med* 2007;357:135-142.

Dekker, GA; de Vries, JIP; Doelitzsch, PM; et al. Underlying disorders associated with severe early-onset preeclampsia. *Am J Obstet Gynecol* 1995;173:1042-1048.

Delange F. Iodine deficiency in Europe. *Thyroid Int* 2002;5:3-18.

Di Gregorio, S; Danilowicz, K; Rubin, Z; Mautalen, C. Osteoporosis with vertebral fractures associated with pregnancy and lactation. *Nutrition* 2000;16:1052-1055.

Dobrzynski, W; Trafikowska, U; Trafikowska, A; Pilecki, A; Szymanski, W; Zachara, BA. Decreased selenium concentration in maternal and cord blood in preterm compared with term delivery. *Analyst* 1998;123:93-97.

Duley, L; Henderson-Smart, D. Reduced salt intake compared to normal dietary salt, or high intake, in pregnancy. Cochrane Database Syst Rev 2002;4:CD001687.

Evans, P; Halliwell, B. Micronutrients: oxidant/antioxidant status. *Br J Nutr* 2001;85:S67-S74.

Fawzi, WW; Msamanga, GI; Spiegelman, D; Urassa, EJ; McGrath, N; Mwakagile, D; Antelman, G; Mbise, R; Herrera, G; Kapiga, S; Willett, W; Hunter, DJ. Randomised trial of effects of vitamin supplements on pregnancy outcomes and T cell counts in HIV-1-infected women in Tanzania. *Lancet* 1998;351:1477-1482.

Fawzi, WW; Msamanga, GI; Spiegelman, D; Wei, R; Kapiga, S; Villamor, E; Mwakagile, D; Mugusi, F; Hertzmark, E; Essex, M; Hunter, DJ. A randomized trial of multivitamin supplements and HIV disease progression and mortality. *N Engl J Med* 2004;351:23-32.

Fawzi, WW; Villamor, E; Msamanga, GI; Antelman, G; Aboud, S; Urassa, W; Hunter, D. Trial of zinc supplements in relation to pregnancy outcomes, hematologic indicators, and T cell counts among HIV-1-infected women in Tanzania. *Am J Clin Nutr* 2005;81:161-167.

Fawzi, WW; Msamanga, GI; Urassa, W; Hertzmark, E; Petraro, P; Willett, WC; Spiegelman, D. Vitamins and perinatal outcomes among HIV-negative women in Tanzania. *N Engl J Med* 2007;356:1423-1431.

Fraser, WD; Audibert, F; Bujold, E; et al. The vitamin E debate: implications for ongoing trials of pre-eclampsia prevention. *BJORG* 2005;112:684-688.

Friis, H; Goma, E; Nyazema, N; et al. Effects of multimicronutrients supplementation on gestational length and birth size: a randomized, placebo-controlled, double-blind effectiveness trial in Zimbabwe. *Am J Clin Nutr* 2004;80:178-184.

Gandley, RE; Tyurin, VA; Huang, W; Arroyo, A; Daftary, A; Harger, G; Jiang, J; Pitt, B; Taylor, RN; Hubel, CA; Kagan, VE. S-nitrosoalbumin-mediated relaxation is enhanced by ascorbate and copper: effects in pregnancy and preeclampsia plasma. *Hypertension* 2005;45:15-17.

Gartner, LM; Greer, FR. Prevention of rickets and vitamin D deficiency: new guidelines for vitamin D intake. *Pediatrics* 2003;111:908-910.

Ghyselinck, NB; Dupe, V; Dierich, A; et al. Role of the retinoic acid receptor beta (RAR beta) during mouse development. *Int J Dev Biol* 1997;41:425-447.

Gillman, MW; Rifas-Shiman, SL; Kleinman, KP; Rich-Edwards, JW; Lipshultz, SE. Maternal calcium intake and offspring blood pressure. *Circulation* 2004;110:1990-1995.

Gillman, MW. Developmental origins of health and disease. *N Engl J Med* 2005;353:1848-1850.

Glinoer, D. The regulation of thyroid function during normal pregnancy: importance of the iodine nutrition status. *Best Pract Res Clin Endocrinol Metab* 2004;18:133-152.

Golub, MS; Hogrefe, CE; Tarantal, AF; Germann, SL; Beard, JL; Georgieff, MK; Calatroni, A; Lozoff, B. Die-induced iron deficiency anemia and pregnancy outcome in rhesus monkeys. *Am J Clin Nutr* 2006;83:647-656.

Gonzales-Reyes, S; Alvarez, L; Diez-Pardo, JA; Tovar, JA. Prenatal vitamin E improves lung and heart hypoplasia in experimental diaphragmatic hernia. *Pediatr Surg Int* 2003;19:331-334.

Groenen, PM; van Rooij, IA; Peer, PG; Gooskens, RH; Zielhuis, GA; Steegers-Theuissen, RP. Marginal maternal vitamin B12 status increases the risk of offspring with spina bifida. *Am J Obstet Gynecol* 2004a ;191:11-17.

Groenen, PM; van Rooij, IA; Peer, PG; Ocke, MC; Zielhuis, GA; Steegers-Theunissen, RP. Low maternal dietary intakes of iron, magnesium, and niacin are associated with spina bifida in the offspring. *J Nutr* 2004b;134:1516-1522.

Gulmezoglu, AM; Hofmeyr, GJ; Oosthuisen, MM. Antioxidants in the treatment of severe preeclampsia: an explanatory randomised trial. *Br J Obstet Gynaecol* 1997;104:689-696.

Gunton, JE; Hams, G; Hitcman, R; McElduff, A. Serum chromium does not predict glucosa tolerance in late pregnancy. *Am J Clin Nutr* 2001;73:99-104.

Gupta, P; Ray, M; Dua, T; Radhakrishnan, G; et al. Multimicronutrient supplementation for undernourished pregnant women and the birth size of their offspring. *Arch Pediatr Adolesc Med* 2007;161:58-64.

Hafeez, A; Mehmood, G; Mazhar, F. Oral zinc supplementation in pregnant women and its effect on birth weight: a randomised colntrolled trial. *Arch Dis Child Fetal Neonatal Ed* 2005;90:F170-171.

Haider, BA; Bhutta, ZA. Multiple-micronutrient supplementation for women during pregnancy. Cochrane Database of Systematic Reviews 2006, Issue 4. Art.No.: CD004905. DOI: 10.1002/14651858.CD004905.pub2.

Hambidge, M. Human zinc deficiency. *J Nutr* 2000;130:1344S-1349S.

Hambridge, KM; Abebe, Y; Gibson, RS; Westcott, JE; Miller, LV; Lei, S; Stoecker, BJ; Arbide, I; Teshome, A; Bailey, KB; Krebs, NF. Zinc absorption during late pregnancy in rural southern Ethiopia. *Am J Clin Nutr* 2006;84:1102-1106.

Hamilton, IMJ; Gilmore, WS; Benzie, IFF; Mulholland, CW. Interactions between vitamin C and E in human subjects. *Br J Nutr* 2000;84:261-267.

Harding, JE. The nutritional basis of the fetal origins of adult disease. *Int J Epidemiol* 2001;30:15-23.

Harvey, LJ; Dainty, JR; Hollands, WJ; Bull, VJ; Hoogewerff, JA; Foxall, RJ; McAnena, L; Strain, JJ; Fairweather-Tait, SJ. Effect of high-dose iron supplements on fractional zinc absorption and status in pregnant women. *Am J Clin Nutr* 2007;85:131-136.

Harville, EW; Schramm, M; Watt-Morse, M; Chantala, K; Anderson, JJ; Hertz-Picciotto. I. Calcium intake during pregnancy among white and African-American pregnant women in the United States. *J Am Coll Nutr* 2004;23:43-50.

Herrmann, W; Hubner, U; Koch, I; Obeid, R; Retzke, U; Geisel, J. Alteration of homocysteine catabolism in pre-eclampsia, HELLP syndrome and placental insufficiency. *Clin Chem Lab Med* 2004;42:1109-1116.

Holick, MF. Vitamin D deficiency. *N Engl J Med* 2007;357:266-281.

Hollis, BW. Circulating 25-hydroxyvitamin D levels indicative of vitamin D sufficiency: implications for establishing a new effective dietary intake recommendation for vitamin D. *J Nutr* 2005;135:317-322.

Hollowell, JG; Staehling, NW; Hannon, WH; et al. Iodine nutrition in the United States. Trends and public health implications: iodine excretion data from National Health and Nutrition Examination Surveys I and III (1971-1974 and 1988-1994). *J Clin Endocrinol Metab* 1998;83:3401-3408.

Holmes, VA; Young, IS; Maresh, MJ; et al. The Diabetes and Pre-eclampsia Intervention Trial. *Int J Gynaecol Obstet* 2004;87:66-71.

Holmes, VA; Walace, JM; Alexander, HD; Gilmor, WS; Bradbury, I; Ward, M; Scott, JM; McFaul, P; McNulty, H. Homocysteine is lower in the third trimester of pregnancy in women with enhanced folate status from continued folic acid supplementation. *Clin Chem* 2005;51:629-634.

Hösli, I; Zanetti-Daellenbach, R; Holzgreve, W; Lapaire, O. Role of omega 3-fatty acids and multivitamins in gestation. *J Perinat Med* 2007;35:S19-S24.

Hubel, CA; Kozlov, AV; Kagan, VE; Evans, RW; et al. Decreased transferrin and increased transferrin saturation in sera of women with preeclampsia: implications for oxidative stress. *Am J Obstet Gynecol* 1996;175:692-700.

Jauniaux, E; Watson, AL; Hempstock, J; et al. Onset of maternal arterial blood flow and placental oxidative stress: a possible factor in human early pregnancy failure. *Am J Pathol* 2000; 157:2111-2122.

Jewell, D; Young, G. Interventions for nausea and vomiting in early pregnancy. *Cochrane Database Syst Rev*. 2003:CD000145.

Kaestel, P; Michaelsen, KF; Aaby, P; Friis, H. Effects of prenatal micronutrient supplements on birth weight and perinatal mortality: a randomised, controlled trial in Guinea-Bissau. *Eur J Clin Nutr* 2005;59:1081-1089.

Kallen, B. Use of folic acid supplementation and risk of dizygotic twining. *Early Hum Dev* 2004;80:143-151.

Kharb, S. Vitamin E and C in preeclampsia. *Eur J Obstet Gynecol Reprod Biol* 2000;93:37-39.

Kingsley, PD; Whitin, JC; Cohen, HJ; Palis, J. Developmental expression of extracellular glutathione peroxidase suggests antioxidant roles in deciduum, visceral yolk sac, and skin. *Mol Reprod Dev* 1998;49:343-355.

Kisters, K; Barenbrock, M; Louwen, F; Hausberg, M; et al. Membrane, intracellular, and plasma magnesium and calcium concentrations in preeclampsia. *Am J Hypertens* 2000;13:765-769.

Koblinsky, MA; Campbell, OMR; Harlow, S. Mother and more: A broader perspective on women's health. In: Koblinsky M, Timyan J, Gay J (Eds). *The health of Women: A Global Perspective*. Westview Press Boulder, CO. 1992:33-62.

Kontic-Vucinic, O; Sulovic, N; Radunovic, N. Micronutrients in women's reproductive Health: I. Vitamins. *Int J Fertil* 2006a; 51: 106-115.

Kontic-Vucinic, O; Sulovic, N; Radunovic, N. Micronutrients in women's reproductive Health: II. Minerals and trace elements. *Int J Fertil* 2006b; 51: 116-124.

Krapels, IP; van Rooij, IA; Ocke, MC; van Cleef, BA; Kuijpers-Jagtman, AM; Steegers-Theunissen, RP. Maternal dietary B vitamin intake, other than the folate, and the association with orofacial cleft in the offspring. *Eur J Nutr* 2004;43:7-14.

Kupka, R; Msamanga, GI; Spiegelman, D; Morris, S; Mugusi, F; Hunter, DJ; Fawzi, WW. Selenium status is associated with accelerated HIV disease progression among HIV-1-infected pregnant women in Tanzania. *J Nutr* 2004;134:2556-2560.

Lao, TT; Tam, KF; Chan, LY. Third trimester iron status and pregnancy outcome in non-anemic women; pregnancy unfavorably affected by maternal iron excess. *Hum Reprod* 2000;15:1843-1848.

Lawlor, DA; Davey Smith, G; Ebrahim, S. Birth weight of offspring and insulin resistance in late adulthood: cross sectional survey. *BMJ* 2002;325:359.

Leeda, M; Riyazi, N; de Vries, JIP; Jakobs, C; van Geijn, HP; Dekker, GA. Effects of folic acid and vitamin B_6 supplementation on women with hyperhomocysteinemia and a history of preeclampsia or fetal growth restriction. *Am J Obstet Gynecol* 1998;79:135-139.

Levine, RJ; Hauth, JC; Curet, LB; Sibai, BM; Catalano, PM; Morris, CD; DerSimonian, R; Esterlitz, JR; Raymond, EG; Bild, DE; Clemens, JD; Cutler, JA. Trial of calcium to prevent preeclampsia. *N Engl J Med* 1997;337:69-76.

Liu, PM; Fang, PC; Huang, CB; Kou, HK; Chung, MY; Yang, YH; Chung, CH. Risk factors of retinopathy of prematurity in premature infants weighing less than 1600gr. *Am J Perinatol* 2005;22:115-120.

Mahomed, K; Williams, MA; Woelk, GB; et al. Leukocyte selenium, zinc, and copper concentration in preeclamptic and normotensive pregnant women. *Biol Trace Elem Res* 2000a ;75:107-118.

Mahomed, K. Follate supplementation in pregnancy. Cochrane Database Syst Rev 2000b;2:CD000183

Mahomed, K. Zinc supplementation during pregnancy. *Cochrane Database Syst Rev* 2000c;2:CD000230.

Makhoul, IR; Sammour, RN; Diamond, E; Shohat, I; Tamir, A; Shamir, R. Selenium concentrations in maternal and umbilical cord blood at 24-42 weeks of gestation: basis for optimization of selenium supplementation to premature infants. *Clin Nutr* 2004;23:373-381.

Makrides, M; Crowther, MA. Magnesium supplementation in pregnancy. *Cochrane Database Syst Rev* 2000;2:CD000937.

Malinow, MR; Rajkovic, A; Duell, PB; Hess, DL; Upson, BM. The relationship between maternal and neonatal umbilical cord plasma homocyst(e)ine suggests a potential role for maternal homocyst(e)ine in fetal metabolism. *Am J Obstet Gynecol* 1998;178:228-233.

McKay, JA; Williams, EA; Mathers, JC. Folate and DNA methylation during in utero development and aging. *Bioch Soc Trans* 2004;32:1006-1007.

Merialdi, M; Caulfield, LE; Zavaleta, N; Figueroa, A; Costigan, KA; Dominici, F; Dipietro, JA. Randomized controlled trial of prenatal zinc supplementation and fetal bone growth. *Am J Clin Nutr* 2004a;79:826-830.

Merialdi, M; Caulfield, LE; Zavaleta, N; Figueroa, A; Dominici, F; Dipietro, JA. Randomized controlled trial of prenatal zinc supplementation and the development of fetal heart rate. *Am J Obstet Gynecol* 2004b;190:1106-1112.

Mikhail, MS; Anyaegbunam, A; Garfinkel, D; Palan,PR; Basu, J; Romney, SL. Preeclampsia and antioxidant nutrients: decreased plasma levels of reduced ascorbic acid, alpha-tocopherol, and beta-carotene in women with preeclampsia. *Am J Obstet Gynecol* 1994;171:150-157.

Mock, DM; Quirk, JG; Mock, NI. Marginal biotin deficiency during normal pregnancy. *Am J Clin Nutr* 2002;75:295-299.

Morley, R; Carlin, JB; Dwyer, T. Maternal calcium supplementation and cardiovascular risk factors in twin offspring. *Int J Epidemiol* 2004;33:1309-1310.

Morreale de Escobar, G; Obregon, MJ; Escobar del Rey, F. Role of thyroid hormone during early brain development. *Eur J Endocrinol* 2004;151:25-37.

Nielsen, FH. Ultratrace minerals. In: Shils M, Olson JA, Shike M, Ross AC (Eds*). Nutrition in Health and Disease.* 9th ed. Baltimore: Williams & Wilkins; 1999: 283-303.

Northrop-Clewes, CA; Thurnham, DI. Monitoring micronutrients in cigarette smokers. *Clin Chim Acta* 2007;377:14-38.

Norwitz, ER; Robinson, JN; Repke, JT. Prevention of preeclampsia: is it possible? *Clin Obstet Gynecol* 1999;42:436-454.

Ohara, N; Tsujino, T; Maruo, T. The role of thyroid hormone in trophoblast function, early pregnancy maintenance, and fetal neurodevelopment. *J Obstet Gynaecol Can* 2004;26:982-990.

Oliver, MH; Jaquiery, AL; Bloomfield, FH; Harding, JE. The effects of maternal nutrition around the time of conception on the health of the offspring. *Soc Reprod Fertil Suppl* 2007;64:397-410.

Osendarp, SJ; van Raaij, JM; Arifeen, SE; Wahed, M; Baqui, AH; Fuchs, GJ. A randomized, placebo-controlled trial of the effect of zinc supplementation during pregnancy on pregnancy outcome in Bangladeshi urban poor. *Am J Clin Nutr* 2000;71:114-119.

Osrin, D; de L.Costello, AM. Maternal nutrition and fetal growth: practical issues in international health. *Semin Neonatol* 2000;5:209-219.

Osrin, D; Vaidya, A; Shrestha, Y; et al. Effects of antenatal multiple micronutrient supplementation on birthweight and gestational duration in Nepal: double-blind, randomised controlled trial. *Lancet* 2005;365:955-962.

Pathak, P; Kapil, U. Role of trace elements zinc, copper and magnesium during pregnancy and its outcome. *Indian J Pediatr* 2004;71:1003-1005.

Pena-Rosas, JP; Viteri, FE. Effects of routine oral iron supplementation with or without folic acid for women during pregnancy. *Cochrane Database Syst Rev* 2006;3: CD004736.

Plessinger, MA; Woods, JR; Miller, RK. Pretreatment of human chorioamnion with vitamins C and E prevents hypochlorous acid-induced damage. *Am J Obstet Gynecol* 2000;183:979-985.

Polyzos, NP; Mauri, D; Tsappi, M; Tzioras, S; Kamposioras, K; Cortinovis, I; Casazza, G. Combined vitamin C and E supplementtaion during pregnancy for preeclampsia prevention: a systematic review. *Obstet Gynecol Surv* 2007;62: 202-206.

Poston, L; Raijmakers, M; Kelly, F. Vitamin E in preeclampsia. *Ann N Y Acad Sci* 2004;1031:242-248.

Poston, L; Briley, AL; Seed, PT; Kelly, FJ; Shennan, AH. Vitamins in Pre-eclampsia (VIP) Trial Consortium. Vitamin C and vitamin E in pregnant women at risk for pre-eclampsia (VIP trial): randomised placebo-controlled trial. *Lancet* 2006;367:1145-1154.

Pressman, EK; Cavanaugh, JI; Mingione, M; Norkus, EP; Woods, JR. Effects of maternal antioxidant supplementation on maternal and fetal antioxidant levels: A randomized, double-blind study. *Am J Obstet Gynecol* 2003;189:1720-1725.

Proskocil, BJ; Sekhon, HS; Clark, JA; Lupo, SL; Jia, Y; Hull, WM; Whitsett, JA; Starcher, BC; Spindel, ER. Vitamin C prevents the effects of prenatal nicotine on pulmonary function in newborn monkey. *Am J Respir Crit Care Med* 2005;171:1032-1039.

Ramakrishnan, U; Manjrekar, R; Rivera, J; Gonzales-Cassio, T; Martorell, R. Micronutrients and pregnancy outcome: A review of the literature. *Nutr Res* 1999;19:103-159.

Ramakrishnan, U; Gonzales-Cossio, T; Neufeld, LM; et al. Multiple micronutrient supplementation during pregnancy does not lead to greater infant birth size than does iron-only supplementation: a randomized controlled trial in a semirural community in Mexico. *Am J Clin Nutr* 2003;77:720-725.

Ramakrishnan, U. Nutrition and low bitrh weight: from research to practice. *Am J Clin Nutr* 2004;79:17-21.

Ramsay, JE; Ferrell, WR; Crawford, L; et al. Maternal obesity is associated with dysregulation of metabolic, vascular, and inflammatory pathways. *J Clin Endocrinol Metab* 2002;87:4231-4237.

Rayman, MP. Dietary selenium: time to act. *BMJ* 1997;314:387-388.

Rayman, MP; Bode, P; Redman, CW. Low selenium status is associated with the occurrence of the pregnancy disease preeclampsia in women from United Kingdom. *Am J Obstet Gynecol* 2003;189:1343-1349.

Ritchie, LD; King, JC. Dietary calcium and pregnancy-induced hypertension: is there a relation? *Am J Clin Nutr* 2000;71:1371S.

Roberts, JM; Redman, CWG. Pre-eclampsia: more than pregnancy-induced hypertension. *Lancet* 1993;341:1447-1451.

Roberts, JM; Hubel, CA. Is oxidative stress the link in the two-stage model of pre-eclampsia? *Lancet* 1999;354:788-789.

Roberts, JM; Balk, JL; Bodnar, LM; Belizan, JM; et al. Nutrient involvement in preeclampsia. *J Nutr* 2003;133:1684S-1692S.

Roberts, JM. National Institute of Child Health and Human Development, Maternal Fetal Medicine Units Network. Combined Antioxidant and Preeclampsia Prediction Studies (CAPPS). (Accessed March 31, 2006, at *http://www.clinicaltrials.gov/ct/show/NCT00135707?order=7.*)

Rodrigo, R; Parra, M; Bosco, C; Fernandez, V; Barja, P; Guajardo, J; Messina, R. Pathophysiological basis for the prophylaxis of preeclampsia through early supplementation with antioxidant vitamins. *Pharmacol Ther* 2005;107:177-197.

Rumbold, A; Crowther, CA. Vitamin C supplementation during pregnancy. *Cochrane Database Syst Rev* 2005a;2:CD004072.

Rumbold, AR; Maats, FH; Crowther, CA. Dietary intake of vitamine C and vitamine E and the development of hypertensive disorders of pregnancy. *Eur J Obstet Gynecol Reprod Biol* 2005b;119:67-71.

Rumbold, A; Crowther, CA. Vitamin E supplementation in pregnancy. *Cochrane Database Syst Rev* 2005c;2:CD004069.

Rumbold, A; Duley, L; Crowther, C; Haslam, R. Antioxidants for preventing pre-eclampsia. *Cochrane Database Syst Rev* 2005d;4:CD004227.

Rumbold, AR; Crowther, CA; Haslam, RR; Dekker, GA; Robinson, JS. Vitamins C and E and the risks of preeclampsia and perinatal complications. *N Engl J Med* 2006;354:1796-1806.

Rumiris, D; Purwosunu, Y; Wibowo, N; et al. Lower rate of preeclampsia after antioxidant supplementation in pregnant women with low antioxidant status. *Hypertens Pregnancy* 2006;25:241-253.

Ruz, M. Zinc supplementation and growth. *Curr Opin Clin Nutr Metab Care* 2006;9:757-762.

Sanchez-Vera, I; Bonet, B; Viana, M; Sanz, C. Relationship between alpha-tocopherol content in the different lipoprotein fractions in term pregnant women and in umbilical cord blood. *Ann Nutr Metab* 2004;48:146-150.

Saugstad, OD. Update on oxygen radical disease in neonatology. *Curr Opin Obstet Gynecol* 2001;13:147-153.

Saunders, C; do Carmo Leal, M; Gomes, MM; Campos, LF; dos Santos Silva, BA; Thiapo de Lima, AP; Ramalho, RA. Gestational nightblindness among women attending a public maternity hospital in Rio de Janeiro, Brazil. *J Health Popul Nutr* 2004;22:348-356.

Scholl, TO; Hediger, ML; Schall, JI; Khoo, CS; Fischer, RL. Dietary and serum folate: their influence on the outcome of pregnancy. *Am J Clin Nutr* 1996;63:520-525.

Scholl, TO; Johnson, WG. Folic acid: influence on the outcome of pregnancy. *Am J Clin Nutr* 2000;71:1295S-1303S.

Scholl, TO. Iron status during pregnancy: setting the stage for mother and infant. *Am J Clin Nutr* 2005;81:1218S-1222S.

Scholl, TO; Chen, X; Sims, M; Stein, TP. Vitamin E: maternal concentrations are associated with fetal growth. *Am J Clin Nutr* 2006;84:1442-1448.

Semba, RD. Overview of the potential role of vitamin A in mother-to-children transmission of HIV-1. *Acta Paediatr* 1997;421:107-112.

Seydoux, J; Girardin, E; Paunier, L; Beguin, F. Serum and intracellular magnesium during normal pregnancy and in patients with pre-eclampsia. *Br J Obstet Gynaecol* 1992;99:207-211.

Shah, D; Sachdev, HP. Zinc deficiency in pregnancy and fetal outcome. *Nutr Rev* 2006;64:15-30.

Shenkin, A. Micronutrients in health and disease. *Postgrad Med J* 2006;82:559-567.

Sibai, BM; Villar, MA; Bray, EAm. Magnesium supplementation during pregnancy: a double blind randomized controlled clinical trial. *J Obstet Gynecol* 1989;161:115-119.

Siega-Riz, AM; Promislow, JH; Savitz, DA; Thorp, JMJr; McDonald, T. Vitamin C intake and the risk of preterm delivery. *Am J Obstet Gynecol* 2003;189: 519-525.

Siega-Riz, AM; Savitz, DA; Zeisel, SH; Thorp, JM; Herring, A. Second trimester folate status and preterm birth. *Am J Obstet Gynecol* 2004;191:1851-1857.

Smith, GC; Pell, JP; Walsh, D. Pregnancy complications and maternal risk of ischaemic heart disease: a retrospective cohort study of 129,290 births. *Lancet* 2001;357:2002-2006.

Song, WO; Wyse, BW; Hansen, RG. Pantothenic acid status of pregnant and lactating women. *J Am Diet Assoc* 1985;85:192-198.

Spears, K; Cheney, C; Zerzan, J. Low plasma retinol concentrations increase the risk of developing broncopulmonary dysplasia and long-term respiratory disability in very-low-birth-weight infants. *Am J Clin Nutr* 2004;80:1589-1594.

Specker, B. Vitamin D requirements during pregnancy. *Am J Clin Nutr* 2004;80:1740S-1747S.

Spinnato, JA. Antioxidant therapy to prevent preeclampsia. (Accessed March 31, 2006, at http://www.clinicaltrials.gov/ct/show/NCT00097110?order=9.)

Staff, AC; Halvorsen, B; Ranheim, T; et al. Elevated level of free 8-iso-prostaglandin F2alpha in the decidua basalis of women with preeclampsia. *Am J Obstet Gynecol* 1999;181:1211-1215.

Stephens, D; Jackson, PL; Gutierrez, Y. Subclinical vitamin A Deficiency: a potential unrecognized problem in the United States. *Pediatr Nurs* 1996;22:377-389.

Stuart, EL; Evans, GS; Lin, YS; Powers, HJ. Reduced collagen and ascorbic acid concentrations and increased proteolytic susceptibility with prelabor fetal membrane rupture in women. *Biol Reprod* 2005;72:230-235.

Thorp, JA; Gaston, L; Caspers, DR; Pal, ML. Current concepts and controversies in the use of vitamin K. *Drugs* 1995;49:376-387.

Traber, MG. Vitamin E. In: Shils M, Olson JA, Shike M, Ross AC (Eds). *Nutrition in Health and Disease*. 9th ed. Baltimore: Williams&Wilkins; 1999;347-362.

United Nations Children's Fund and World Health Organization. Low birth weight: country, regional and global estimates. New York, NY: UNICEF;2004.

Vahratian, A; Siega-Riz, AM; Savitz, DA; Thorp, JM. Multivitamin use and the risk of preterm birth. *Am J Epidemiol* 2004;160:886-892.

van Rooij, IA; Swinkels, DW; Blom, HJ; Merkus, HM; Steegers-Theunissen, RP. Vitamin and homocystein status of mothers and infants and the risk of nonsyndromic orofacial clefts. *Am J Obstet Gynecol* 2003;189:1155-1160.

Vermiglio, F; Lo Presti, VP; Moleti, M; Sidoti, M; Tortorella, G; Scaffidi, G; Castagna, MG; Mattina, F; Violi, MA; Crisa, A; Artemisia, A; Trimarchi, F. Attention deficit and hyperactivity disorders in the offspring of mothers exposed to mild-moderate iodine deficiency: a possible novel iodine deficiency disorder in developed countries. *J Clin Endocrinol Metab* 2004;89:6054-6060.

von Mandach, U; Huch, R; Huch, A. Maternal and cord serum vitamin E levels in normal and abnormal pregnancy. *Int J Vit Nutr Res* 1994;64:26-32.

Wacker, J; Fruhauf, J; Schulz, M; Chiwora, FM; Volz, J; Becker, K. Riboflavin deficiency and preeclampsia. *Obstet Gynecol* 2000;96:38-44.

Wedner, SH; Ross, DA; Congdon, N; Balira, R; Spitzer, V; Foster, A. Validation of night blidness reports among children and women in a vitamin A deficient population in rural Tanzania. *Eur J Clin Nutr* 2004;58:409-419.

Weiss, R; Fogelman, Y; Bennett, M. Severe vitamin B12 deficiency in an infant associated with a maternal deficiency and a strict vegetarian diet. *J Pediatr Hematol Oncol* 2004;26:270-271.

Werler, MM; Lammer, EJ; Rosenberg, L; Mitchell, AA. Maternal vitamin A supplementation in relation to selected bitrh defects. *Teratology* 1990;42:497-503.

Werler, MM; Louik, C; Shapiro, S; et al. Prepregnant weight in relation to risk of neural tube defects. *JAMA* 1996;275:1089-1092.

West, KPJr; Katz, J; Khatry, SK; LeClerq, SC; Pradhan, EK; Shrestha, SR; Connor, PB; Dali, SM; Christian, P; Pokhrel, RP; Sommer, A; on behalf of the NNIPS-2 Study Group. Double blind, cluster randomized trial of low dose supplementation with vitamin A or beta-carotene on mortality related to pregnancy in Nepal. *Br Med J* 1999;318:570-575.

WHO. Make every mother and child count. World Health Report, 2005. Geneva: World Health Organization, 2005.

Wilcox, AJ; Lie, RT; Solvoll, K; Taylor, J; McConnaughey, DR; Byholm, F; Vindenes, H; Vollset, SE; Drevon, CA. Folic acid supplements and risk of facial cleft: national population based case-control study. *BMJ* 2007;334:464-469.

Woods, JRJr; Plessinger, MA; Miller, RK. Vitamins C and E: missing links in preventing preterm premature rupture of membranes? *Am J Obstet Gynecol* 2001; 185: 5-10.

World Health Organization. Revised 1990 Estimates of Maternal Mortality: A New Approach of by WHO and UNICEF. 1996. Geneva: WHO Publications.

Zeni, SN; Ortela Soler, CR; Lazzari, A; Lopez, L; Suarez, M; Di Gregorio, S; Somoza, JI; de Portela, ML. Interrelationship between bone turnover markers and dietary calcium intake in pregnant women: a longitidunal study. *Bone* 2003;33:606-613.

Zetterberg, H. Methylenetetrahydrofolate reductase and trascobalamin genetic polymorphisms in human spontaneous abortion: biological and clinical implications. *Reprod Biol Endocrinol* 2004;2:7.

Ziaei, S; Norrozi, M; Faghihzadeh, S; Jafarbegloo, E. A randomised placebo-controlled trial to determine the effect of iron supplementation on pregnancy outcome in pregnant women with haemoglobin > or = 13.2 g/dl. *BJOG* 2007;114:684-688.

Zimmermann, M; Delange, F. Iodine supplementation of pregnant women in Europe: a review and recommendation. *Eur J Clin Nutr* 2003;58:979-984.

In: Micronutrients and Health Research
Editor: Takumi Yoshida, pp. 147-179

ISBN: 978-1-60456-056-5
© 2008 Nova Science Publishers, Inc.

Chapter IV

MICRONUTRIENTS THAT DECREASE ENDOGENOUS TOXINS, A STRATEGY FOR DISEASE PREVENTION

Flore Depeint, W. Robert Bruce, Owen Lee,
Rhea Mehta and Peter J. O'Brien

Faculty of Pharmacy and Dept. of Nutritional Sciences, Faculty of Medicine,
University of Toronto, Toronto, Ontario, M5S 3M2 Canada.

ABSTRACT

A number of health disorders may find their cause in the formation, accumulation and damaging effect of endogenous toxins. The disorders appear to include the metabolic syndrome, diabetes, hypertension, cardiovascular disease, Alzheimer's disease, colorectal and possibly other epithelial cancers. The identification of the endogenous toxins and the development of preventive strategies is difficult, however, as the toxins cannot be readily isolated and identified. To surmount this problem we have developed cell systems that model *in vivo* tissue cytotoxicity associated with known endogenous toxins and tested the relative ability of micronutrients to mitigate their cytotoxic effects. The toxins evaluated were: 1) Oxidative stress, i.e. superoxide, hydrogen peroxide, hypochlorite and nitric oxide, that can result for example from inflammatory processes such as bacterial infection and from hypoxia:reoxygenation injury of endothelial and astrocyte cells; 2) Carbonyls from the autoxidation or metabolism of unsaturated fatty acids or phospholipids to form advanced lipid endproducts (ALE); 3) Dicarbonyls from the autoxidation or metabolism of glucose/ fructose to form advanced glycation endproducts; and 4) Fatty acids from fat and/or carbohydrate overload that can result in the metabolic syndrome and related disease processes. In studies of combined endogenous toxins we observed a marked synergism in the cytotoxicity of oxidative stress (H_2O_2) and exposure to carbonyls (associated with fructose) and increased cytotoxicity of fatty acids (polyunsaturated fatty acids). The micronutrients, evaluated and ranked for their ability to prevent cytotoxicity *in vitro*, included vitamins, minerals and plant-derived antioxidants and scavengers of reactive oxygen species (ROS). The results demonstrate marked differences in the ranking of the micronutrients with the different endogenous toxins. They thus suggest that mitigation studies with micronutrients could provide an assessment of the association of endogenous toxins with disease and a systematic strategy for testing the role of micronutrients on oxidative stress and disease prevention.

1. ENDOGENOUS TOXINS IN CHRONIC HEALTH DISORDERS

Many of the health disorders that afflict populations of the developed world are thought to be a consequence of environmental exposure- that is, to non-genetic factors including diet, the physical environment, social and lifestyle factors. The importance of such factors is evident both in the markedly higher rates for many chronic diseases in developed countries, and in the marked increase of these diseases in populations during periods of rapidly increasing economic development. For example, colon cancer mortality in Japan was long considered amongst the lowest in the world (Segi et al. 1966) but this rate increased markedly from the 1960s to the 1990s, almost ten-fold for Japanese males (Parkin et al. 2005). Death rates from ischemic heart disease and cerebral infarction were also low in the 1960s and increased to a similar degree through this period (Kida et al. 1999). Presumably, changes in environmental exposures associated with economical development increased the outcome of health disorders through an increase in exposure to chemical or biochemical toxins associated with the environment. In principle it would seem to be feasible to identify the toxins, to reduce their concentration, and to prevent the disorders.

Exogenous toxins, such as the genotoxic polycyclic hydrocarbons and arylamines formed in food preparation, could account for some of the environmental risk. Endogenous toxins, however, could be more important. Epidemiological evidence suggests that risk for many of the chronic diseases is associated with more general dietary factors, such as increased caloric intake, reduced exercise, and the consumption of refined foods. These apparently non-specific dietary factors can have many effects. Refining of carbohydrates and fats, for instance, can reduce the concentrations of specific micronutrients, reducing thiamin and choline to marginal or deficient concentrations (World Cancer Research Fund and American Institute for Cancer Research 1997). Refining, increased caloric intake and reduced exercise can also have significant effects on energy metabolism, exposing the liver, muscle, fat and other tissues to high levels of energy substrates. Red meat, iron and cooked foods can increase oxidative stress and ROS. Thus there would appear to be many conditions which could result in the formation of endogenous toxins, cyto- and genotoxicity and chronic disease.

In 2000 the U.S. Institute of Medicine cautioned, however, that a relation between reactive species and chronic disease was far from established. "... *Although vitamin C, vitamin E and selenium have been shown to decrease the concentrations of some of the biomarkers associated with oxidative stress, the relationship between such observations and chronic disease remain to be elucidated. ...*" (Institute of Medicine 2000). Several more recent developments have suggested ways by which the relationship between environment and disease could be better elucidated. 1) The results of large cohort studies with diverse populations such as those of the EPIC program have now become available (Riboli et al. 2002). They provide blood samples collected prior to the appearance of symptoms of disease. Assessment of risk markers through the disease process similarly permit a clarification of disease development. 2) Data relating to genetic polymorphisms have also become available. These have demonstrated clear associations of risk with metabolic pathways in many cases, challenging the investigators to establish the details of the mechanisms involved. 3) Epidemiological studies have demonstrated a remarkable similarity in the risk factors for type 2 diabetes (T2D) and the metabolic syndrome (MetS, a cluster of risk factors characterized by insulin resistance and predictive of T2D) with cardiovascular disease, non-alcoholic steatohepatitis and some cancers (McKeown-Eyssen 1994; Giovannucci 2003; Jenab et al. 2007). The associations have been attributed to the proliferative effect of elevated concentrations of insulin as in insulin resistance (Tran et al. 2006; Giovannucci and Michaud 2007) or elevated concentrations of glucose as in T2D. They could perhaps be more readily explained as a consequence of a common exposure to endogenous toxins. 4) Biomarkers of oxidative stress have been shown to be decreased by many factors in addition to vitamin C, vitamin E and selenium. For instance, calcium can decrease oxidative stress through its effect on the solubility and absorption of iron (Pierre et al. 2003). Lipoic acid and CoQ can restore levels of vitamin E (Paker et al. 1997), whilst uric acid can conserve vitamin C (Ames et al. 1981).

The results of the recent studies cited in Table 1 suggest that many chronic health disorders may be associated with endogenous toxins. The metabolic syndrome (MetS) (considered here with type 2 diabetes (T2D)), cardiovascular disease, non-alcoholic steatohepatitis (NASH) and cancers (including colorectal cancer) may be associated with reactive oxygen species (ROS), dicarbonyls and excess intracellular free fatty acids (FFAs). Similarly neurodegenerative diseases such as Alzheimer's may be associated with increased catecholamine-derived aldehydes whilst Sjogren-Larsson syndrome and other metabolic syndromes could be associated with increased aldehydes (Jansen et al. 2001; Vangala and Tonelli 2007).

It is well known that diets deficient in thiamin can result in exposure to endogenous toxins (the dicarbonyls, methylglyoxal and deoxyglucosone) and to the Wernike-Korsakoff syndrome and beriberi. It seems reasonable to suppose that diets in developed countries, with their high levels of fat, refined carbohydrates, meat, and cooked foods, could result in exposure to endogenous toxins and, in the absence of specific micronutrients to many of the health disorders afflicing populations of the developed world. What endogenous toxins are formed with our diet? What micronutrients could mitigate their toxicity? What dietary changes are necessary to reduce endogenous toxins and the development of disease?

2. THE FORMATION OF ENDOGENOUS TOXINS

The studies cited above suggest that consideration should be given first to the formation of the endogenous toxins - of endogenous ROS, carbonyls, dicarbonyls, and excess intracelluar free fatty acids (FFAs).

Table 1. Endogenous Toxins Associated with Chronic Health Disorders

Health disorder	Endogenous toxin	Recent examples of evidence	Reference
Metabolic syndrome (MetS) and Type 2 Diabetes (T2D)	ROS as H_2O_2	Excess iron as ferritin in patients subsequentaly developing T2D.	(Forouhi et al. 2007)
	ROS	Excess iron as non-transferrin iron in patients with newly diagnosed T2D.	(Lee et al. 2006)
	ROS	Deficiency of Mg, excess malondialdehyde in patients developing MetS.	(Guerrero-Romero and Rodriguez-Moran 2006)
	ROS or Dicarbonyls	N-acetyl cysteine, taurine, resveratrol prevent insulin resistance in the rat.	(Haber et al. 2003; Baur et al. 2006)
	Dicarbonyls	Methylglyoxal adduct concentration elevated in T2D.	(Kilhovd et al. 2003)
	Dicarbonyls	AGE formation is increased by GLOX1 or aldose reductase inhibitors or GSH depletion in T2D complications.	(Thornalley 1994; Thornalley 2003; Vander Jagt and Hunsaker 2003)
	Mitochondrial FFAs	Increased O_2^- in T2D complications.	(Brownlee 2001)
	Mitochondrial FFAs	Defective UPC2 polymorhisms associated with insulin resistance, T2D.	(D'Adamo et al. 2004; Wang et al. 2004)
Cardiovascular disease (CVD) and Coronary heart disease (CHD)	As above (MetS)	CVD risk clearly associated with risk of MetS.	(Galassi et al. 2006; Wang et al. 2007)
	ROS	Plasma markers of oxidative stress associated with CHD in T2D.	(Stephens et al. 2006)
	Dicarbonyls	Serum pentosidine associated with CHD and heart failure.	(Koyama et al. 2007)
	Dicarbonyls	Endothelial cells in vivo sensitive to glucose, protected by thiamin.	(Beltramo et al. 2004)
	Mitochondrial FFAs	Defective UPC2 polymorphisms associated with oxidative stress, CHD.	(Dhamrait et al. 2004)
Non alcoholic steatohepatitis (NASH)	As above (MetS)	NASH risk clearly associated with risk of MetS.	(Neuschwander-Tetri 2005)
	ROS	Iron overload in choline deficient rat increases liver inflammation and necrosis.	(Kirsch et al. 2006)
	Mitochondrial FFAs	Diet-induced NASH in rat results in mitochondrial dysfunction.	(Begriche et al. 2006)
Cancer	As above (MetS)	Colon cancer risk associated with risk of MetS.	(McKeown-Eyssen 1994; Giovannucci 2003)
	ROS	NAD(P)H:quinone oxidoreductase 1 polymorphism associated with colon cancer.	(Begleiter et al. 2006)

Table 1. Continued

Health disorder	Endogenous toxin	Recent examples of evidence	Reference
Cancer	ROS	Increased intake of heme iron in subjects subsequently developing colon cancer.	(Lee et al. 2004; Larsson et al. 2005)
	ROS	Polymorphisms in oxidative stress pathway associated with non-Hodgkins lymphoma.	(Lan et al. 2007)
	ROS	Polymorphisms in MnSOD and myeloid leukemia.	(Vineis et al. 2007)
	ROS	Polymorphisms in NQO1 and lung cancer.	(Vineis et al. 2007)
	ROS	Choline deficiency in the rat increase ROS with liver carcinogenesis.	(Floyd et al. 2002)
	ROS	Heme iron in rat increases oxidative stress, colon cancer promotion.	(Sesink et al. 2001; Pierre et al. 2003)
	Dicarbonyls	Thiamin deficiency in rat induces formation of putative colon cancer precursor.	(Bruce et al. 2003)
Schizophrenia	ROS	Glutamate cysteine ligase modifier gene defect associated with disease.	(Tosic et al. 2006)
	Mitochondria FFAs	Defective UCP2 and 4 associated with disease.	(Yasuno et al. 2007)
	Mitochondia function	Altered mitochondrial gene expression in disease.	(Iwamoto et al. 2005)
Alzheimer's disease	Dicarbonyls	Co-localization of areas of ferritin, cell death in rat brain with thiamin deficiency.	(Calingasan et al. 1998; Karuppagounder et al. 2007)
	Catecholamine-derived aldehydes	Reduced activity of aldehyde dehydrogenase (ALDH) results in increased neurotoxic aldehydes.	(Marchitti et al. 2007)
Multiple sclerosis	Dicarbonyls	Polymorphisms of glyoxylase 1 A111E, paraoxonase 1 Q192R associated with disease.	(Sidoti et al. 2007)
Sjogren-Larsson Syndrome	Catecholamine-derived aldehydes	Reduced activity od ALDH results in increased neurotoxic aldehydes. Many inborn errors of metabolism may result in the formation of endogenous toxins.	(Marchitti et al. 2007)

2.1. Endogenous Reactive Oxygen Species

2.1.1. Nox Family of NADPH Oxidases

Superoxide radicals are formed by membrane located NADPH oxidases in most cells (Bedard and Krause 2007). The most active oxidases are the NADPH oxidase (Nox2) specific to phagocytic immune cells such as leukocytes, eosinophils, monocytes and some macrophages. The latter includes hepatic Kupffer cells in which phagocytosis is triggered by bacterial products and cytokines via cytosolic kinases. The phagocytosis triggers the translocation of the kinases to the phagosome membrane where they phosphorylate and thus activate Nox2 resulting in a cyanide resistant "respiratory burst". The superoxide radicals formed in this reaction caused death and destruction of the microbes in the phagosome. Patients with chronic granulomatous disease lack Nox2 or have defects in the activating kinases and the disease is associated with severe recurring bacterial and fungal infections. The non-phagocytic NADPH oxidase (Nox1) is activated by lipopolysaccharide or TGFβ and is highly expressed in the colon epithelial cells (particularly at the luminal surface) than other cells. Oxidative stress resulting from excessive ROS formed by colonic Nox1 has been implicated in the pathogenesis of colon inflammation e.g. inflammatory bowel disease, Crohn's disease, ulcerative colitis and colon cancer. Nox2 of infiltrating leukocytes may also contribute to these pathologies. NADPH oxidases Nox4-5 are located in intracellular organelles of fibroblasts, endothelial cells, vascular smooth muscle, tumor cells, hepatocytes, neurons, kidney. The family also includes DUOX1 and 2, located in the thyroid with a dual function of H_2O_2 formation and thyroid peroxidase activity required for thyroxine synthesis. In enterocytes they also likely have a dual defence function associated with H_2O_2 formation and lactoperoxidase activity.

2.1.2. Intracellular organelle and cytosolic ROS formation

a) Cells normally produce low level ROS from their intracellular organelles and cytosol fraction (Siraki et al. 2002). Presumably this ROS formation is used by the cell for signaling functions as they do not affect the viability of the cell and are rapidly removed by various antioxidant enzymes located in these compartments. Signaling functions could be mediated by ERK, MAPK, JNK, NF-kB resulting in cell proliferation (protein and DNA synthesis) or inflammation. On the other hand oxidative DNA damage by ROS could cause cell transformation (carcinogenesis) or cell death (apoptosis) (Orrenius et al. 2007). Enzymes involved in ROS or H_2O_2 formation are mostly confined to cellular organelles.

b) Nuclear oxidase Nox4 is induced by phorbol-12-myristate-13-acetate (PMA) in human vascular endothelial cells and prevented by Nox4 silencing, suggesting that superoxide regulates gene expression (Kuroda et al. 2005). Some GSH peroxidase and GSH reductase activity has been located in the nucleus (Rogers et al. 2002). Overexpression of peroxiredoxin 5, a thioredoxin peroxidase that reduces H_2O_2 or hydroperoxides, can prevent nuclear DNA damage by H_2O_2 (Banmeyer et al. 2004). Surprisingly ROS removal is less effective in the nuclei than mitochondria (Vartanyan et al. 2000). A phospholipid hydroperoxide GSH peroxidase is also located in the nucleus, mitochondria, and cytosol of testes cells.

c) Peroxisomal oxidases include fatty acyl CoA oxidase required for β-oxidation, glycolate oxidase for glycolate metabolism and xanthine and uric acid oxidases required for adenine catabolism. Peroxisomal H2O2 though is readily removed by catalase and GSH peroxidase.

d) Lysosomal oxidases includes a membrane NADH oxidase and CoQ which acts as a proton translocator for regulating acidification of the lysosomal matrix (Gille and Nohl 2000). The ROS removal enzymes are not known.

e) Mitochondrial ROS is formed when mitochondria electron transport (required for ATP formation) is slowed down but the ROS formed is usually readily removed by GSH peroxidase and thioredoxin reductase.

f) Endoplasmic reticular NAD(P)H oxidase also involves an electron transport system but consists of a P450 reductase and reduced cytochrome P450 which carries out the oxidative metabolism of steroids and endogenous toxins) but the ROS removal enzymes are not known and are less active in the cytoplasm than mitochondria (Vartanyan et al. 2000).

g) Most cytotosolic oxidases are located in organelles except xanthine oxidase which is located in the cytoplasm of endothelial cells and hepatocytes as well as in the matrix and core of peroxisomes in hepatocytes (Frederiks and Vreeling-Sindelarova 2002). Peroxiredoxins are located in the cytosol, mitochondria, peroxisomes, nuclei and reduce H_2O_2 or hydroperoxides. The cytoplasm of all cells though contains several highly active ROS detoxifying enzymes (GSH peroxidase, catalase) presumably to minimize plasma membrane damage by xanthine oxidase and any ROS released by organelles.

In addition to the endogenous sources, cells can be exposed to oxidative stress from activated immune cells as a result of viral or bacterial infections. Endotoxin produced by Gram-negative bacteria in the intestine can often translocate across the intestinal mucosa into the portal vein circulation and can then activate resident immune cells (liver Kupfer cells) or cause other immune cells (neutrophils) to infiltrate liver and other tissues. The net result is a release by the immune cells of ROS and proinflammatory mediators which cause tissue exogenous oxidative stress. This is a normal but episodic response in some individuals and often occurs without symptoms. It can also be triggered by diet, alcohol, GI distress, liver disease, anesthesia, surgery, drugs etc (Roth et al. 2003). Rat experiments have shown that low amounts of endotoxin markedly increased in vivo liver susceptibility to idiosyncratic drugs. Furthermore endotoxin added to cocultures of Kupffer cells and hepatocytes also increased hepatocyte cytotoxicity induced by hepatotoxic drugs (Tukov et al. 2006).

2.2. Endogenous Carbonyls

These toxins (Figure 1) are formed from oxidized polyunsaturated fatty acids or unsaturated phospholipids and bind to proteins to form advanced lipoxidation products (ALE). ALE levels are mostly determined by the levels of cellular aldehydes formed from the decomposition of lipid peroxides. The intracellular levels of medium/long chain alkanals or alkenals but not short chain alkanals, such as acetaldehyde or alkenals e.g. acrolein or crotonaldehyde, are mostly determined by oxidative detoxification by peroxisome/microsomal fatty aldehyde dehydrogenase ALDH 3A2. ALDH 3A2 expression, induced by insulin treatment of hepatocytes or adipocytes, prevented ROS formation, induced by 4-hydroxynonenal. Further hepatotoxic lipid peroxidation aldehyde products are likely accumulated in the diabetic rat liver because detoxifying enzymes (e.g. ALDH 3A2) were overcome (Demozay et al. 2004). This dehydrogenase is also a component of fatty alcohol:NAD oxidoreductase, which catalyses the oxidation of pristanal, an -oxidation intermediate of phytanic acid metabolism. ALDH 3A2 also detoxifies aromatic or medium/long-chain aliphatic aldehydes (Wanders and Tager 1998; Di Paola et al. 2006). Enzymes detoxifying 4-hydroxynonenal in the liver include Glo-1, ADH, ALDH2 and AKR. The cysteine of the endoplasmic reticulum chaperone protein disulfide isomerase was targeted by 4-hydroxynonenal in ethanol fed rats (Carbone et al. 2005). Proteins targeted by acrolein were identified by proteomics as tropomyosins of the cytoskeletal system (Mello et al. 2007). Enzymes targeted and inactivated by acrolein were mitochondrial pyruvate and ketoglutarate dehydrogenases, both enzymes that require thiamine for their activity (Pocernich and Butterfield 2003).

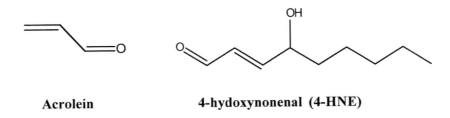

Acrolein   **4-hydoxynonenal (4-HNE)**

Figure 1. Examples of endogenous carbonyl toxins.

2.3. Endogenous Dicarbonyls

Autoxidation or rapid metabolism of glucose/ fructose can form the dicarbonyls glyoxal or methylglyoxal respectively (Figure 2) which can bind to proteins to form advanced glycation end-products (Wanders and Tager 1998). AGE levels can be increased as a result of a partial thiamine deficiency.

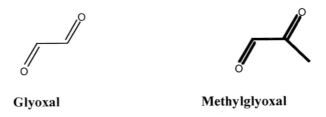

Glyoxal   **Methylglyoxal**

Figure 2. Examples of endogenous dicarbonyl toxins.

Up to 0.3% of consumed glucose is converted to methylglyoxal (MG) by cells as a result of a nonenzymic dephosphorylation of dihydroxyacetone phosphate and glyceraldehyde phosphate and/or catalysed by the enzyme MG synthase or triose phosphate isomerase. However MG is readily detoxified by cytosolic MG reductase that uses NADPH to reduce MG to L-lactaldehyde; by cytosolic glyoxalase I and mitochondrial glyoxalase II that uses GSH to reduce MG to D-lactic acid; and by aldose reductase that uses NADPH to reduce MG in a two-step reaction to acetol and 1,2-propanediol. Increased MG increases glyoxalase I and aldose reductase expression (O'Brien et al. 2005).

Interestingly, MG caused cellular ATP depletion, inhibited glycolysis and inhibited Complex I of the mitochondria respiratory chain of tumor cells (human leukemia leukocytes, Ehrlich ascites carcinoma cells) and cardiac tissue but not of other normal tissue (Biswas et al. 1997; Ray et al. 1997). MG, being an electrophile, can covalently bind to the DNA nucleophilic base guanine to form a tricyclic compound; can covalently bind to protein arginine, lysine, cysteine residues to form advanced glycation endproducts; can inhibit DNA replication by crosslinking DNA guanine with lysine and cysteine of the DNA polymerase binding site; and can interfere with protein synthesis, thereby preventing initiation of DNA replication (Murata-Kamiya and Kamiya 2001).

MG however increased ROS formation by phagocytes as it activated p38 mitogen-activated protein kinase (MAPK) thereby increasing the phagocyte basal respiratory burst that forms H_2O_2 and O_2^{-}. MG also further increased the respiratory burst induced by Staphylococcus aureus and formyl-methionyl-leucyl-phenylalanine (Ward and McLeish 2004). MG could therefore contribute to tissue oxidative stress toxicity associated with phagocyte infiltration such as renal failure induced by uraemic toxin.

MG can be generated by bacteria when their energy source is glycerol or a poor sugar such as ribose, arabinose or xylose. This enables bacteria to survive for a short time until they find glucose but if they do not they will eventually die from the accumulated intracellular MG. Temporary survival occurs because the MG formed from dihydroxyacetone can form glucose by gluconeogenesis even though MG bypasses the two ATP forming steps of glycolysis. This occurs as MG is metabolized to D-lactate, catalysed by GLOX1 and GLOX II, thereby releasing GSH. The D-lactate can then be oxidized by NAD, catalysed by D-lactate dehydrogenase, to form pyruvate which is then converted to glucose by gluconeogenesis (Booth et al. 2003). Although D-lactate dehydrogenase was thought to be mostly in bacteria and yeast, it has recently been found in human mitochondria along with a D-lactate mitochondrial transporter (Ewaschuk et al. 2005). An alternative minor pathway could also involve MG reduction by NAD(P)H to acetol catalysed by aldehyde reductase and then reduction to 1,2 propanediol . The latter would then be oxidised to L-lactaldehyde by NAD catalysed by alcohol dehydrogenase followed by oxidation to L-lactate by NAD catalysed by aldehyde dehydrogenase. L-lactate would then be oxidized to pyruvate by NAD catalysed by lactate dehydrogenase. Plasma L-lactate is usually 100 times that of D-lactate levels. Diabetes increased both plasma L-and D- lactate levels whereas sepsis and trauma mostly increased D-lactate. The MG bypass proposed for E.coli may also occur in mammalian cells and the glucose formed may similarly enable the cells to adapt to a glucose energy deficit. MG is readily metabolized by murine hepatocytes to glucose so that MG could act as an energy source to offset mitochondrial toxicity without risking MG induced "cell death by misadventure" as occurs with E coli (Booth et al. 2003).

2.4. Endogenous excess of intracellular Free Fatty acids

2.4.1. Lipotoxicity

High dietary energy intake, from fat or carbohydrate, increases the risk of type 2 diabetes, cardiovascular diseases, NASH and cancers. Some drugs also cause fatty liver (steatosis) that can progress to NASH or liver cancer as they inhibit mitochondrial fatty acid oxidation, sequester CoA or inhibit hepatic triglyceride export (O'Brien PJ et al. in preparation). Non-esterified fatty acids are bound to specific or unspecific fatty acid-binding proteins e.g. serum albumin. A small part is associated with membranes and only a minute part remains free. Nonetheless, an elevation of plasma saturated free fatty acids (FFA; Figure 3) resulting from high dietary fat intake, is associated with ventricular myocyte toxicity (de Vries et al. 1997). There is also increased insulin resistance in muscles and a release of proinflammatory cytokines. Increased fasting plasma free fatty acid levels have also been associated with a higher risk of type 2 diabetes and NASH.

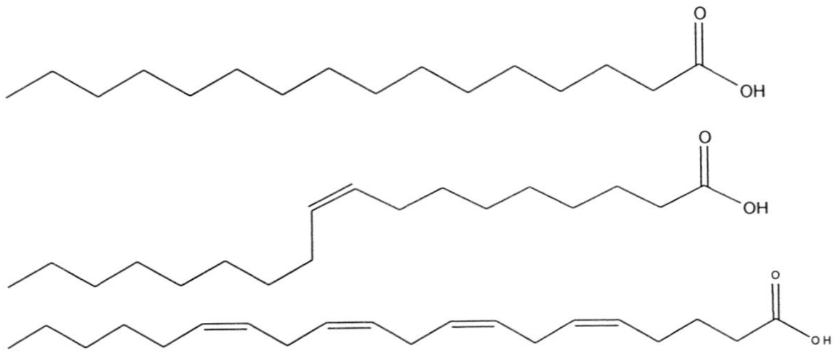

Palmitic acid

Oleic acid

Arachidonic acid

Figure 3. Examples of free fatty acids.

Seven activation mechanisms (a. to g.) have been proposed to explain the toxicity of free fatty acids:

a. *Mitochondrial uncoupling and reactive oxygen species induced by saturated/unsaturated fatty acids.* Addition of micromolar concentrations of long chain free fatty acids e.g. oleate, palmitate to respiring mitochondria decreased transmembrane potential, increased state 4 respiration with a smaller decrease in state 3 respiration, decreased the respiratory control ratio and decreased the ADP to oxygen ratio (ADP/O). Fatty acids can thus act as protonophores and natural uncouplers which by speeding up electron transport would decrease reactive oxygen species formation in the resting state (Di Paola and Lorusso 2006). Furthermore, when calcium loaded mitochondria are exposed to micromolar free fatty acids, ROS is generated at coupling sites I and II (Di Paola and Lorusso 2006). This increases the permeability of the inner membrane opening the permeability transition pore, causing matrix swelling, rupture of the outer membrane and release of proapoptotic proteins.

b. *Inhibition of mitochondrial adenine nucleotide translocator (ANT) by long chain acyl-CoA (LCAC).* It has long been known that the function of ANT is compromised by LCAC and that diabetes is also associated with an increase in the concentration of LCAC, suggesting that the toxicity of FFA involves the inhibition of ANT (Wanders et al. 1984). Isolated rat liver mitochondria experiments showed that addition of an LCAC (5uM palmitoyl-CoA) caused ROS production formed by the inhibition of the ATP-consuming module ANT/hexokinase (Ciapaite et al. 2006). A high fat diet fed to rats induced a 24% increase in hepatic LCAC (mostly C18) and increased hepatocyte cytosolic CML, a protein AGE (glyoxal adducts of protein lysine) and oxidative stress biomarker. Body weight did not increase and glucose tolerance was impaired after a glucose load. The mitochondria number per liver cell was not affected but cytochrome c was decreased (an apoptosis indicator). Oxidative phosphorylation, however, was not affected, suggesting that it had not adapted to these metabolic changes and that ANT had been inhibited. It was hypothesized that oxidative stress resulting from the inhibition of ANT by LCAC underlies the mechanism associating the cellular dysfunction of obesity with type 2 diabetes (Ciapaite et al. 2007). We suggest that this same mechanism for increased oxidative stress could also be involved in the development of NASH, cardiovascular risk and some forms of carcinogenesis.

c. Mitochondrial toxicity by unsaturated fatty acid autoxidation. A third hypothesis is that the accumulation of unsaturated fatty acids in hepatocytes contributes to the progression of steatosis to NASH. These fatty acids could undergo oxidation to form toxic radicals and carbonyls that may inhibit mitochondrial respiration resulting in ROS formation. In turn this could promote inflammation or induce fibrogenesis. The three enzymes that catalyse the oxidation of unsaturated fatty acid toxins include cyclooxygenases, lipoxygenases and cytochrome P450. Hepatic P450 CYP2E1 was also induced in NASH and generated ROS and increased cellular endogenous ROS formation (Weltman et al. 1998). CYP2E1 also readily catalysed unsaturated fatty acid oxidation, induced oxidative stress which released calcium from intracellular stores and caused mitochondrial toxicity (Caro and Cederbaum 2007). The CYP2E1 requirement was presumably to generate ROS that catalysed the arachidonate oxidation. Release of calcium from mitochondrial or endoplasmic reticular calcium stores by oxidative stress was part of the cytotoxic mechanism and cytotoxicity could be prevented by inhibitors of the calcium activated phospholipase A_2. Calcium activation of phospholipase A_2 would cause arachidonate release and further increase mitochondrial toxicity. The mitochondrial toxicity signaling pathway involved activation of p38 MAPK whereas the transcription factor Nrf2 pathway prevented toxicity, likely by increasing hepatocyte GSH levels. Calcium loaded mitochondria are particularly susceptible to arachidonate by a mechanism involving the permeability transition with hepatocyte mitochondria and ANT with heart mitochondria (Di Paola et al. 2006).

d. Drug induced inhibition of mitochondrial fatty acid oxidation causing ROS formation. Most of the ATP generated in cells arises from the β-oxidation of fatty acids. The first step of the β-oxidation of fatty acids located in the mitochondrial matrix is catalysed by the FAD cofactor of acyl-CoA dehydrogenase which oxidizes fatty acyl CoA, thereby reducing FAD to FADH2 which is then reoxidized by electron transfer protein (ETF) located in the inner membrane. The reduced ETF then transfers its electrons to CoQ and then via Complex III and complex IV to oxygen, forming water and 2ATP for each C2 of the fatty acids. Inhibition of acyl-CoA dehydrogenase by drugs would be expected to slow mitochondrial respiration and thereby increase ROS formation.

e. Peroxisomal fatty acid oxidation causing ROS formation. Beta-oxidations of saturated and unsaturated fatty acids are carried out by mitochondria and peroxisomes. Mitochondria though are unable to oxidize fatty acids C22:1 and longer chains are oxidized by peroxisomes. The first enzyme of this metabolic pathway is fatty acyl CoA oxidase, which is located in peroxisomes and, unlike the mitochondrial oxidase, forms H_2O_2 which is mostly detoxified by catalase, also located in the peroxisomes (Wanders and Tager 1998). However environmental and drug peroxisome proliferators induce fatty acyl CoA oxidase activity up to 30 fold whereas catalase activity is only induced 1.6 fold. Because of this, liver cancer induced in rodents by these non- mutagenic peroxisome proliferators has been attributed to oxidative DNA damage induced by H_2O_2 released by peroxisomes metabolizing fatty acids (Varanasi et al. 1994). Whilst rat hepatic ROS is increased by proliferators in vivo, hepatic lipid peroxidation is decreased, probably because of the 3-4 fold induction of peroxisomal and microsomal aldehyde dehydrogenases which have a broad aldehyde specificity including long-chain aliphatic aldehydes (Antonenkov et al. 1985; Nicholls-Grzemski et al. 2000). This dehydrogenase is likely fatty aldehyde dehydrogenase ALDH10, a component of fatty alcohol:NAD oxidoreductase, which catalyses the oxidation of pristanal, an α-oxidation intermediate of phytanic acid metabolism.

f. Mitochondrial or lysosomal lipoapoptosis induced by saturated fatty acids. i) Saturated fatty acids incubated with mouse hepatocytes were more effective than monounsaturated fatty acids at causing a sustained activation of JNK1 which mediated mitochondrial apoptosis involving mitochondrial membrane depolarization, cytochrome c release and caspase activation. JNK activation may engage the core mitochondrial proapoptotic machinery with Bim-mediated Bax activation. Small interfering RNA targeted knock-down of Bim decreased Bax activation and cell death (Malhi et al. 2006). JNK inhibitors could prove useful in preventing NASH and end stage liver disease. ii) Saturated long chain fatty acids bound to serum albumin when incubated with hepatocytes caused a translocation of cytosolic Bax to lysosomes which destabilized (permeabilised) their membrane. This released the protease cathepsin B into the cytosol and signaled a TNF-α cascade induced apoptosis. Genetic or pharmacological inhibition of cathepsin B also prevented fatty liver disease in mice induced by a sucrose diet (Feldstein et al. 2004). Bax inhibitors also prevented fatty acid induced hepatocyte apoptosis (Feldstein et al. 2006). Lipoapoptosis, in β-cells of the islets resulting in diabetes or, in heart resulting in myopathy, was prevented by caloric restriction, thiazolidinedione treatment or by iNOS inhibitors (Unger 2002).

g. Saturated fatty acid iron complexes. Palmitic acid was shown to facilitate iron translocation into endothelial cells through a transferrin-receptor independent mechanism resulting in extracellular oxidative stress, plasma membrane lysis and cell death. Palmitic acid also translocated iron into the mitochondria of the endothelial cell. Higher vascular iron deposition was also observed in mice administered a high fat diet (Yao et al. 2005).

2.4.2. Glucotoxicity

Chronic exposures to diets high in sucrose or fructose diets can result in fatty livers and indeed such exposures are used in an animal model for non-alcoholic steatoheatitis (NASH). Presumably the effects are a consequence of the high energy substrate through mechanisms similar to those observed with high fat diets.

Acute exposures to fructose can be protective and will prevent hepatocyte cytotoxicity induced by mitochondrial respiration inhibitors or hypoxia by acting as a glycolytic ATP source. However, acute exposures to a bolus dose of 10mM fructose, unlike glucose, results in initial ATP depletion and death, as cells first need ATP to form fructose 1-phosphate catalysed by fructokinase which is over 12 times more active than glucokinase in hepatocytes.

ATP slowly recovers and cell viability is not affected. Fructose though caused cytotoxicity if the hepatocytes were exposed to low level H_2O_2 generated by glucose/glucose oxidase at doses that did not affect hepatocyte GSH levels or viability. The fructose metabolites glyceraldehyde and dihydroxyacetone were more cytotoxic than fructose and cell death induced by the three agents was attributed to oxidative stress and mitochondrial toxicity. The endogenous toxic reactive species were likely carbon radicals and dicarbonyls formed by the H_2O_2 catalysed autoxidation of glyceraldehyde and dihydroxyacetone (Lee and O'Brien in preparation). Glyceraldehyde incubated with erythrocytes caused GSH depletion and oxidative stress that was attributed to autoxidation (Thornalley and Stern 1984).

3. SOME MICRONUTRIENTS THAT MAY MITIGATE THE EFFECTS OF ENDOGENOUS TOXINS

We present here a small range of micronutrients that have been shown to modulate oxidative stress markers. Some structures are represented in Figure 4.

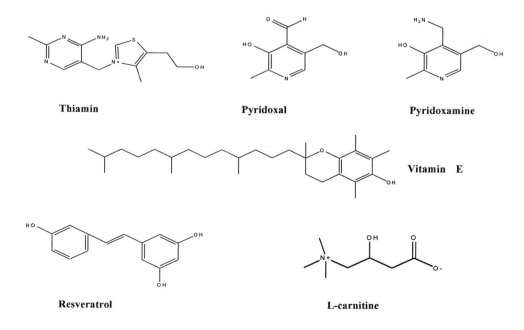

Figure 4. Selected nutrient with antioxidant potential.

3.1. Vitamin B Micronutrients

3.1.1. Vitamin B1 (Thiamin)

Thiamin has been considered for treatment of epilepsy (Ranganathan and Ramaratnam 2005), and other neurodegenerative disorders (Balk et al. 2006; Thomson and Marshall 2006), even though the underlying mechanims involved were often unclear. Its use for preventing diabetic complications has also been well documented (Bakker et al. 2000; Ascher et al. 2001; Thornalley et al. 2001; Ahmed and Thornalley 2007).

Thiamin is a coenzyme for transketolase and restored the activity of erythrocyte transketolase that had been decreased in erythrocytes when they were incubated with 50mM glucose. The increased triose phosphate and MG levels induced by this treatment was also restored by the thiamin supplement (Thornalley et al. 2001). Partial thiamin deficiency increased dicarbonyl protein adducts in F344 rats (Shangari et al. 2005) that was associated with aberrant crypt foci formation (Bruce et al. 2003). Thiamin supplementation could restore those oxidative markers in the rat plasma to control level (Depeint et al. in preparation) while supplementation in hemodialysis patients did not show an improvement in oxidative status (Nascimento et al. 2006). The role of thiamin in reversing protein carbonyl formation has also been observed with acetaldehyde exposure (Aberle et al. 2004)

Thiamin is also a coenzyme for ketoglutarate and pyruvate dehydrogenases that are part of the multienzyme complexes which form part of the Citric Acid cycle. Glyoxals also inactivated these dehydrogenases and thiamin pyrophosphate restored their activity. The inactivation was attributed to the glycation of two arginine residues at the substrate binding site (Nemerya et al. 1984; Eswaran et al. 1995; Ostrovtsova 1998).

Copper induced cytotoxicity of neuroblastoma cells was also prevented by thiamin in vivo or in vitro by acting as a coenzyme for mitochondrial ketoglutarate and pyruvate dehydrogenase activity. These dehydrogenase activities that had been inhibited as a result of ROS formation by copper (Sheline and Choi 2004; Sheline and Wei 2006). A similar protective effect against lead toxicity was observed with a combination of thiamin and vitamin C on lead toxicity (Wang et al. 2006), but the authors also raised the potential problem of toxicity associated with excessive dosage of the vitamins.

3.1.2. B6 Vitamers

Vitamin B6 as a therapeutic agent has been described in relation to diabetes (Jain 2007), epilepsy (Gaby 2007), or cardiovascular disease (Wierzbicki 2007). These and other authors have long been considering the antioxidant and radical scavenging properties of the B6 vitamers, for example in reducing oxidative stress markers associated with homocysteinemia (Mahfouz and Kummerow 2004) or in preventing ROS formation and lipid peroxidation in a cellular model (Kannan and Jain 2004). Although the role of the vitamers in one-carbon transfer has not been neglected, combination trials with folate and vitamin B12 (Cook and Hess 2005; Lonn et al. 2006) have shown unclear results.

B6 vitamers are coenzymes for cytosolic and mitochondrial transaminases which prevented the inactivation of these transaminase by low levels of the endogenous acetaldehyde toxin (Crouch and Solomon 1989). Glycation of aspartate transaminase (Bakker et al.) was attributed to increased endogenous MG formation in diabetics. This glycated transaminase also persisted longer than unglycated enzymes in diabetic tissue (Okada et al. 1997). MG added to AAT glycated 6 lysine residues, inhibited the enzyme and changed the protein conformation (Seidler and Kowalewski 2003).

3.2. Antioxidants

3.2.1. Vitamin E, Vitamin C

Vitamin E has been considered for treatment of chonic liver damage (Di Sario et al. 2007), prostate cancer (Crispen et al. 2007), or even type 2 diabetes (Dogru Pekiner et al. 2003; Wu et al. 2007), both as an antioxidant and anti-inflammatory agent (Singh and Devaraj 2007) but often with mixed effects. It was recently reported that the various natural forms of vitamin E may prove to have specific and unique antioxidant and health benefits (Sen et al. 2007), and this may lead to new discoveries about the role of vitamin E in health protection. Vitamin E seems to act by augmenting the activity of antioxidant enzymes such as superoxide dismutase (SOD) or glutathione peroxidase (GPx) as well as total antioxidant levels (Mahmoud and Hijazi 2007) as well as reducing lipid peroxidation markers, but this function requires both optimal doses of vitamin E and C (Traber 2007).

Ascorbic acid (vitamin C) has been considered, alone or in combination with vitamin E and other antioixdant nutrients, in the treatment of respiratory disorders (Riccioni et al. 2007), cardiovascular diseases (Witte and Clark 2006; Riccioni et al. 2007), and cancers (McKeown-Eyssen et al. 1988; Greenberg et al. 1994; Block and Mead 2003). Vitamin C has been shown to reduce oxidative stress by maintening glutathione oxidoreduction balance (Bryer and Goldfarb 2006) or preventing protein carbonylation or lipid peroxidation following intensive exercise regimen (Close et al. 2006). Vitamin C also reduced nitric oxide formation and iNOS activity in an hypoxia/reoxygenation exercise (Sureda et al. 2004). This vitamin has also been shown to reduce damage related to cigarette smoking by modulating VEGF-dependent activities (Stadler et al. 2007) and inflammation markers (Majewicz et al. 2005), suggesting that it can protect against smoking-induced oxidative stress. As with any antioxidant molecule, but more specifically because of its role in modulating the redox state of beta-carotene and alpha-tocopherol, however there is also the risk that under specific circumstances it has prooxidant properties(Black 2004; Bailey et al. 2006).

Oxidative stress induced by hydroperoxides, acrolein or dichromate caused depletion of hepatocyte GSH, protein thiols and depleted 60% of the micronutrient Vitamin C with a nearly complete depletion of vitamin E. Added Vitamin E 100uM prevented oxidative stress cytotoxicity and restored endogenous Vitamin E and Vitamin C levels (Susa et al. 1996). Interestingly rat hepatocyte GSH depletion alone can cause a compensatory doubling of cell ascorbate levels which markedly increased resistance to hydroperoxide induced cytotoxicity (Chan et al. 2005).

3.2.2. Plant antioxidants, e.g. Resveratrol

Recently high doses of resveratrol, a polyphenolic phytoalexin found in grape skins were successful in preventing mouse obesity induced by a high fat diet by increasing the aerobic capacity of the obese mice as shown by doubling their running endurance and increasing oxygen consumption in muscle fibres (Lagouge et al. 2006). The mechanism involved activating the protein deacetylase, SIRT1 which increased the number of mitochondria in the cell (mitochondrial biogenesis) and thereby increased fatty acid oxidation. In another study, resveratrol by preventing obesity also extended the life span of mice fed a high fat diet by increased insulin sensitivity, decreased insulin-like growth factor-1 and increased AMP-activated protein kinase and peroxisome proliferator-activated PGC-1α. There was also an increased mitochondria number per cell and improved motor function (Baur et al. 2006).

3.3. ROS Scavengers

Coenzyme Q10 (coQ10) has been tested to modulate symptoms in thalassemia patients (Kalpravidh et al. 2005), a case of cerebellar ataxia (Artuch et al. 2006), and generally with cardiovascular disorders (Belardinelli et al. 2005; Witte and Clark 2006). The nutrient also seems to be of some promise in the treatment of neurodegenerative diseases such as Parkinson's (Weber and Ernst 2006). Its effect in decreasing the lipid peroxidation marker, malondialdehyde, was observed by other researchers (Singh et al. 2005). CoQ10 was also shown to delay formation of oxidative DNA damage such as 8-hydroxydeoxy-guanosine in lymphocytes (Niklowitz et al. 2007). CoQ10 activity is both a ROS scavenger and mitochondrial enzyme cofactor to the electron transport chain (Sandhu et al. 2003).

The micronutrient carnitine is metabolised to acetyl-L-carnitine which facilitates the mitochondrial transport and beta-oxidation of long chain fatty acids. It also suppresses the mitochondrial permeability transition thereby inhibiting apoptosis induced by mitochondrial toxicity (Furuno et al. 2001). Acetyl-L-carnitine readily crosses the blood brain barrier. Acetylcarnitine also promotes energy metabolism by supplying acetyl CoA to the Krebs cycle. L-carnitine also acts as a lipid antioxidant , ROS scavenger and a ferrous iron chelator (Gulcin 2006). Pyrroloquinoline quinone (PQQ) is another essential nutrient acting as a ROS scavenger, mostly against superoxide formation (Hara et al. 2007). Vitamin E described earlier is another example of ROS scavenger nutrient (Kir et al. 2005).

Lipoic acid requires a transporter to enter cells or to cross the brain barrier and is reduced in all tissues by NADH and lipoamide dehydrogenase to dihydrolipoate which scavenges ROS, NO, Cu and prevents H_2O_2 or Cd toxicity. It can also restore reduced vitamins C and E, CoQ and thioredoxin by reducing their one electron oxidation product. Reduced CoQ in turn can restore vitamin E. In this way lipoic acid can prevent vitamin C or vitamin E deficiency (Packer et al. 1997).

4. IDENTIFICATION OF MICRONUTRIENTS THAT DECREASE ENDOGENOUS TOXINS

Diets to reduce caloric intake and physical exercise to increase calorie requirement are thought to have beneficial effects on NASH, MeS, T2D, CVD and on the development of many cancers. Both diet and exercise improve insulin sensitivity in muscles, liver and adipose tissue by increasing AMP-activated protein kinase (AMPK) which removes fatty acids by increasing fatty acid oxidation. Antidiabetic drug therapy could also be beneficial particularly if they activated liver AMPK activity, inhibited gluconeogenesis and improved liver insulin sensitivity e.g. the antidiabetic drugs metformin or thiazolidinediones. Hypolipidemic drugs such as bezafibrate or gemfibrozil but not clofibrate also prevented the progression of NASH (Medina et al. 2004). Increasing fatty acid oxidation by natural means e.g. carnitine or β-aminoisobutyric acid (a thymine catabolite) have also been successful (Begriche et al. 2006). The observations made in section 3 above suggest that micronutrients could also be usefull.

4.1. The in Vitro Rat Hepatocyte Model

Our approach was to identify micronutients that decrease endogenous toxins associated with, and possibly the cause of, disease. We chose to identify protective micronutrients with an in vitro model because of the large number of endogenous toxins and micronutrients to evaluate. We chose the liver as our souce of cells because hepatocytes are available in large numbers, they are exposed to the full effect of the diet, and they are known to be affected by micronutrient deficiency (e.g. choline deficiency) and energy excess (e.g. the metabolic syndrome, fatty liver disease and steatohepatitis). Other cells in the body are exposed to the same endogenous toxins and micronutrients, but the effects on hepatocytes would provide a primary eassessment of cytotoxicity and protection.

We used the in vitro hepatocyte model to evaluate the oxidative damage associated with the four endogenous toxins, reactive oxygen and nitrogen species, carbonyls, dicarbonyls, and the free fatty acids associated with energy substrate overload. In addition we evaluated combinations of endogenous toxins. Isolated hepatocytes were collected following collagen perfusion of the liver (Moldeus et al. 1978). Isolated hepatocytes were suspended in Krebs-Henseleit buffer (pH7.4) containing 12.5mM Hepes in continually rotating round-bottom flasks, under an atmosphere of 95% O_2 and 5% CO_2 in a waterbath at 37°C. The ROS-generating system was achieved with a glucose/glucose oxidase mixture, generating a constant supply of H_2O_2. The other 3 models were based on the addition of the toxins directly to the hepatocyte suspension. For each system, doses of the toxins were used that induced about 50% cell death (as measured by trypan blue uptake) at 2 hours incubation. For combination experiments, sub-toxic doses were used to allow for synergestic cytotoxicity. The micronutrients, at non-toxic doses, were added with or prior to the endogenous toxin and ranked for their ability to prevent the *in vitro* cytotoxicity with each of the toxins.

4.2. Results Obtained with the Model

4.2.1. ROS Exposure

Multiple aliquots of freshly prepared hepatocytes treated with various vitamins were exposed to intracellular ROS generated by an extracellular H_2O_2 generating system consisting of glucose and glucose oxidase (Table 2). The order of effectiveness of B6 vitamers at preventing ROS-induced hepatocyte cytotoxicity was pyridoxal = pyridoxal phosphate >

pyridoxamine > pyridoxine. Thiamin and thiamin pyrophosphate were equally active as pyridoxal and pyridoxamine, while lipoic acid, nicotinamide, pantothenic acid, and folic acid were not succesfull at protecting the hepatocytes against ROS-induced cytotoxicity. The ranking also correlated with their effectiveness at inhibiting hepatocyte ROS formation. This shows that different vitamins, even different vitamers of the same vitamin, have varied effects against a specific toxin.

4.2.2. The Example of B6 Vitaminers Against a Range of Endogenous Threats

Similar aliquots of hepatocytes treated with vitamins were exposed to oxidative stress induced by iron, glyoxal or acrolein. The same order of effectiveness of the B6 vitamers was again observed for the prevention of hepatocyte cytotoxicity and lipid peroxidation. Interestingly the B6 vitamers also protected against copper or cyanide-induced hepatocyte cytotoxicity and for ROS formation. These observations suggest that B6 vitamers can act as intracellular lipid antioxidants and iron chelators; that they prevented mitochondrial toxicity by acting as cofactors for mitochondrial enzymes; and that they acted as copper chelators and likely also as cofactors for mitochondrial dehydrogenases (Mehta and O'Brien 2007; Mehta et al. 2007).

Table 2. Example of a nutrient protection screening

	% Cytotoxicity (trypan blue uptake)			% ROS
	60min	120min	180min	90min
Control-hepatocytes	22 ± 3	23 ± 3	24 ± 3	100
+ H$_2$0$_2$ Generating System	40 ± 4	47 ± 5	54 ± 5	148 ± 12
+ Thiamin 3mM	32 ± 3	30 ± 3	41 ± 4	112 ± 7
+ Thiamin 3mM (pre inc 1h)	21 ± 6	25 ± 6	40 ± 6	99 ± 8
+ Thiamin pyrophosphate 3 mM (pre inc 1h)	25	31	43	73
+ Nicotinamide 5mM	37 ± 2	52 ± 3	58 ± 3	128 ± 6
+ Pantothenic acid 5mM	47 ± 4	53 ± 5	54 ± 5	132 ± 13
+ Pyridoxal Phosphate 3mM	23 ± 1	23 ± 1	28 ± 2	101 ± 5
+ Pyridoxal 3mM	22 ± 2	22 ± 2	24 ± 2	99 ± 8
+ Pyridoxine 5mM	37 ± 3	47 ± 4	47 ± 4	109 ± 11
+ Pyridoxamine 5mM	24 ± 1	31 ± 2	42 ± 3	104 ± 6
+ Folic Acid 5mM	41 ± 3	52 ± 4	59 ± 4	125 ± 6
+ Vit.E 0.2mM	39	45	55	151

This shows cytoprotection of certain vitamins against hydrogen peroxide toxicity, associated with the inhibition of ROS formation (Mehta et al. in preparation).

4.2.3. The example of thiamin protection against carbonyls and dicarbonyls

Glyoxal added to hepatocytes caused ATP depletion and a collapse of the mitochondrial membrane potential that was partly attributed to inhibiton of the citric acid cycle dehydrogenases (Shangari et al. 2005).

Thiamin even at at 3mM was not very effective at preventing hydroperoxide-, chloroacetaldehyde- or iron- induced hepatocyte cytotoxicity and lipid peroxidation. This indicates that thiamin was a poor lipid antioxidant and iron chelator.

Thiamin however was effective at preventing formaldehyde or acrolein induced cytotoxicity and partly prevented lipid peroxidation. This suggested that thiamin, in addition to acting as a vitamin and can prevent mitochondrial oxidative stress toxicity caused by formaldehyde or acrolein. Thiamin was also the most effective of the B1 and B6 vitamers at preventing copper induced cytotoxicity and ROS formation (Mehta and O'Brien 2007; Mehta et al. 2007).

Table 3 presents a summary of the ranking of B1 and B6 vitamins against a range of endogenous toxins. It shows once again that specific functions of the vitamins are needed against different tyes of oxidative stress, represented here as oxygen species formation versus lipid peroxidation. Figure 5 shows the possible mechanisms by which B vitamins can generate such a wide array of protective effects.

Table 3. Cross-comparison and nutrient ranking

	Cytotoxicity 60 min	Cytotoxicity 120 min	ROS formation 90 min	Lipid peroxidation 90 min
Control Hepatocytes	**19 (3)**	**21 (3)**	**99 (5)**	**0.24 (0.01)**
+ H2O2	**40 (4)**	**47 (5)**	**148 (12)**	
+ Thiamin	+	++	++	
+ Thiamin pyrophosphate	++	++	+++	
+ Pyridoxal	+++	+++	+++	
+ Pyridoxal phosphate	+++	+++	+++	
+ Pyridoxine	-	-	+++	
+ Pyridoxamine	+++	++	+++	
+ Acrolein	**24 (1)**	**51 (1)**		**2.71 (0.24)**
+ Thiamin	+++	++		+++
+ Thiamin pyrophosphate	-	-		-
+ Pyridoxal	+++	++		+++
+ Pyridoxal phosphate	-	+		++
+ Pyridoxine	+++	++		-
+ Pyridoxamine	+++	+		++
+ Glyoxal	**42 (4)**	**58 (7)**	**240 (12)**	
+ Thiamin	+++	++	+++	
+ Thiamin pyrophosphate	+++	+	++	
+ Pyridoxal	+++	+++	+++	
+ Pyridoxal phosphate	+++	++	++	
+ Pyridoxine	+	+	++	
+ Pyridoxamine	++	++	+++	

Vitamins are ranked for each endogenous toxin according to the intendity of the protective effect, from none (-) or low protection (+) to a near complete recovery of the system (+++). The table was chelated from data obtained in our laboratory (Mehta et al. 2007). Cytotoxicity was expressed as percentage cell death at each time point; ROS as percentage of the control ROS levels (FU); Lipid peroxidation was measured at 532nm as TBAR metabolites.

4.2.4. Combined Energy Substrate Overload and Oxidative Stress

Surprisingly fructose, but not glucose, killed hepatocytes when these hepatocytes were subjected to nontoxic oxidative stress. Freshly prepared hepatocytes were little affected by either fructose (50mM) or H_2O_2 (1mM per h, generated with a glucose oxidase system) but suffered a marked decrease in survival within 2 h when exposed to both fructose (10mM) and H_2O_2. Interestingly, ATP recovery was inhibited and AMP levels were markedly increased

(Lee et al. in preparation). The micronutrient ROS scavenger dihydrolipoic acid or carnitine protected the cells against this cytotoxicity.

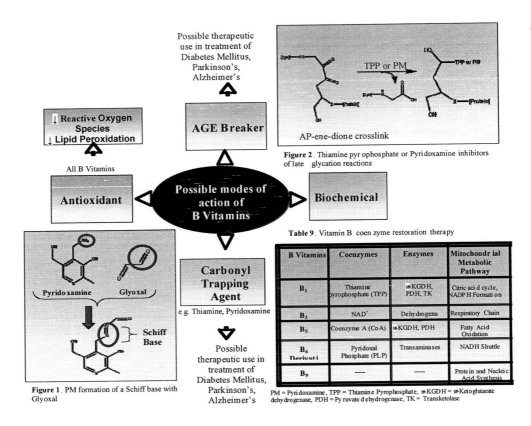

Figure 5. Possible roles of B vitamins in the protection against endogenous toxins.

4.3. Interpretation of Results

1. Reactive oxygen stress endogenous toxin (represented by hydrogen peroxide) was decreased by pyridoxal, carnitine and choline. Reactive oxygen stress resulting from iron and copper was decreased by the micronutrient B6 vitamers, likely through chelating effects.

2. Carbonyl endogenous toxins (represented by glyoxal, acrolein) was decreased by micronutrients pyridoxal, carnitine, choline or vitamin E.

3. Fructose cytotoxicity to hepatocytes exposed to low nontoxic H_2O_2 was prevented by thiamine, pyridoxal, dehydroascorbate, reduced lipoic acid, carnitine and the ferric chelator desferoxamine.

4. Unsaturated fatty acid toxicity (resulting from fat and carbohydrate energy substrate overload) was markedly increased by hydroperoxide induced oxidative stress and lipid peroxidation. This was decreased by micronutrient lipoic acid (reduced), vitamin E or carnitine and iron chelators.

5. CONCLUSION

It is evident from the evidence presented in Table 1 that many health disorders may find their cause in the effects of endogenous toxins. The isolation and identification of these toxins poses a major challenge. We noted, however, that the toxins can be formed in many ways and their formation and action mitigated by a wide range of micronutrients. This suggested that their identification might be made without isolation, by identifying micronutrients that inhibit their cytotoxicity.

We have described an in vitro cellular model that can be used to test a wide range of micronutrients, for their efficacy at reducing the toxicity of endogenous toxins. The early results obtained with this model show that the interaction can be quite complex, but identifies as effective a number of micronutrient inc;uding alpha-lipoic acid, that is proving of interest in the prevention of diabetes and obesity, possibly through its effect on AMP-activated protein kinase (Targonsky et al. 2006). The model thus promises to provide a cost-effective system for assessing micronutrients for their efficacy and systematically classifying them based on their favoured oxidative targets. The model may thus provide an effective response to the current problems of oxidative stress assessment posed by the Institute of Medicine (2001) as cited above.

A possible weakness of the proposed in vitro model is that it is based on analyses of effects on a mature, non-proliferating cells from a single organ, the liver. Further studies will be needed to determine to what degree the results obtained with this model also apply to cells from other organs or to less differentiated or proliferating cells. However, the marked similarity of the risk factors for non-alcoholic steatohepatitis, the metabolic syndrome, type 2 diabetes, cardiovascular disease and some epithelial cancers, suggests that the underlying toxicological mechanisms invovled for each may be very similar. The strength of the approach is that it provides a simple and inexpensive method to define mechanisms important in the etiology of chronic health disorders. Application of this method could lead to testable hypotheses, to the design of intervention studies, and thus to a strategy for disease prevention.

ACKNOWLEDGEMENTS

We thank Gail McKeown-Eyssen, University of Toronto, for her careful reading of the manuscript. We also would like to acknowledge funding, for the work presented here, from the National Cancer Institute of Canada, the Canadian Cancer Research Society and a Marie Curie grant from the European Union.

REFERENCES

Aberle, N.S., 2nd, Burd, L., Zhao, B.H. and Ren, J. (2004). "Acetaldehyde-induced cardiac contractile dysfunction may be alleviated by vitamin B1 but not by vitamins B6 or B12." *Alcohol Alcohol 39*(5): 450-4.

Ahmed, N. and Thornalley, P.J. (2007). "Advanced glycation endproducts: what is their relevance to diabetic complications?" *Diabetes Obes Metab 9*(3): 233-45.

Ames, B.N., Cathcart, R., Schwiers, E. and Hochstein, P. (1981). "Uric acid provides an antioxidant defense in humans against oxidant- and radical-caused aging and cancer: a hypothesis." *Proc Natl Acad Sci U S A 78*(11): 6858-62.

Antonenkov, V.D., Pirozhkov, S.V. and Panchenko, L.F. (1985). "Intraparticulate localization and some properties of a clofibrate-induced peroxisomal aldehyde dehydrogenase from rat liver." *Eur J Biochem 149*(1): 159-67.

Artuch, R., Brea-Calvo, G., Briones, P., Aracil, A., Galvan, M., Espinos, C., Corral, J., Volpini, V., Ribes, A., Andreu, A.L., Palau, F., Sanchez-Alcazar, J.A., Navas, P. and Pineda, M. (2006). "Cerebellar ataxia with coenzyme Q10 deficiency: diagnosis and follow-up after coenzyme Q10 supplementation." *J Neurol Sci 246*(1-2): 153-8.

Ascher, E., Gade, P.V., Hingorani, A., Puthukkeril, S., Kallakuri, S., Scheinman, M. and Jacob, T. (2001). "Thiamine reverses hyperglycemia-induced dysfunction in cultured endothelial cells." *Surgery 130*(5): 851-8.

Bailey, D.M., Raman, S., McEneny, J., Young, I.S., Parham, K.L., Hullin, D.A., Davies, B., McKeeman, G., McCord, J.M. and Lewis, M.H. (2006). "Vitamin C prophylaxis promotes oxidative lipid damage during surgical ischemia-reperfusion." *Free Radic Biol Med 40*(4): 591-600.

Bakker, S.J., ter Maaten, J.C. and Gans, R.O. (2000). "Thiamine supplementation to prevent induction of low birth weight by conventional therapy for gestational diabetes mellitus." *Med Hypotheses 55*(1): 88-90.

Balk, E., Chung, M., Raman, G., Tatsioni, A., Chew, P., Ip, S., Devine, D. and Lau, J. (2006). "B vitamins and berries and age-related neurodegenerative disorders." *Evid Rep Technol Assess (Full Rep)*(134): 1-161.

Banmeyer, I., Marchand, C., Verhaeghe, C., Vucic, B., Rees, J.F. and Knoops, B. (2004). "Overexpression of human peroxiredoxin 5 in subcellular compartments of Chinese hamster ovary cells: effects on cytotoxicity and DNA damage caused by peroxides." *Free Radic Biol Med 36*(1): 65-77.

Baur, J.A., Pearson, K.J., Price, N.L., Jamieson, H.A., Lerin, C., Kalra, A., Prabhu, V.V., Allard, J.S., Lopez-Lluch, G., Lewis, K., Pistell, P.J., Poosala, S., Becker, K.G., Boss, O., Gwinn, D., Wang, M., Ramaswamy, S., Fishbein, K.W., Spencer, R.G., Lakatta, E.G., Le Couteur, D., Shaw, R.J., Navas, P., Puigserver, P., Ingram, D.K., de Cabo, R. and Sinclair, D.A. (2006). "Resveratrol improves health and survival of mice on a high-calorie diet." *Nature 444*(7117): 337-42.

Bedard, K. and Krause, K.H. (2007). "The NOX family of ROS-generating NADPH oxidases: physiology and pathophysiology." *Physiol Rev 87*(1): 245-313.

Begleiter, A., Hewitt, D., Maksymiuk, A.W., Ross, D.A. and Bird, R.P. (2006). "A NAD(P)H:quinone oxidoreductase 1 polymorphism is a risk factor for human colon cancer." *Cancer Epidemiol Biomarkers Prev 15*(12): 2422-6.

Begriche, K., Igoudjil, A., Pessayre, D. and Fromenty, B. (2006). "Mitochondrial dysfunction in NASH: causes, consequences and possible means to prevent it." *Mitochondrion 6*(1): 1-28.

Belardinelli, R., Mucaj, A., Lacalaprice, F., Solenghi, M., Principi, F., Tiano, L. and Littarru, G.P. (2005). "Coenzyme Q10 improves contractility of dysfunctional myocardium in chronic heart failure." *Biofactors 25*(1-4): 137-45.

Beltramo, E., Berrone, E., Buttiglieri, S. and Porta, M. (2004). "Thiamine and benfotiamine prevent increased apoptosis in endothelial cells and pericytes cultured in high glucose." *Diabetes Metab Res Rev 20*(4): 330-6.

Biswas, S., Ray, M., Misra, S., Dutta, D.P. and Ray, S. (1997). "Selective inhibition of mitochondrial respiration and glycolysis in human leukaemic leucocytes by methylglyoxal." *Biochem J 323 (Pt 2)*: 343-8.

Black, H.S. (2004). "Mechanisms of pro- and antioxidation." *J Nutr 134*(11): 3169S-70S.

Block, K.I. and Mead, M.N. (2003). "Vitamin C in alternative cancer treatment: historical background." *Integr Cancer Ther 2*(2): 147-54.

Booth, I.R., Ferguson, G.P., Miller, S., Li, C., Gunasekera, B. and Kinghorn, S. (2003). "Bacterial production of methylglyoxal: a survival strategy or death by misadventure?" *Biochem Soc Trans 31*(Pt 6): 1406-8.

Brownlee, M. (2001). "Biochemistry and molecular cell biology of diabetic complications." *Nature 414*(6865): 813-20.

Bruce, W.R., Furrer, R., Shangari, N., O'Brien, P.J., Medline, A. and Wang, Y. (2003). "Marginal dietary thiamin deficiency induces the formation of colonic aberrant crypt foci (ACF) in rats." *Cancer Lett 202*(2): 125-9.

Bryer, S.C. and Goldfarb, A.H. (2006). "Effect of high dose vitamin C supplementation on muscle soreness, damage, function, and oxidative stress to eccentric exercise." *Int J Sport Nutr Exerc Metab 16*(3): 270-80.

Calingasan, N.Y., Park, L.C., Calo, L.L., Trifiletti, R.R., Gandy, S.E. and Gibson, G.E. (1998). "Induction of nitric oxide synthase and microglial responses precede selective cell death induced by chronic impairment of oxidative metabolism." *Am J Pathol 153*(2): 599-610.

Carbone, D.L., Doorn, J.A., Kiebler, Z. and Petersen, D.R. (2005). "Cysteine modification by lipid peroxidation products inhibits protein disulfide isomerase." *Chem Res Toxicol 18*(8): 1324-31.

Caro, A.A. and Cederbaum, A.I. (2007). "Role of intracellular calcium and phospholipase A2 in arachidonic acid-induced toxicity in liver cells overexpressing CYP2E1." *Arch Biochem Biophys 457*(2): 252-63.

Chan, T.S., Shangari, N., Wilson, J.X., Chan, H., Butterworth, R.F. and O'Brien, P.J. (2005). "The biosynthesis of ascorbate protects isolated rat hepatocytes from cumene hydroperoxide-mediated oxidative stress." *Free Radic Biol Med 38*(7): 867-73.

Ciapaite, J., Bakker, S.J., Diamant, M., van Eikenhorst, G., Heine, R.J., Westerhoff, H.V. and Krab, K. (2006). "Metabolic control of mitochondrial properties by adenine nucleotide translocator determines palmitoyl-CoA effects. Implications for a mechanism linking obesity and type 2 diabetes." *Febs J 273*(23): 5288-302.

Ciapaite, J., Bakker, S.J., Van Eikenhorst, G., Wagner, M.J., Teerlink, T., Schalkwijk, C.G., Fodor, M., Ouwens, D.M., Diamant, M., Heine, R.J., Westerhoff, H.V. and Krab, K. (2007). "Functioning of oxidative phosphorylation in liver mitochondria of high-fat diet fed rats." *Biochim Biophys Acta 1772*(3): 307-16.

Close, G.L., Ashton, T., Cable, T., Doran, D., Holloway, C., McArdle, F. and MacLaren, D.P. (2006). "Ascorbic acid supplementation does not attenuate post-exercise muscle soreness following muscle-damaging exercise but may delay the recovery process." *Br J Nutr 95*(5): 976-81.

Cook, S. and Hess, O.M. (2005). "Homocysteine and B vitamins." *Handb Exp Pharmacol*(170): 325-38.

Crispen, P.L., Uzzo, R.G., Golovine, K., Makhov, P., Pollack, A., Horwitz, E.M., Greenberg, R.E. and Kolenko, V.M. (2007). "Vitamin E succinate inhibits NF-kappaB and prevents the development of a metastatic phenotype in prostate cancer cells: implications for chemoprevention." *Prostate 67*(6): 582-90.

Crouch, J.Y. and Solomon, L.R. (1989). "Inhibition of rat liver transaminases by low levels of acetaldehyde and the pharmacologic effects of B6 vitamers." *Biochem Pharmacol 38*(20): 3431-7.

D'Adamo, M., Perego, L., Cardellini, M., Marini, M.A., Frontoni, S., Andreozzi, F., Sciacqua, A., Lauro, D., Sbraccia, P., Federici, M., Paganelli, M., Pontiroli, A.E., Lauro, R., Perticone, F., Folli, F. and Sesti, G. (2004). "The -866A/A genotype in the promoter of the human uncoupling protein 2 gene is associated with insulin resistance and increased risk of type 2 diabetes." *Diabetes 53*(7): 1905-10.

de Vries, J.E., Vork, M.M., Roemen, T.H., de Jong, Y.F., Cleutjens, J.P., van der Vusse, G.J. and van Bilsen, M. (1997). "Saturated but not mono-unsaturated fatty acids induce apoptotic cell death in neonatal rat ventricular myocytes." *J Lipid Res 38*(7): 1384-94.

Demozay, D., Rocchi, S., Mas, J.C., Grillo, S., Pirola, L., Chavey, C. and Van Obberghen, E. (2004). "Fatty aldehyde dehydrogenase: potential role in oxidative stress protection and regulation of its gene expression by insulin." *J Biol Chem 279*(8): 6261-70.

Dhamrait, S.S., Stephens, J.W., Cooper, J.A., Acharya, J., Mani, A.R., Moore, K., Miller, G.J., Humphries, S.E., Hurel, S.J. and Montgomery, H.E. (2004). "Cardiovascular risk in healthy men and markers of oxidative stress in diabetic men are associated with common variation in the gene for uncoupling protein 2." *Eur Heart J 25*(6): 468-75.

Di Paola, M. and Lorusso, M. (2006). "Interaction of free fatty acids with mitochondria: coupling, uncoupling and permeability transition." *Biochim Biophys Acta 1757*(9-10): 1330-7.

Di Paola, M., Zaccagnino, P., Oliveros-Celis, C. and Lorusso, M. (2006). "Arachidonic acid induces specific membrane permeability increase in heart mitochondria." *FEBS Lett 580*(3): 775-81.

Di Sario, A., Candelaresi, C., Omenetti, A. and Benedetti, A. (2007). "Vitamin E in chronic liver diseases and liver fibrosis." *Vitam Horm 76*: 551-73.

Dogru Pekiner, B., Das Evcimen, N., Ulusu, N.N., Bali, M. and Karasu, C. (2003). "Effects of vitamin E on microsomal Ca(2+) -ATPase activity and calcium levels in streptozotocin-induced diabetic rat kidney." *Cell Biochem Funct 21*(2): 177-82.

Eswaran, D., Ali, M.S., Shenoy, B.C., Korotchkina, L.G., Roche, T.E. and Patel, M.S. (1995). "Arginine-239 in the beta subunit is at or near the active site of bovine pyruvate dehydrogenase." *Biochim Biophys Acta 1252*(2): 203-8.

Ewaschuk, J.B., Naylor, J.M. and Zello, G.A. (2005). "D-lactate in human and ruminant metabolism." *J Nutr 135*(7): 1619-25.

Feldstein, A.E., Werneburg, N.W., Canbay, A., Guicciardi, M.E., Bronk, S.F., Rydzewski, R., Burgart, L.J. and Gores, G.J. (2004). "Free fatty acids promote hepatic lipotoxicity by stimulating TNF-alpha expression via a lysosomal pathway." *Hepatology 40*(1): 185-94.

Feldstein, A.E., Werneburg, N.W., Li, Z., Bronk, S.F. and Gores, G.J. (2006). "Bax inhibition protects against free fatty acid-induced lysosomal permeabilization." *Am J Physiol Gastrointest Liver Physiol 290*(6): G1339-46.

Floyd, R.A., Kotake, Y., Hensley, K., Nakae, D. and Konishi, Y. (2002). "Reactive oxygen species in choline deficiency induced carcinogenesis and nitrone inhibition." *Mol Cell Biochem 234-235*(1-2): 195-203.

Forouhi, N.G., Harding, A.H., Allison, M., Sandhu, M.S., Welch, A., Luben, R., Bingham, S., Khaw, K.T. and Wareham, N.J. (2007). "Elevated serum ferritin levels predict new-onset type 2 diabetes: results from the EPIC-Norfolk prospective study." *Diabetologia 50*(5): 949-56.

Frederiks, W.M. and Vreeling-Sindelarova, H. (2002). "Ultrastructural localization of xanthine oxidoreductase activity in isolated rat liver cells." *Acta Histochem 104*(1): 29-37.

Furuno, T., Kanno, T., Arita, K., Asami, M., Utsumi, T., Doi, Y., Inoue, M. and Utsumi, K. (2001). "Roles of long chain fatty acids and carnitine in mitochondrial membrane permeability transition." *Biochem Pharmacol 62*(8): 1037-46.

Gaby, A.R. (2007). "Natural approaches to epilepsy." *Altern Med Rev 12*(1): 9-24.

Galassi, A., Reynolds, K. and He, J. (2006). "Metabolic syndrome and risk of cardiovascular disease: a meta-analysis." *Am J Med 119*(10): 812-9.

Gille, L. and Nohl, H. (2000). "The existence of a lysosomal redox chain and the role of ubiquinone." *Arch Biochem Biophys 375*(2): 347-54.

Giovannucci, E. (2003). "Nutrition, insulin, insulin-like growth factors and cancer." *Horm Metab Res 35*(11-12): 694-704.

Giovannucci, E. and Michaud, D. (2007). "The role of obesity and related metabolic disturbances in cancers of the colon, prostate, and pancreas." *Gastroenterology 132*(6): 2208-25.

Greenberg, E.R., Baron, J.A., Tosteson, T.D., Freeman, D.H., Jr., Beck, G.J., Bond, J.H., Colacchio, T.A., Coller, J.A., Frankl, H.D., Haile, R.W. and et al. (1994). "A clinical trial of antioxidant vitamins to prevent colorectal adenoma. Polyp Prevention Study Group." *N Engl J Med 331*(3): 141-7.

Guerrero-Romero, F. and Rodriguez-Moran, M. (2006). "Hypomagnesemia, oxidative stress, inflammation, and metabolic syndrome." *Diabetes Metab Res Rev 22*(6): 471-6.

Gulcin, I. (2006). "Antioxidant and antiradical activities of L-carnitine." *Life Sci 78*(8): 803-11.

Haber, C.A., Lam, T.K., Yu, Z., Gupta, N., Goh, T., Bogdanovic, E., Giacca, A. and Fantus, I.G. (2003). "N-acetylcysteine and taurine prevent hyperglycemia-induced insulin resistance in vivo: possible role of oxidative stress." *Am J Physiol Endocrinol Metab 285*(4): E744-53.

Hara, H., Hiramatsu, H. and Adachi, T. (2007). "Pyrroloquinoline quinone is a potent neuroprotective nutrient against 6-hydroxydopamine-induced neurotoxicity." *Neurochem Res 32*(3): 489-95.

Institute of Medicine (2000). Dietary reference intakes for vitamin C, vitamin E, selenium, and carotenoids. Washington, DC, National Academy Press.

Iwamoto, K., Bundo, M. and Kato, T. (2005). "Altered expression of mitochondria-related genes in postmortem brains of patients with bipolar disorder or schizophrenia, as revealed by large-scale DNA microarray analysis." *Hum Mol Genet 14*(2): 241-53.

Jain, S.K. (2007). "Vitamin B6 (pyridoxamine) supplementation and complications of diabetes." *Metabolism 56*(2): 168-71.

Jansen, G.A., van den Brink, D.M., Ofman, R., Draghici, O., Dacremont, G. and Wanders, R.J. (2001). "Identification of pristanal dehydrogenase activity in peroxisomes: conclusive evidence that the complete phytanic acid alpha-oxidation pathway is localized in peroxisomes." *Biochem Biophys Res Commun 283*(3): 674-9.

Jenab, M., Riboli, E., Cleveland, R.J., Norat, T., Rinaldi, S., Nieters, A., Biessy, C., Tjonneland, A., Olsen, A., Overvad, K., Gronbaek, H., Clavel-Chapelon, F., Boutron-Ruault, M.C., Linseisen, J., Boeing, H., Pischon, T., Trichopoulos, D., Oikonomou, E., Trichopoulou, A., Panico, S., Vineis, P., Berrino, F., Tumino, R., Masala, G., Peters, P.H., van Gils, C.H., Bueno-de-Mesquita, H.B., Ocke, M.C., Lund, E., Mendez, M.A., Tormo, M.J., Barricarte, A., Martinez-Garcia, C., Dorronsoro, M., Quiros, J.R., Hallmans, G., Palmqvist, R., Berglund, G., Manjer, J., Key, T., Allen, N.E., Bingham, S., Khaw, K.T., Cust, A. and Kaaks, R. (2007). "Serum C-peptide, IGFBP-1 and IGFBP-2 and risk of colon and rectal cancers in the European Prospective Investigation into Cancer and Nutrition." *Int J Cancer 121*(2): 368-76.

Kalpravidh, R.W., Wichit, A., Siritanaratkul, N. and Fucharoen, S. (2005). "Effect of coenzyme Q10 as an antioxidant in beta-thalassemia/Hb E patients." *Biofactors 25*(1-4): 225-34.

Kannan, K. and Jain, S.K. (2004). "Effect of vitamin B6 on oxygen radicals, mitochondrial membrane potential, and lipid peroxidation in H2O2-treated U937 monocytes." *Free Radic Biol Med 36*(4): 423-8.

Karuppagounder, S.S., Shi, Q., Xu, H. and Gibson, G.E. (2007). "Changes in inflammatory processes associated with selective vulnerability following mild impairment of oxidative metabolism." *Neurobiol Dis 26*(2): 353-62.

Kida, K., Ito, T. and Yang, S.W. (1999). Preventive nutrition; The comprehensive guide for health professionals: Effects of western diet on risk factors of chronic dsease in Asia. Totawa, New Jersey, Humana Press.

Kilhovd, B.K., Giardino, I., Torjesen, P.A., Birkeland, K.I., Berg, T.J., Thornalley, P.J., Brownlee, M. and Hanssen, K.F. (2003). "Increased serum levels of the specific AGE-compound methylglyoxal-derived hydroimidazolone in patients with type 2 diabetes." *Metabolism 52*(2): 163-7.

Kir, H.M., Dillioglugil, M.O., Tugay, M., Eraldemir, C. and Ozdogan, H.K. (2005). "Effects of vitamins E, A and D on MDA, GSH, NO levels and SOD activities in 5/6 nephrectomized rats." *Am J Nephrol 25*(5): 441-6.

Kirsch, R., Sijtsema, H.P., Tlali, M., Marais, A.D. and Hall Pde, L. (2006). "Effects of iron overload in a rat nutritional model of non-alcoholic fatty liver disease." *Liver Int 26*(10): 1258-67.

Koyama, Y., Takeishi, Y., Arimoto, T., Niizeki, T., Shishido, T., Takahashi, H., Nozaki, N., Hirono, O., Tsunoda, Y., Nitobe, J., Watanabe, T. and Kubota, I. (2007). "High serum level of pentosidine, an advanced glycation end product (AGE), is a risk factor of patients with heart failure." *J Card Fail 13*(3): 199-206.

Kuroda, J., Nakagawa, K., Yamasaki, T., Nakamura, K., Takeya, R., Kuribayashi, F., Imajoh-Ohmi, S., Igarashi, K., Shibata, Y., Sueishi, K. and Sumimoto, H. (2005). "The superoxide-producing NAD(P)H oxidase Nox4 in the nucleus of human vascular endothelial cells." *Genes Cells 10*(12): 1139-51.

Lagouge, M., Argmann, C., Gerhart-Hines, Z., Meziane, H., Lerin, C., Daussin, F., Messadeq, N., Milne, J., Lambert, P., Elliott, P., Geny, B., Laakso, M., Puigserver, P. and Auwerx, J. (2006). "Resveratrol improves mitochondrial function and protects against metabolic disease by activating SIRT1 and PGC-1alpha." *Cell 127*(6): 1109-22.

Lan, Q., Zheng, T., Shen, M., Zhang, Y., Wang, S.S., Zahm, S.H., Holford, T.R., Leaderer, B., Boyle, P. and Chanock, S. (2007). "Genetic polymorphisms in the oxidative stress pathway and susceptibility to non-Hodgkin lymphoma." *Hum Genet 121*(2): 161-8.

Larsson, S.C., Rafter, J., Holmberg, L., Bergkvist, L. and Wolk, A. (2005). "Red meat consumption and risk of cancers of the proximal colon, distal colon and rectum: the Swedish Mammography Cohort." *Int J Cancer 113*(5): 829-34.

Lee, D.H., Anderson, K.E., Harnack, L.J., Folsom, A.R. and Jacobs, D.R., Jr. (2004). "Heme iron, zinc, alcohol consumption, and colon cancer: Iowa Women's Health Study." *J Natl Cancer Inst 96*(5): 403-7.

Lee, D.H., Liu, D.Y., Jacobs, D.R., Jr., Shin, H.R., Song, K., Lee, I.K., Kim, B. and Hider, R.C. (2006). "Common presence of non-transferrin-bound iron among patients with type 2 diabetes." *Diabetes Care 29*(5): 1090-5.

Lonn, E., Yusuf, S., Arnold, M.J., Sheridan, P., Pogue, J., Micks, M., McQueen, M.J., Probstfield, J., Fodor, G., Held, C. and Genest, J., Jr. (2006). "Homocysteine lowering with folic acid and B vitamins in vascular disease." *N Engl J Med 354*(15): 1567-77.

Mahfouz, M.M. and Kummerow, F.A. (2004). "Vitamin C or Vitamin B6 supplementation prevent the oxidative stress and decrease of prostacyclin generation in homocysteinemic rats." *Int J Biochem Cell Biol 36*(10): 1919-32.

Mahmoud, K.Z. and Hijazi, A.A. (2007). "Effect of vitamin A and/or E on plasma enzymatic antioxidant systems and total antioxidant capacity of broiler chickens challenged with carbon tetrachloride." *J Anim Physiol Anim Nutr (Berl) 91*(7-8): 333-40.

Majewicz, J., Rimbach, G., Proteggente, A.R., Lodge, J.K., Kraemer, K. and Minihane, A.M. (2005). "Dietary vitamin C down-regulates inflammatory gene expression in apoE4 smokers." *Biochem Biophys Res Commun 338*(2): 951-5.

Malhi, H., Gores, G.J. and Lemasters, J.J. (2006). "Apoptosis and necrosis in the liver: a tale of two deaths?" *Hepatology 43*(2 Suppl 1): S31-44.

Marchitti, S.A., Deitrich, R.A. and Vasiliou, V. (2007). "Neurotoxicity and metabolism of the catecholamine-derived 3,4-dihydroxyphenylacetaldehyde and 3,4-dihydroxyphenyl-glycolaldehyde: the role of aldehyde dehydrogenase." *Pharmacol Rev 59*(2): 125-50.

McKeown-Eyssen, G., Holloway, C., Jazmaji, V., Bright-See, E., Dion, P. and Bruce, W.R. (1988). "A randomized trial of vitamins C and E in the prevention of recurrence of colorectal polyps." *Cancer Res 48*(16): 4701-5.

McKeown-Eyssen, G. (1994). "Epidemiology of colorectal cancer revisited: are serum triglycerides and/or plasma glucose associated with risk?" *Cancer Epidemiol Biomarkers Prev 3*(8): 687-95.

Medina, J., Fernandez-Salazar, L.I., Garcia-Buey, L. and Moreno-Otero, R. (2004). "Approach to the pathogenesis and treatment of nonalcoholic steatohepatitis." *Diabetes Care 27*(8): 2057-66.

Mehta, R. and O'Brien, P.J. (2007). "Therapeutic intracellular targets for preventing cell death with B vitamins or drugs." Weiner H., Maser E., Lindahl R., Plapp B. (Eds) *Enzymology and molecular biology of carbonyl metabolism, 13th Ed*, Purdue University Press: 113-120.

Mehta, R., Shangari, N. and O'Brien, P.J. (2007). "Preventing cell death induced by carbonyl stress, oxidative stress or mitochondrial toxins with vitamin B anti-AGE agents." *Molecular Nutrition and Food Research* (In press).

Mello, C.F., Sultana, R., Piroddi, M., Cai, J., Pierce, W.M., Klein, J.B. and Butterfield, D.A. (2007). "Acrolein induces selective protein carbonylation in synaptosomes." *Neuroscience 147*(3): 674-9.

Moldeus, P., Hogberg, J. and Orrenius, S. (1978). "Isolation and use of liver cells." *Methods Enzymol 52*: 60-71.

Murata-Kamiya, N. and Kamiya, H. (2001). "Methylglyoxal, an endogenous aldehyde, crosslinks DNA polymerase and the substrate DNA." *Nucleic Acids Res 29*(16): 3433-8.

Nascimento, M.M., Suliman, M.E., Murayama, Y., Nihi, M., Hayashi, S.Y., Stenvinkel, P., Riella, M.C. and Lindholm, B. (2006). "Effect of high-dose thiamine and pyridoxine on advanced glycation end products and other oxidative stress markers in hemodialysis patients: a randomized placebo-controlled study." *J Ren Nutr 16*(2): 119-24.

Nemerya, N.S., Khailova, L.S. and Severin, S.E. (1984). "Arginine residues in the active centers of muscle pyruvate dehydrogenase." *Biochem Int 8*(3): 369-76.

Neuschwander-Tetri, B.A. (2005). "Nonalcoholic steatohepatitis and the metabolic syndrome." *Am J Med Sci 330*(6): 326-35.

Nicholls-Grzemski, F.A., Belling, G.B., Priestly, B.G., Calder, I.C. and Burcham, P.C. (2000). "Clofibrate pretreatment in mice confers resistance against hepatic lipid peroxidation." *J Biochem Mol Toxicol 14*(6): 335-45.

Niklowitz, P., Sonnenschein, A., Janetzky, B., Andler, W. and Menke, T. (2007). "Enrichment of coenzyme Q10 in plasma and blood cells: defense against oxidative damage." *Int J Biol Sci 3*(4): 257-62.

O'Brien, P.J., Siraki, A.G. and Shangari, N. (2005). "Aldehyde sources, metabolism, molecular toxicity mechanisms, and possible effects on human health." *Crit Rev Toxicol* 35(7): 609-62.

Okada, M., Murakami, Y. and Miyamoto, E. (1997). "Glycation and inactivation of aspartate aminotransferase in diabetic rat tissues." *J Nutr Sci Vitaminol (Tokyo) 43*(4): 463-9.

Orrenius, S., Gogvadze, V. and Zhivotovsky, B. (2007). "Mitochondrial oxidative stress: implications for cell death." *Annu Rev Pharmacol Toxicol 47*: 143-83.

Ostrovtsova, S.A. (1998). "Chemical modification of lysine and arginine residues of bovine heart 2-oxoglutarate dehydrogenase: effect on the enzyme activity and regulation." *Acta Biochim Pol 45*(4): 1031-6.

Packer, L., Tritschler, H.J. and Wessel, K. (1997). "Neuroprotection by the metabolic antioxidant alpha-lipoic acid." *Free Radic Biol Med 22*(1-2): 359-78.

Parkin, D.M., Bray, F., Ferlay, J. and Pisani, P. (2005). "Global cancer statistics, 2002." *CA Cancer J Clin 55*(2): 74-108.

Pierre, F., Tache, S., Petit, C.R., Van der Meer, R. and Corpet, D.E. (2003). "Meat and cancer: haemoglobin and haemin in a low-calcium diet promote colorectal carcinogenesis at the aberrant crypt stage in rats." *Carcinogenesis 24*(10): 1683-90.

Pocernich, C.B. and Butterfield, D.A. (2003). "Acrolein inhibits NADH-linked mitochondrial enzyme activity: implications for Alzheimer's disease." *Neurotox Res 5*(7): 515-20.

Ranganathan, L.N. and Ramaratnam, S. (2005). "Vitamins for epilepsy." *Cochrane Database Syst Rev*(2): CD004304.

Ray, S., Biswas, S. and Ray, M. (1997). "Similar nature of inhibition of mitochondrial respiration of heart tissue and malignant cells by methylglyoxal. A vital clue to understand the biochemical basis of malignancy." *Mol Cell Biochem 171*(1-2): 95-103.

Riboli, E., Hunt, K.J., Slimani, N., Ferrari, P., Norat, T., Fahey, M., Charrondiere, U.R., Hemon, B., Casagrande, C., Vignat, J., Overvad, K., Tjonneland, A., Clavel-Chapelon, F., Thiebaut, A., Wahrendorf, J., Boeing, H., Trichopoulos, D., Trichopoulou, A., Vineis, P., Palli, D., Bueno-De-Mesquita, H.B., Peeters, P.H., Lund, E., Engeset, D., Gonzalez, C.A., Barricarte, A., Berglund, G., Hallmans, G., Day, N.E., Key, T.J., Kaaks, R. and Saracci, R. (2002). "European Prospective Investigation into Cancer and Nutrition (EPIC): study populations and data collection." *Public Health Nutr 5*(6B): 1113-24.

Riccioni, G., Barbara, M., Bucciarelli, T., di Ilio, C. and D'Orazio, N. (2007). "Antioxidant vitamin supplementation in asthma." *Ann Clin Lab Sci 37*(1): 96-101.

Riccioni, G., Bucciarelli, T., Mancini, B., Corradi, F., Di Ilio, C., Mattei, P.A. and D'Orazio, N. (2007). "Antioxidant vitamin supplementation in cardiovascular diseases." *Ann Clin Lab Sci 37*(1): 89-95.

Rogers, L.K., Gupta, S., Welty, S.E., Hansen, T.N. and Smith, C.V. (2002). "Nuclear and nucleolar glutathione reductase, peroxidase, and transferase activities in livers of male and female Fischer-344 rats." *Toxicol Sci 69*(1): 279-85.

Roth, R.A., Luyendyk, J.P., Maddox, J.F. and Ganey, P.E. (2003). "Inflammation and drug idiosyncrasy--is there a connection?" *J Pharmacol Exp Ther 307*(1): 1-8.

Sandhu, J.K., Pandey, S., Ribecco-Lutkiewicz, M., Monette, R., Borowy-Borowski, H., Walker, P.R. and Sikorska, M. (2003). "Molecular mechanisms of glutamate neurotoxicity in mixed cultures of NT2-derived neurons and astrocytes: protective effects of coenzyme Q10." *J Neurosci Res 72*(6): 691-703.

Segi, M., Kurihara, M. and Tskahara, Y. (1966). Cancer mortality for selected sites in 24 countries. Sendai, Japan, Department of Public Health, Tohoku University School of Medicine.

Seidler, N.W. and Kowalewski, C. (2003). "Methylglyoxal-induced glycation affects protein topography." *Arch Biochem Biophys 410*(1): 149-54.

Sen, C.K., Khanna, S., Rink, C. and Roy, S. (2007). "Tocotrienols: the emerging face of natural vitamin E." *Vitam Horm 76*: 203-61.

Sesink, A.L., Termont, D.S., Kleibeuker, J.H. and Van der Meer, R. (2001). "Red meat and colon cancer: dietary haem-induced colonic cytotoxicity and epithelial hyperproliferation are inhibited by calcium." *Carcinogenesis 22*(10): 1653-9.

Shangari, N., Depeint, F., Furrer, R., Bruce, W.R. and O'Brien, P.J. (2005). "The effects of partial thiamin deficiency and oxidative stress (i.e., glyoxal and methylglyoxal) on the levels of alpha-oxoaldehyde plasma protein adducts in Fischer 344 rats." *FEBS Lett 579*(25): 5596-602.

Sheline, C.T. and Choi, D.W. (2004). "Cu2+ toxicity inhibition of mitochondrial dehydrogenases in vitro and in vivo." *Ann Neurol 55*(5): 645-53.

Sheline, C.T. and Wei, L. (2006). "Free radical-mediated neurotoxicity may be caused by inhibition of mitochondrial dehydrogenases in vitro and in vivo." *Neuroscience 140*(1): 235-46.

Sidoti, A., Antognelli, C., Rinaldi, C., D'Angelo, R., Dattola, V., Girlanda, P., Talesa, V. and Amato, A. (2007). "Glyoxalase I A111E, paraoxonase 1 Q192R and L55M polymorphisms: susceptibility factors of multiple sclerosis?" *Mult Scler 13*(4): 446-53.

Singh, R.B., Niaz, M.A., Kumar, A., Sindberg, C.D., Moesgaard, S. and Littarru, G.P. (2005). "Effect on absorption and oxidative stress of different oral Coenzyme Q10 dosages and intake strategy in healthy men." *Biofactors 25*(1-4): 219-24.

Singh, U. and Devaraj, S. (2007). "Vitamin E: inflammation and atherosclerosis." *Vitam Horm 76*: 519-49.

Siraki, A.G., Pourahmad, J., Chan, T.S., Khan, S. and O'Brien, P.J. (2002). "Endogenous and endobiotic induced reactive oxygen species formation by isolated hepatocytes." *Free Radic Biol Med 32*(1): 2-10.

Stadler, N., Eggermann, J., Voo, S., Kranz, A. and Waltenberger, J. (2007). "Smoking-induced monocyte dysfunction is reversed by vitamin C supplementation in vivo." *Arterioscler Thromb Vasc Biol 27*(1): 120-6.

Stephens, J.W., Gable, D.R., Hurel, S.J., Miller, G.J., Cooper, J.A. and Humphries, S.E. (2006). "Increased plasma markers of oxidative stress are associated with coronary heart disease in males with diabetes mellitus and with 10-year risk in a prospective sample of males." *Clin Chem 52*(3): 446-52.

Sureda, A., Batle, J.M., Tauler, P., Aguilo, A., Cases, N., Tur, J.A. and Pons, A. (2004). "Hypoxia/reoxygenation and vitamin C intake influence NO synthesis and antioxidant defenses of neutrophils." *Free Radic Biol Med 37*(11): 1744-55.

Susa, N., Ueno, S., Furukawa, Y. and Sugiyama, M. (1996). "Protective effect of vitamin E on chromium (VI)-induced cytotoxicity and lipid peroxidation in primary cultures of rat hepatocytes." *Arch Toxicol 71*(1-2): 20-4.

Targonsky, E.D., Dai, F., Koshkin, V., Karaman, G.T., Gyulkhandanyan, A.V., Zhang, Y., Chan, C.B. and Wheeler, M.B. (2006). "alpha-lipoic acid regulates AMP-activated protein kinase and inhibits insulin secretion from beta cells." *Diabetologia 49*(7): 1587-98.

Thomson, A.D. and Marshall, E.J. (2006). "The treatment of patients at risk of developing Wernicke's encephalopathy in the community." *Alcohol Alcohol 41*(2): 159-67.

Thornalley, P.J. and Stern, A. (1984). "The effect of glyceraldehydes on red cells. Haemoglobin status, oxidative metabolism and glycolysis." *Biochim Biophys Acta* 804: 308-23.

Thornalley, P.J. (1994). "Methyglyoxal, glyoxalases and the development of diabetic complications." *Amino Acids 6*: 15-23.

Thornalley, P.J., Jahan, I. and Ng, R. (2001). "Suppression of the accumulation of triosephosphates and increased formation of methylglyoxal in human red blood cells during hyperglycaemia by thiamine in vitro." *J Biochem (Tokyo) 129*(4): 543-9.

Thornalley, P.J. (2003). "Glyoxalase I--structure, function and a critical role in the enzymatic defence against glycation." *Biochem Soc Trans 31*(Pt 6): 1343-8.

Tosic, M., Ott, J., Barral, S., Bovet, P., Deppen, P., Gheorghita, F., Matthey, M.L., Parnas, J., Preisig, M., Saraga, M., Solida, A., Timm, S., Wang, A.G., Werge, T., Cuenod, M. and Do, K.Q. (2006). "Schizophrenia and oxidative stress: glutamate cysteine ligase modifier as a susceptibility gene." *Am J Hum Genet 79*(3): 586-92.

Traber, M.G. (2007). "Heart disease and single-vitamin supplementation." *Am J Clin Nutr 85*(1): 293S-9S.

Tran, T.T., Naigamwalla, D., Oprescu, A.I., Lam, L., McKeown-Eyssen, G., Bruce, W.R. and Giacca, A. (2006). "Hyperinsulinemia, but not other factors associated with insulin resistance, acutely enhances colorectal epithelial proliferation in vivo." *Endocrinology 147*(4): 1830-7.

Tukov, F.F., Maddox, J.F., Amacher, D.E., Bobrowski, W.F., Roth, R.A. and Ganey, P.E. (2006). "Modeling inflammation-drug interactions in vitro: a rat Kupffer cell-hepatocyte coculture system." *Toxicol In Vitro 20*(8): 1488-99.

Unger, R.H. (2002). "Lipotoxic diseases." *Annu Rev Med 53*: 319-36.

Vander Jagt, D.L. and Hunsaker, L.A. (2003). "Methylglyoxal metabolism and diabetic complications: roles of aldose reductase, glyoxalase-I, betaine aldehyde dehydrogenase and 2-oxoaldehyde dehydrogenase." *Chem Biol Interact 143-144*: 341-51.

Vangala, S. and Tonelli, A. (2007). "Biomarkers, metabonomics and drug development: can inborne errors of metabolism hrlp us understand drug toxicity?" *In Press*.

Varanasi, U., Chu, R., Chu, S., Espinosa, R., LeBeau, M.M. and Reddy, J.K. (1994). "Isolation of the human peroxisomal acyl-CoA oxidase gene: organization, promoter analysis, and chromosomal localization." *Proc Natl Acad Sci U S A 91*(8): 3107-11.

Vartanyan, L.S., Gurevich, S.M., Kozachenko, A.I., Nagler, L.G., Lozovskaya, E.L. and Burlakova, E.B. (2000). "Changes in superoxide production rate and in superoxide dismutase and glutathione peroxidase activities in subcellular organelles in mouse liver under exposure to low doses of low-intensity radiation." *Biochemistry (Mosc) 65*(4): 442-6.

Vineis, P., Veglia, F., Garte, S., Malaveille, C., Matullo, G., Dunning, A., Peluso, M., Airoldi, L., Overvad, K., Raaschou-Nielsen, O., Clavel-Chapelon, F., Linseisen, J., Kaaks, R., Boeing, H., Trichopoulou, A., Palli, D., Crosignani, P., Tumino, R., Panico, S., Bueno-De-Mesquita, H., Peeters, P., Lund, E., Gonzalez, C., Martinez, C., Dorronsoro, M., Barricarte, A., Navarro, C., Quiros, J., Berglund, G., Jarvholm, B., Day, N., Key, T., Saracci, R., Riboli, E. and Autrup, H. (2007). "Genetic susceptibility according to three metabolic pathways in cancers of the lung and bladder and in myeloid leukemias in nonsmokers." *Ann Oncol.*

Wanders, R.J., Groen, A.K., Van Roermund, C.W. and Tager, J.M. (1984). "Factors determining the relative contribution of the adenine-nucleotide translocator and the ADP-regenerating system to the control of oxidative phosphorylation in isolated rat-liver mitochondria." *Eur J Biochem 142*(2): 417-24.

Wanders, R.J. and Tager, J.M. (1998). "Lipid metabolism in peroxisomes in relation to human disease." *Mol Aspects Med 19*(2): 69-154.

Wang, C., Zhang, Y., Liang, J., Shan, G., Wang, Y. and Shi, Q. (2006). "Impacts of ascorbic acid and thiamine supplementation at different concentrations on lead toxicity in testis." *Clin Chim Acta 370*(1-2): 82-8.

Wang, H., Chu, W.S., Lu, T., Hasstedt, S.J., Kern, P.A. and Elbein, S.C. (2004). "Uncoupling protein-2 polymorphisms in type 2 diabetes, obesity, and insulin secretion." *Am J Physiol Endocrinol Metab 286*(1): E1-7.

Wang, J., Ruotsalainen, S., Moilanen, L., Lepisto, P., Laakso, M. and Kuusisto, J. (2007). "The metabolic syndrome predicts cardiovascular mortality: a 13-year follow-up study in elderly non-diabetic Finns." *Eur Heart J 28*(7): 857-64.

Ward, R.A. and McLeish, K.R. (2004). "Methylglyoxal: a stimulus to neutrophil oxygen radical production in chronic renal failure?" *Nephrol Dial Transplant 19*(7): 1702-7.

Weber, C.A. and Ernst, M.E. (2006). "Antioxidants, supplements, and Parkinson's disease." *Ann Pharmacother 40*(5): 935-8.

Weltman, M.D., Farrell, G.C., Hall, P., Ingelman-Sundberg, M. and Liddle, C. (1998). "Hepatic cytochrome P450 2E1 is increased in patients with nonalcoholic steatohepatitis." *Hepatology 27*(1): 128-33.

Wierzbicki, A.S. (2007). "Homocysteine and cardiovascular disease: a review of the evidence." *Diab Vasc Dis Res 4*(2): 143-50.

Witte, K.K. and Clark, A.L. (2006). "Micronutrients and their supplementation in chronic cardiac failure. An update beyond theoretical perspectives." *Heart Fail Rev 11*(1): 65-74.

World Cancer Research Fund and American Institute for Cancer Research (1997). *Food, nutrition and the prevention of cancer: a global perspective.* Washington, DC, American Institute for Cancer Research.

Wu, J.H., Ward, N.C., Indrawan, A.P., Almeida, C.A., Hodgson, J.M., Proudfoot, J.M., Puddey, I.B. and Croft, K.D. (2007). "Effects of alpha-tocopherol and mixed tocopherol supplementation on markers of oxidative stress and inflammation in type 2 diabetes." *Clin Chem 53*(3): 511-9.

Yao, D., Shi, W., Gou, Y., Zhou, X., Yee Aw, T., Zhou, Y. and Liu, Z. (2005). "Fatty acid-mediated intracellular iron translocation: a synergistic mechanism of oxidative injury." *Free Radic Biol Med 39*(10): 1385-98.

Yasuno, K., Ando, S., Misumi, S., Makino, S., Kulski, J.K., Muratake, T., Kaneko, N., Amagane, H., Someya, T., Inoko, H., Suga, H., Kanemoto, K. and Tamiya, G. (2007). "Synergistic association of mitochondrial uncoupling protein (UCP) genes with schizophrenia." *Am J Med Genet B Neuropsychiatr Genet 144*(2): 250-5.

In: Micronutrients and Health Research
Editor: Takumi Yoshida, pp. 181-205

ISBN: 978-1-60456-056-5
© 2008 Nova Science Publishers, Inc.

Chapter V

ADDRESSING CLINICAL QUERIES FOR MICRONUTRIENT SUPPLEMENTATION IN THE MANAGEMENT OF DISEASES AND MEDICAL CONDITIONS: *WHAT CAN I TELL MY PATIENT?*

Deborah Ellen (Boyko) Wildish
ARAMARK Canada Ltd. at the Toronto Rehabilitation Institute, Toronto, ON

ABSTRACT

The high prevalence of research related to micronutrients (i.e. vitamins and minerals) warrants attention, especially when current scientific guidelines such as dietary reference intakes (DRIs) for micronutrient requirements are geared to healthy populations. This poses a dilemma for health professionals who care for individuals with various diseases and medical conditions which are further complicated by treatments. Answers for many clinical queries about micronutrient supplementation remain ambiguous and health care recipients are caught in the middle while the media exacerbates the situation. Clinical efficacy for (safe) supplementation with micronutrients requires sufficient evidence, relevant to the specific clinical situation and tailored for a given individual. It requires weighing risks versus benefits. Since studies are not typically powered to assess risks, potential harm may be under-assessed or shared as anecdotal reports or singular case studies. Any purported benefits must translate into meaningful clinical outcomes, rather than endpoints (e.g. intermediate biochemical markers) of questionable significance. Megadoses of individual micronutrients require special consideration as they can cause relative deficiency of other micronutrients and result in detrimental health effects. Health professionals must ensure that their sources of evidence meet high standards of credibility because they are accountable for their micronutrient recommendations. Evidence for micronutrient supplementation must be sought from multiple perspectives, including disease etiology, treatment and prognosis. This chapter describes a learning journey, with five central goals: 1. constructing clinical queries related to micronutrients. 2. locating relevant and high quality evidence. 3. assessing whether there is sufficient evidence for micronutrient supplementation. 4. identifying and bridging gaps in the existing body of knowledge. 5. applying knowledge when counseling a patient about micronutrient supplements.

INTRODUCTION

This chapter consists of a collection of dietitian experiences and insights derived from engagement in projects that reviewed the literature to answer specific treatment questions about micronutrients for the care of adult patients. Some of these projects have been published; while other projects have been cited as *unpublished reviews* (to date).

It is essential to understand that only glimpses of these projects have been included to illustrate various points within this chapter. Whenever references have been cited, these references should only be viewed as examples and *not* as the most recent, best reference(s) or an exhaustive set of supporting references.

The author's role in all of these projects has varied, often working with dietitians to brainstorm micronutrient projects with potential applications to their area of patient practice. Oftentimes the role involved providing advice and direction, especially when barriers arose (e.g. developing the project plan or how to limit the project's scope).

Gray and Gray [1] have described the steps in locating the best evidence: formulating the clinical query; performing a literature review; appraising the evidence; applying the results and assessing the outcome. It has been estimated that up to 40% of clinical decision-making is not supported by research evidence [2].

Constructing Clinical Queries Related to Micronutrients

The first step is to construct a clinical query that is of *intense interest* to the health professional undertaking the project. If the clinical query is not sufficiently intriguing to sustain the effort required, the project may be abandoned. The most enlightening clinical queries arise from daily clinical practice. Every day, health professionals struggle with gaps in knowledge which impact clinical decision-making and dialogue with patients. With respect to micronutrients, many clinical queries remain unanswered or study results are conflicting. Dietary reference intakes (DRIs) are primarily geared to healthy populations [3]; therefore, much is to be learned about micronutrient supplementation for prevention or management of diseases and medical conditions.

Secondly, the clinical query must be *relevant* and *applicable* to patients in the practice setting. This will help ensure that the time investment yields useful results which can be implemented in patient care, for both treatment and education. The focus is measurable outcomes, which will satisfy organizational requirements for effectiveness. Such projects may be supported as quality enhancement projects or professional development activities, which can be linked to corporate reporting frameworks.

Different types of clinical queries have been matched with the most appropriate study design and begin with formulating PICO questions [1, 2, 4-6].

P = **population with a clinical problem**
I = **intervention or exposure**
C = **comparator intervention or exposure (may not apply)**
O = **outcomes**

Table 1 provides two examples of PICO questions for vitamin E and vitamin C.

Table 1. Examples of PICO Questions Related to Treatment

Example 1:
Should vitamin E supplements be recommended for *secondary* prevention of heart attack or stroke?
    P = Patients who have suffered a heart attack or stroke
    I = Vitamin E supplement (in addition to diet)
    C = No Vitamin E supplement (diet alone)
    O= Decreased, increased or no effect on incidence of recurrent heart attack or stroke

Example 2:
Are vitamin C supplements required for *chronic* wound healing?
    P = Patients who present with chronic wounds
    I = Vitamin C supplement (in addition to diet)
    C = No Vitamin C supplement (diet alone)
    O = Decreased, increased or no effect on wound healing time

These PICO questions form the basis of the micronutrient project plan (refer to Table 2).

The test of a *focused* clinical query is its precision in locating evidence. The clinical query should be as *narrow* as possible to locate *available* evidence. Wilk's initial scan of the literature found several topics related to vitamin D: diabetes, kidney function, colon cancer, obesity, cardiovascular function, hypertension, bone health, osteoporosis, and falls and fractures [7]. Wilk decided to narrow her project focus to vitamin D and falls prevention which enabled her to link with a corporate best practice initiative involving elderly patients undergoing active rehabilitation.

Sometimes too narrow a focus will result in negligible information. For example, Dawson [8] had questions about zinc supplementation for wound healing in patients requiring hemodialysis. This clinical query appears appropriately narrow and specific. However, following a literature review, no studies were located with any relevance to the clinical query and only three editorials were found [9-11]. In such instances, the clinical query needs to be broadened. For example, the clinical query was expanded to capture zinc supplementation for wound healing in the *general* patient population. This approach did result in locating studies related to zinc supplements and wound healing that reported mixed results [12-20].

The highest quality evidence for zinc supplementation was located in a Cochrane review, wherein six randomized controlled trials met the strict criteria for appraisal [12]. Although heterogenous designs did not allow pooling of data, two of the randomized controlled trials had analyzed the results based on serum zinc levels [13, 14]. Both of these studies used doses of zinc above the 40 mg tolerable upper intake level (UL), providing 600 mg zinc sulphate (135 mg elemental zinc) daily, divided into three doses. Neither study reported a statistically significant decrease in healing time with zinc supplements. Therefore, the Cochrane review [12] concluded that only weak evidence existed to support the benefit of oral zinc supplements for healing of leg ulcers in people with low serum zinc levels. Further research is required to determine a serum zinc concentration, below which supplemental zinc of a defined dose and duration would be of benefit to patients with leg ulcers.

This Cochrane review suggests that zinc supplements may only be beneficial for the healing of leg ulcers *when* low serum zinc levels exist. However, the next challenge is how to interpret this general evidence for potential application in a specific patient population. For patients requiring hemodialysis, various factors associated with end-stage renal disease need to be considered. For example: renal disease, hemodialysis and drug treatment may change zinc requirements and impact serum zinc levels, which have been reported to be lower among hemodialysis patients [21-24]. Several studies, of varying quality, have suggested a combination of contributing factors: poor nutritional intake [25-27], decreased zinc absorption [28-30], increased zinc excretion [31] and altered body zinc distribution [26].

Posing clinical queries is an iterative cycle of inductive and deductive reasoning. It begins with formulating broad questions which are broken down into a specific set of answerable queries. It is common for new questions to emerge, just when the health professional thought the project was complete. However, these new questions can form the basis of the next project. "Stoppers" must be plugged in at various points to prevent the project from becoming unmanageable. A sample micronutrient project plan has been outlined to illustrate the many angles of questioning that a health professional must address (see Table 2).

Locating Relevant and High Quality Evidence

All micronutrient projects should begin with a thorough review of the dietary reference intakes chapter specific to that micronutrient [3, 33, 37-40]. This will help answer many of the questions in the micronutrient project plan (Table 2) and provide a framework for pursuing the micronutrient project.

This chapter will not address how to conduct a comprehensive literature review because many health professionals are fortunate to have librarian assistance. However, one important point of emphasis is that *multiple databases* should be searched, beginning with high quality databases (e.g. Best Evidence database) [41].

Table 2. Micronutrient Project Plan for Vitamin C Supplementation in Patients Requiring *Chronic* Wound Healing

Main Clinical Query:
Are vitamin C supplements required for *chronic* wound healing?

Definition: Chronic wounds encompass: diabetic ulcers, venous stasis and arterial ulcers, and pressure sores [32].

Potential Treatment Effect: a tangible clinical benefit for chronic wound healing is decreased healing time with vitamin C supplementation.

Subset of Clinical Queries:

What are the indications and contraindications for vitamin C supplementation?

1. What is the role of vitamin C? (Essential background information.)
a) For general health maintenance?
b) For prevention of infection?
c) For various adult age groups e.g. changes in metabolism with aging?
Review the dietary reference intakes (DRIs) for Vitamin C [3, 33].

2. What is the best biochemical measure to assess vitamin C status?
Collaborate with an expert to determine the best measures of vitamin C status.

3. Under what conditions is vitamin C supplementation indicated?
a) When there is a measured deficit in vitamin C stores?
b) When a patient is eating poorly and has an inadequate oral vitamin C intake?
   Liaise with a dietitian who can perform a comprehensive nutritional assessment[34].
c) When other factors result in an increased vitamin C requirement? (Clarify each factor.)
   For example: Studies have indicated that smokers have a higher metabolic turnover of vitamin C (due to increased oxidative stress) and their recommended dietary allowance (RDA) is higher [3].
d) When a patient presents with chronic wounds, what ulcer stages (if any) might be responsive to vitamin C supplementation?
e) When would a change in practice be warranted (i.e. outcome of sufficient magnitude)?
   For example: Vitamin C supplements decrease wound healing time by at least 3 days.

Table 2. Micronutrient Project Plan for Vitamin C Supplementation in Patients Requiring *Chronic* Wound Healing (continued)

4. Under what conditions is vitamin C supplementation contraindicated?

a) When vitamin C stores are *normal* <u>and</u> the patient is eating well?

b) For safety, what is the tolerable upper intake level (UL) for vitamin C?

c) What potential adverse effects might occur and under what conditions?

> *For example: large doses of vitamin C have been reported to negatively impact both copper and vitamin B12 status [3].*

d) Are specific patient populations at particular risk?

> *For example: the tradition of restricting vitamin C supplements for individuals prone to kidney stones (to below 100 mg daily) was reviewed and only weak evidence was located to support this practice [35].*

5. What is the best type of vitamin C supplement?

a) Oral supplement? (versus intravenous)

b) Does potency of supplements vary according to their forms or sources?

c) Should vitamin C be supplemented alone or in combination with other nutrients?

d) Do these nutrients promote or impede vitamin C absorption or retention?

Collaborate with a pharmacist to integrate their expertise.

6. What dose of vitamin C is recommended?

a) What is the *minimum* dose of vitamin C that can produce the desired treatment effect?

b) Is this dose within the dietary reference intakes (DRIs) range or is this a megadose?

c) What conditions promote or impede effectiveness of vitamin C supplementation?

> *For example: independent of vitamin C intake, proton pump inhibitors have been reported to reduce bioavailability of vitamin C [36].*

d) When are dose adjustments required?

> *For example: is the patient receiving other supplements containing vitamin C (e.g. multiple vitamins with minerals) or enteral supplements fortified with vitamin C?*

7. What duration of vitamin C supplementation is required?

a) What is the *minimum* duration of vitamin C supplementation required?

b) Will wounds recur without continued vitamin C supplementation?

8. How can these findings be applied to patient practice?

a) Are the findings important and relevant to my patients?

b) Is it feasible to apply these findings to my patients (e.g. budget for supplements)?

In collaboration with the health professional team, formulate recommendations for implementation in patient care and develop guidelines for patient education.

A systematic literature review involves filtering literature. Since this process is quite complex and can be very subjective, it is recommended that full abstracts be reviewed, rather than a simplistic review of titles. The goal is to carefully select the most appropriate information sources for thorough review.

It may be helpful to have two or more individuals determine whether a given abstract should lead to retrieval and review of the full article or study. The pairing of reviewers may decrease the rate of false-negative responses for article selection [42]. Sometimes, it is necessary to retrieve the full article before a definitive decision can be made regarding its potential relevance to the micronutrient project plan. As well, articles often provide enlightening discussions or helpful secondary references.

Table 3 provides a template, which can be further customized to the micronutrient project plan, to assist with the screening and selection of appropriate articles.

Various weaknesses are common to micronutrient studies. Potential *confounding factors* arise whenever more than one micronutrient is studied within the same treatment. In such instances, it is difficult to draw conclusions about the impact of a single micronutrient. For example, when the author reviewed the literature to determine the impact of antioxidants on the effectiveness of oncology treatment (radiation or chemotherapy), antioxidants were frequently studied as a group of micronutrients and treatments varied between studies [32]. Therefore, it is not surprising that conflicting evidence was reported, as to whether antioxidants decrease [43-45] or increase [46-49] the effectiveness of and tolerance to oncology treatment.

Complementary or inverse relationships between micronutrients, may require that more than one micronutrient be studied simultaneously. Wilk [7] attempted to review vitamin D supplementation in isolation from calcium supplementation for bone health and falls prevention. However, the literature review located many studies whose treatments combined vitamin D and calcium supplements [50-62]. One study has suggested that vitamin D plus calcium - not vitamin D alone, prevents osteoporotic fractures in the elderly [63]. The micronutrient relationships in bone health could be further expanded to include many other nutrients. For example, vitamin K is essential for the function of bone proteins and one observational study has reported an association between high levels of dietary vitamin K and a decreased risk of hip fracture [64, 65]. However, the findings of subsequent randomized controlled trials of vitamin K are limited because they did not examine calcium or vitamin D intake in the treatment or control groups [65].

Measurement of nutritional status is very important when determining the effects of micronutrient supplementation. For example, a malnourished patient is suspected to present with decreased stores of all micronutrients. Therefore, it would be anticipated that such patients would have greater benefit from micronutrient supplementation, if no metabolic aberrations exist (e.g. inflammatory responses associated with disease and injury). All micronutrient studies should begin with a *comprehensive* nutritional assessment [34] by a registered dietitian. At minimum, the baseline assessment must include a diet history, weight history and relevant biochemical measures for each subject, prior to study commencement. Knowledge of recent and marked changes in weight or appetite, in the weeks or months prior to the study, may warrant that the subject be excluded from the proposed study. Such patients may exhibit a heightened response to micronutrient supplementation, and biochemical measures alone may be inadequate, especially if the subject presents just below the threshold for detection of low micronutrient stores. High quality studies will also incorporate intermittent nutritional assessments at defined intervals, to assess any changes in nutritional status that may impact clinical outcomes. All studies should conclude with a nutritional assessment, so that comparisons can be drawn between baseline, intermittent and final assessments relative to any conclusions about treatment effects.

Table 3. Template for Article Selection

Factors to Review	Inclusion Criteria	Exclusion Criteria
Classify the resource according to type of article and review inclusion and exclusion criteria	Systematic Reviews of Randomized Controlled Trials (e.g. Best Evidence database)	None
	Meta-Analysis	Aggregated the results of weak studies or studies with heterogeneous designs
	Randomized Controlled Trial	Serious design flaws
	Review Article supported by evidence	Review articles based on weak evidence (e.g. older books, commentaries) or expert opinion
	Observational Studies e.g. cohort or case-control studies	Weak study designs
	Case Studies describing potential risk of harm, adverse events, or complications	Case studies related to benefits (stronger research designs should have been utilized)
	Formal guidelines or scientific reports (e.g. dietary reference intakes) [3, 33, 37-40]	Statements or conclusions that are not supported by evidence
Relevant to Micronutrient Under Study	The name of the micronutrient is in the title of the article e.g. vitamin E or alpha-tocopherol	The project plan may exclude studies involving a group of micronutrients e.g. antioxidants
Study Population is Similar to Target Population	Studies of patients who are similar to your practice increases the likelihood of potential applications and improves the ability to generalize results	Studies involving unique groups (e.g. specific ethnicity), healthy people, a different age group, or with different medical conditions
Identifies Important and Measurable Outcomes	Focus on clinical outcomes (e.g. decreased morbidity or mortality) and tangible clinical benefits (e.g. enhanced recovery from illness)	Only examines changes in intermediate biochemical markers that cannot be linked to tangible clinical outcomes
Identifies Potential Risks	Captures any risk of harm if inappropriate supplementation (e.g. toxicity) or failure to provide adequate supplementation	None
Provides Relevant Information	May provide important background information or raise new questions	Major diversion from the micronutrient project plan

Studies of short duration may not have the capability to demonstrate any treatment effects. The author's review of the literature found that improvement in biochemical markers of micronutrient status may occur within two or three months of micronutrient supplementation; however, the most significant and complete effects were observed after six months of supplementation [32]. This suggests that the duration of micronutrient treatment (in studies) should last for a few months and perhaps much longer, to observe any significant effects.

After reviewing studies for a given micronutrient topic, it becomes readily apparent which *biochemical measurement* is considered to be a gold standard. Any other studies deviating from this gold standard may produce less valid results. For example, Gottschalk's aggregate literature review [66] determined that *plasma* retinyl esters were directly correlated with *supplemental* intake of vitamin A [67-70]. However, one study [71] was located that utilized *serum* retinol, an inferior marker, to assess biochemical changes associated with either dietary or supplemental vitamin A intake. Another point for consideration is that plasma retinyl is the gold standard for supplemental vitamin A intake; however, this same measure is *not* sensitive to changes in *dietary* intake of vitamin A [67-70].

Defined clinical endpoints that translate into tangible beneficial outcomes are the hallmark of a well-constructed, informative study. When research studies earmark intermediate clinical endpoints (e.g. some biochemical measures) these may not translate into meaningful outcomes that correlate with any real benefits.

The strength of evidence is grounded in study design and the degree to which its results are significant, important and relevant to the health professional's target patient population. Potential study errors, weaknesses or limitations must be carefully reviewed. Statistically significant results ($p < .05$) are of particular interest. Table 4 provides a checklist to help assess study quality and the strength of its findings. More importantly, it helps reviewers identify and weed out weaker studies.

Systematic reviews of randomized controlled clinical trials (e.g. Best-Evidence database), provide the strongest evidence to guide treatment decisions [4]. However, such high quality information is not widely available to answer clinical queries about micronutrients. Well-designed observational studies (e.g. cohort) provide other important information, especially when seeking information about disease prevention. Observational studies may also reveal potential adverse effects of treatment, no treatment or inappropriate treatment, all of which cannot be adequately captured in randomized controlled trials.

Assessing Whether There Is Sufficient Evidence for Micronutrient Supplementation

A hierarchy of strength of evidence has been developed for various types of clinical queries [1, 4, 72-76] . To add rigor, evidence for micronutrient supplementation should be sought from multiple perspectives, including: treatment, prognosis, risk of harm and etiology.

Table 4. Checklist to Identify Factors that Negatively Impact the Strength of Study Design and the Quality of Evidence [4, 72-76]:

o   Small sample size (inadequately powered study)
o   Study not randomized
o   Study not double-blinded
o   Diverse study groups (e.g. broad age range)
o   Unique study groups (i.e. findings cannot be generalized to your target group)
o   Major pre-treatment differences between control and intervention groups
o   Poor description of proposed treatment (failure to report and control dietary intake of micronutrients)
o   Different types or length of treatment for control and intervention groups
o   Other differences in how the groups were treated
o   Subjects were not analyzed in the group to which they were assigned
o   Baseline, intermittent and final nutritional assessment were not performed and integrated with the results
o   Failure to capture and report pre-treatment events (e.g. no mention of screening for pre-treatment events, such as subjects with major weight loss who should be excluded from the study)
o   Poorly defined research goals
o   Failure to focus goals on clinically important outcomes (e.g. benefits or risks)
o   Retrospective linking of micronutrient findings to study goals
o   Failure to utilize existing gold standard for outcome measurement
o   High dropout rates or dropouts not accounted for
o   Short duration of micronutrient treatment (compare against minimum length of micronutrient supplementation required to effect or observe changes in measurement)
o   Manipulated more than 1 treatment variable (varied doses of related micronutrients within the same treatment e.g. vitamin D, calcium, phosphorus)
o   Presence of confounding variables that may influence the treatment effects (e.g. intake of natural health products rich in the studied micronutrient)
o   Results are not statistically significant ($p<.05$)
o   Wide confidence intervals (greater likelihood of chance)
o   Small treatment effect (i.e. large number needed to treat to prevent one bad outcome)
o   Results do not link to tangible clinical outcomes (e.g. measure intermediate biochemical markers of unknown clinical value)
o   Results do not link to important clinical benefits (e.g. insufficient clinical outcome with micronutrient supplementation, such as a small decrease in wound healing time)
o   Findings do not flow from study results i.e. extrapolation and expert opinion
o   Results not relevant to your target patient population (e.g. healthy, free-living people versus sick, hospitalized patients)
o   Treatment is not practical and cannot be implemented in daily practice (e.g. strict regime) ·
o   Study biases exist (e.g. observational studies are more prone to bias)
o   Major study limitations are reported (e.g. high frequency of non-compliance with treatment)

Various systems can be utilized to assess the quality of evidence and assign a level or grade to each study [1]. High quality sources of evidence (e.g. Best Evidence Database) have already been appraised for validity [5, 77]. However, articles obtained through other databases (e.g. Medline) will need to be appraised for validity (see Table 4).

After assessing the quality of evidence for individual studies, findings from various studies must be summarized into an aggregate picture. It is not an easy task to summarize studies with different study goals, populations, treatment regimes, and measurements.

Study factors that should be summarized include:

a) study goal(s);
b) sample size (n);
c) description of study population;
d) description of intervention (treatment) e.g. type, dosage and duration;
e) description of control (if applicable);
f) description of measurements;
g) main findings relevant to micronutrient project mandate; and,
h) potential errors, weaknesses or limitations (e.g. in discussion section).

For each factor, strands of information need to be combined and summarized into concluding statements. Applying these study factors to a "hypothetical" review of vitamin C supplementation, one might conclude:

- the study goals were to link vitamin C supplementation to decreased incidence or duration of the common cold;
- the studies had sample sizes that ranged from 10 to 30 subjects (i.e. small studies);
- the study populations were limited to healthy, free-living adults;
- the treatments ranged from 500 mg to 2000 mg vitamin C over the course of two or three weeks;
- no important differences were revealed between the treatment and control groups;
- only three of 10 studies reported significant results, one study showed a decreased incidence of the common cold and two showed a decreased duration of infection;
- baseline nutritional assessment was only performed in five studies, none of the studies performed intermittent or end-of-study nutritional assessments; and,
- the duration of vitamin C supplementation may have been inadequate to demonstrate any consistent treatment effects.

From the aggregate data above, one could conclude that only small studies have been conducted in healthy people. Among the three studies reporting significant results, two of these studies did not perform a baseline nutritional assessment. The one study that performed a baseline nutritional assessment reported that one subject who habitually consumed instant breakfast (fortified with vitamin C), was asked to refrain from consuming this product over the study period. In this hypothetical example: due to insufficient evidence, conclusions cannot be drawn to provide specific guidance to patients about vitamin C supplements and the common cold.

How much evidence is considered sufficient to draw conclusions? The answers are not clear-cut. The opinion of this author is: more evidence is required to demonstrate benefits of supplementation and less evidence is required when there is potential risk of harm. For example, the literature was reviewed to determine the safety of vitamin A supplementation in the elderly population [32, 66]. Four articles of B level evidence [67-69, 78] were considered sufficient to conclude that only ½ the tolerable upper intake level (UL) for vitamin A (1500 μg retinol versus 3000 μg) should be recommended for *safe* supplementation in elderly patients because of the consistent findings of potential adverse effects on liver function or skeletal turnover [32].

Identifying and Bridging Gaps in the Existing Body of Knowledge

A systematic approach to reviewing relevant articles and their secondary references, identifies concerning gaps in the body of evidence. It is important to scrutinize references that are cited repeatedly, for strength of evidence. Hirano [79] found that there is insubstantial evidence to draw any conclusions about the efficacy of vitamin C supplements for the treatment of chronic wounds. An informative review by North and Booth [80], entitled: "Why appraise the evidence? A case study of vitamin C and the healing of pressure sores," provides an excellent example. These reviewers located *only* two randomized controlled trials related to vitamin C supplements for chronic wound healing (e.g. pressure ulcers). One study was published in 1974 [81] and reported that 500 mg vitamin C administered twice daily, reduced healing time of pressure ulcers. Despite this study's design flaws, many review articles cite this study's findings to support the case for vitamin C supplementation in chronic wound healing. It is noteworthy that the second randomized controlled trial located by North and Booth is not widely known [80]. This study was published in 1995 [82], it refuted Taylor's findings and concluded that vitamin C supplementation is of no benefit in the treatment of pressure ulcers.

It is not necessary to locate research evidence when stating well-known facts. When specific criteria for multiple vitamins with minerals were developed, it was not necessary to cite references to support some of the indications for supplementation [32]. For example, it is widely accepted that when patients consume a poor quality diet (excluding one or more food groups) or when patients experience chronic malabsorption, diarrhea or vomiting (i.e. resulting in long-term micronutrient losses), supplementation with multiple vitamins with minerals is indicated [32].

After the evidence-based literature review is complete, a health professional may be able to bridge gaps in evidence with good clinical judgment. For example, clinical judgment was exercised when dietitians developed a practice guideline for supplementing tube feeding regimes that provide <100% of the recommended dietary allowances (RDAs) for micronutrients [32]. The RDAs were set with a safety factor (above usual requirements) and in practice, it is not feasible to supplement *all* patients who might fall short of 100% micronutrient requirements. Calculations determined the criterion for micronutrient supplementation and a decision was made to supplement tube fed patients receiving <90% of the RDAs, with multiple vitamins with minerals.

Applying Knowledge When Counseling a Patient About Micronutrient Supplements

Disease processes or treatments may change a patient's nutritional requirements and response to micronutrient supplementation [83-87]. The potential risk of harm is directly proportional to the supplement dose, especially when the dose exceeds the tolerable upper intake level (UL). Many therapeutic doses of micronutrients, utilized to cure deficiencies or treat medical conditions, are above the tolerable upper intake level (UL) [88, 89] and the length of treatment requires close medical monitoring.

The health professional must distill the evidence to convey clear and accurate messages, tailored to each patient's clinical situation. Wilk's [7] review of vitamin D required sorting studies into homogeneous groups, to further distinguish and interpret study findings. Studies of free-living people were separated from studies of hospitalized patients. Studies of subjects at high risk for osteoporosis or who were undergoing active treatment, formed another sub-group. Other variables impacting skin vitamin D synthesis (wherein endogenous cholecalciferol, active vitamin D_3, is produced from skin 7-dehydrocholesterol) were also identified. Subjects with lower endogenous production of vitamin D included those: with minimal exposure to sunlight, living in northern geographic regions, with darker skin pigmentation, with higher percentage of body fat and of older age [90, 91]. The complexity of this topic is demonstrated by Looker [91] who found inversely proportional relationships between lower serum 25-hydroxyvitamin D (reflecting vitamin D stores) and percentage of body fat. Although black women have been reported to be more obese and have poorer vitamin D status than white women [92], the impact of body fat on lowering 25-hydroxyvitamin D was found to be more pronounced in younger, white women.

It is imperative to identify specific populations or groups which may be potentially vulnerable and require a cautious approach to micronutrient supplementation. A literature review was undertaken to determine patient populations of concern at the Toronto Rehabilitation Institute [32, 66]. The elderly were found to be at increased risk for toxicity due to changes in vitamin A metabolism, secondary to increased vitamin A absorption and a concomitant decrease in retinyl ester clearance [67, 68, 70]. As well, a cautionary intake of vitamin A has been advised for women of child-bearing age, to prevent potential teratogenic effects [88].

Megadoses of individual micronutrients require special consideration as they can cause relative deficiency of other micronutrients. Dawson's review [8] of zinc underlined the interaction between zinc and copper: when zinc is supplemented, copper absorption declines. The tolerable upper intake level (UL) for zinc is 40 mg per day [3] and studies using 50 mg of elemental zinc supplements daily (for 6 to10 weeks) have shown changes in intermediate biomarkers, a copper-dependent enzyme (erythrocyte superoxide dismutase) [93, 94]. A review article reported that 100 to 400 mg of elemental zinc daily may impair immune function [95].

It is quite obvious that whenever the potential risk of micronutrient supplementation outweighs the benefits - supplementation is not advised. Risks of potential harm (i.e. adverse effects and complications) of micronutrient supplementation are under-reported in the literature or appear to be largely unknown [96]. Studies are typically powered to demonstrate treatment effectiveness [97]. This suggests that the safety of micronutrient supplementation may be overestimated. Therefore, even singular reports or individual case studies of potential harm associated with micronutrient supplementation should be considered.

One published case study, reported onset of acute hepatitis secondary to megadoses of multiple vitamins with minerals, in an elderly patient residing in a long-term care facility [98]. Another case study, reported iron overload in a 61 year old female with a 27 year history of supplementation with 325 mg ferrous sulfate twice daily, combined with 15,000 mg supplemental vitamin C [99]. The latter supplement was patient-initiated prophylaxis against recurrent upper respiratory tract infections [99], which far exceeds the tolerable upper intake level (UL) for vitamin C set at 2000 mg [3].

Caution must be exercised when recommending individual micronutrient supplements because high potency supplements are readily available in pharmacies, without a prescription. This is alarming because many supplement users exceed the tolerable upper intake level (UL) for safety [89]. This underscores the important role of health professionals in communicating the potential, and unknown risks associated with micronutrient supplements. Common myths exist surrounding the safety of micronutrients, which are often viewed as harmless and "more is better than less". Patients need to understand that micronutrient toxicities are usually caused by supplements, not by dietary intake [88, 100].

Health professionals who recommend micronutrient supplements must be aware of patient populations who require special formulations. For example, patients with end-stage renal disease should not receive standard multiple vitamins with minerals [32] and most formulations for end-stage renal disease are incomplete [101, 102]. The specific requirements for micronutrients in renal disease have not been fully elucidated and alterations in metabolism (secondary to impaired kidney function) may result in toxicity [21, 22, 101, 102].

Vitamin E is purported to have several protective effects in relation to cardiovascular disease. Studies have suggested that as an antioxidant, vitamin E reduces the oxidation of low density lipoprotein particles and it may exert influences on both enzymes and gene expression in the pathogenesis of atherosclerosis [103, 104].

Observational studies [105-107] with a focus on *primary prevention*, have reported a protective effect against coronary artery disease. However, randomized controlled trials to confirm these protective effects - are lacking. For example, no benefit was reported with 600 IU vitamin E (every other day) over the course of 10 years [108].

Ricupero [109] conducted a literature review to examine the efficacy and safety of vitamin E supplementation in *secondary* prevention of heart attack or stroke. Emerging reports of serious adverse effects and even increased mortality - with high doses of vitamin E supplements - was the impetus for reviewing the evidence. A meta-analysis of vitamin E supplementation found an increase in all-cause mortality in high risk cardiac patients, including: patients with coronary artery bypass graft, diabetes, percutaneous transluminal coronary angioplasty or prior myocardial infarction [110]. The increase in all-cause mortality was directly proportional to the vitamin E dose. A broad range of vitamin E supplements has been studied, 150 IU supplemental vitamin E is the lowest dose at which adverse effects have been observed and serious effects such as a significant increase in all cause mortality have been associated with dosages ≥400 IU daily [110]. Another secondary prevention trial [111] reported no benefit with 400 IU supplemental vitamin E over a median duration of seven years, and a concerning statistically significant increase in heart failure was reported.

There appears to be insufficient evidence to conclude whether vitamin E supplements should be recommended for primary prevention of cardiovascular disease and a cautionary approach is advised for secondary prevention. The recommended dietary allowance (RDA) for vitamin E in adults is 15 mg (22 IU) and the tolerable upper intake level (UL) is set at 1000 mg (1500 IU) [3]. Clearly, this tolerable upper intake level (UL) is not geared to secondary prevention of cardiovascular disease, for it is at least triple the level reported to cause serious adverse effects i.e. mortality.

Greenberg [112] states that vitamin E is the most widely utilized supplement, a daily intake of 400 IU (as alpha-tocopherol) is common in available supplements. He challenged the evidence for vitamin E supplements and offered this advice:

"..Thus, our message to the public must be clear on this point: vitamin E supplements won't help, and might harm, so save your money."

However, he concluded that many users of supplements reported they would continue to take supplements - despite the lack of evidenced benefit [113].

Whenever counseling patients about micronutrient supplementation, a written handout will help the patient remember the specific instructions, to enhance their understanding and to disseminate the information to significant others involved in their care. Table 5 is a template for patient education about micronutrient supplementation.

Whenever health professionals recommend micronutrient supplements, they assume accountability for nutritional assessment and counseling, as well as follow-up and reassessment of the continuing need for micronutrient supplementation [32]. Studies suggest that it is often not economical or practical to monitor biochemistry to determine whether micronutrient deficiencies exist or have been corrected [114, 115]. Therefore, a comprehensive nutritional assessment [34] and evaluation of other clinical goals (e.g. recovery from diseases or conditions) must be undertaken.

CONCLUSION

In the absence of diseases and conditions that require clinical nutrition therapy, encouraging a well-balanced diet, rich in naturally occurring sources of micronutrients - is the safest advice. However, if a patient must take a supplement... low potency, broad-spectrum multiple vitamins with minerals – is the next best approach [32, 88].

Health professionals who provide advice about micronutrient supplementation should be familiar with how the dietary reference intakes (DRIs) were developed for each micronutrient [3]. For example, insufficient data were available to establish an Estimated Average Requirement (EAR) for vitamin D, which made it impossible to calculate a recommended dietary allowance (RDA) for vitamin D [3]. Therefore, an average intake (AI) for vitamin D was developed, which assumes no vitamin D is available from skin exposure to ultraviolet B sunlight [3]. Health professionals must also understand the differences between available supplements and their potential potency. For example, the potency of vitamin D_3 (cholecalciferol) supplements, can be 1.7 times higher than vitamin D_2 (erogocalciferol) supplements [116]. Many controversies exist with respect to micronutrient supplementation. Vitamin D supplementation is currently a highly debated topic in North America [117]. Several media releases followed one study which reported a significant impact on all-cancer risk reduction with a high dose of supplemental vitamin D [50]. This has prompted some groups to recommend a high dose of supplemental vitamin D at 25 µg (1000 IU). Hypervitaminosis D may occur with intakes above the tolerable upper intake level (UL) for safety set at 50 µg (2000 IU) [3].

The efficacy and safety for vitamin D supplementation has been scheduled for review by both Health Canada and the United States Institute of Medicine (IOM). In Canada, it is recommended that all adults consume 16 fluid ounces (500 mL) vitamin D-fortified milk daily providing 5 µg (200 IU) and over the age of 50, a daily vitamin D supplement containing 10 µg (400 IU) is advised [117, 118]. For management and prevention of osteoporosis to reduce the risk of bone fractures, 20 µg (800 IU) daily is recommended – which is twice the AI for vitamin D for people above age 50 [65]. Other high risk groups including people with fat malabsorption (secondary to several medical conditions) or impaired vitamin D metabolism (e.g. renal or liver disease), may also require supplemental vitamin D [3]. Calvo and Whiting et al [119] suggest that vitamin D fortification in Canada and the United States requires reconsideration and augmentation.

This collective review of the micronutrient literature reveals an ongoing need for more high quality studies that directly link micronutrient supplementation to measurable, important and relevant clinical outcomes. Further research is required that defines specific clinical endpoints for optimal vitamin and mineral provision in various disease states, severely injured patients, and institutionalized adults including the elderly [32, 83-87, 120].

In light of insufficient evidence to answer many clinical queries, health professionals must rely on good clinical judgment. However, this judgment is impacted by the health professional's educational background and experience. Therefore, collaboration within a team of health professional experts is the best approach to ensure delivery of current best practice. Physicians and other health professionals who specialize in micronutrient therapy - dietitians and pharmacists, must collaborate with researchers to advance the practice of micronutrient therapy for health promotion, disease prevention and in the management and control of diseases and conditions.

Although the science and practice of nutrition and dietetics is highly complex, the general messages are clear and simple (to SEE):

Select a variety of foods within each food group
Exercise moderation and a balanced approach to nutrition
Eat more fruits and vegetables.

Table 5

MICRONUTRIENT SUPPLEMENTATION

Name of Patient: _____ Date: _____

Health Professional: _____ Phone:_____

SUMMARY:

Vitamins and minerals are important for your health. Your health professional has recommended that one or more micronutrient supplements are indicated, in addition to your normal, healthy diet.

The micronutrient(s) recommended: _____

Do not select a higher potency formulation.

This supplement is available in the form of: _____

YOUR ROUTINE:

Dosage: _____

Duration: _____

If you plan to take other supplements, please confer with your dietitian, pharmacist or physician.

Why You Need This Supplement (Health Professional to check the appropriate box (es) -

☐   Poor variety of food eaten_____

☐   Unable to eat enough food _____

☐   Weight loss _____

☐   Digestion problems _____

☐   Wound healing _____

Special Instructions

☐   If you have dysphagia: Using a pill crusher, crush the pill and mix with 15 mL (1 tablespoon) unsweetened applesauce.

☐   If you are on a tube feeding: Using a pill crusher, crush the pill and flush it through the tube with 50-100mL (1/3 cup) of warm water.

☐   Special instructions: if you are taking an enteral nutrition supplement fortified with the targeted vitamin(s) or mineral(s):

_____

However, for a variety of medical (e.g. food allergies, intolerances, therapeutic diet restrictions) and non-medical reasons (e.g. food dislikes, psychosocial and lifestyle factors), not all people can achieve a healthy diet - without micronutrient supplementation. Over half of American adults have been reported to use micronutrient supplements [113, 121]. The high prevalence of micronutrient supplement usage to prevent and treat disease, positions micronutrients as an important area for further research [83, 88, 122, 123].

REFERENCES

[1]   Gray EG, Gray LK. Evidence-based medicine: Applications in dietetic practice. *J Am Diet Assoc.* 2002;102(9):1263-1272.

[2]   Greenhalgh T. *How to Read a Paper: The Basics of Evidence Based Medicine 2nd ed.* London: BMJ Books; 2001.

[3]   Institute of Medicine, *DRI Dietary Reference Intakes: The Essential Guide to Nutrient Requirements.* Washington, DC: The National Academies Press. 2006.

[4]   Sackett DL, Strauss SE, Richardson WS, Rosenberg W, Haynes RB. *Evidence-Based Medicine: How to Practice and Teach EBM 2nd ed.* New York: Churchhill Livingstone; 2000.

[5]   McKibbon A, Hunt D, Richardson WS, Hayward R, Wilson M, Jaeschke R, Haynes B, Wyer P, Craig J, Guyatt G. Finding the evidence. In: *Guyatt G, Rennie D, eds. Users' Guides to the Medical Literature: A Manual for Evidence-Based Clinical Practice.* Chicago: AMA Press; 2002:13-53.

[6]   Dawes M. Formulating a question. In: *Dawes M, Davies P, Gray A, Mant J, Seers K, Snowball R. Evidence-Based Practice: A Primer for Health Professionals.* New York: Churchill Livingstone; 1999:9-13.

[7]   Wilk H. Researching the role of vitamin D in the elderly as a PEN pathway. *Practice, Dietitians of Canada.* 2005;32(3).

[8]   Dawson K. Zinc and wound healing for patients requiring hemodialysis. Unpublished literature review: Toronto Rehabilitation Institute; 2007.

[9]   Cotton A, Beemer. Feeding the patient on dialysis with wounds to heal. *Nephrology Nursing Journal.* 2005;32(4):555-557.

[10]   Gomez NJ. Wound care management in the end-stage renal disease population. *Advances in Renal Replacement Therapy.* 1997;4(4):390-396.

[11]   Winkler MF. Should vitamin C and zinc be administered as supplement for wound healing? Are there contraindications to vitamin C and zinc supplementation in renal failure? *Support Line, Dietitians in Nutrition Support.* 2000;22(4):20-21.

[12]   Wilkinson EAJ, Hawke C. Oral zinc for arterial and venous leg ulcers (Cochrane Review). In: The Cochrane Library. Oxford: Update Software; 2003:1-21.

[13]   Hallbrook T, Lanner E. Serum zinc and healing of venous ulcers. *Lancet.* 1972;2(7781):780-782.

[14]   Haeger K, Lanner E. Oral zinc sulphate and ischaemic leg ulcers. *Journal of Vascular Diseases.* 1974;3(1):77-81.

[15] Brewer RD, Mihaldzic N, Dietz A. The effect of oral zinc sulfate on the healing of decubitus ulcers in spinal cord injured patients. *Proceedings: Clinical Spinal Cord Injury Conference.* 1967;September 27;16:70-72.

[16] Norris J, Reynolds R. The effect of oral zinc sulfate therapy on decubitus ulcers. *Journal of the American Geriatrics Society.* 1971;19(9):793-797.

[17] Phillips A, Davidson M, Greaves MW. Venous leg ulceration: Evaluation of zinc treatment, serum zinc and rate of healing. *Clinical and Experimental Dermatology.* 1977;2(4):395-399.

[18] Pories WJ, Henzel JH, Rob CG, Strain WH. Acceleration of healing with zinc sulfate. *Ann Surg.* 1967;165(3):432-436.

[19] Barcia PJ. Lack of acceleration of healing with zinc sulfate. *Ann Surg.* 1970;172(6):1048-1050.

[20] Flynn A, Pories WJ, Strain WH, Hill OA. Zinc deficiency with altered adrenocortical function and its relation to delayed wound healing. *Lancet.* 1973;1(7807):789-790.

[21] Zima T, Tesar V, Mestek O, Nemecek K. Trace elements in end-stage renal disease. *Blood Purification.* 1999;17:187-198.

[22] Kalantar-Zadeh K, Kopple J. Trace elements and vitamins in maintenance dialysis patients. *Advances in Renal Replacement Therapy.* 2003;10(3):170-182.

[23] Hsieh Y, Shen W, Lee L, Wu T, Ning H, Sun C. Long term changes in trace elements in patients undergoing chronic hemodialysis. *Biological Trace Element Research.* 2006;109:115-121.

[24] Bozalioglu S, Ozkan Y, Turan M, Simsek B. Prevalence of zinc deficiency and immune response in short term hemodialysis. *Journal of Trace Elements in Medicine and Biology.* 2005;18:243-249.

[25] Rocco M, Poole DP, P, Jordan J, Burkart J. Intake of vitamins and minerals in stable hemodialysis patients as determined by 9-day food records. *Journal of Renal Nutrition.* 1997;7(1):17-24.

[26] Reid D, Barr S, Leichter J. Effects of folate and zinc supplementation on patients undergoing chronic hemodialysis. *J Am Diet Assoc.* 1992;92(5):574-579.

[27] Muirhead N, Kertesz A, Flanagan P, Hodsman A, Hollomby D, Valberg L. Zinc metabolism in patients on maintenance hemodialysis. *Am. J. Nephrol.* 1986;6:422-426.

[28] Abu-Hamdan D, Mahajan S, Migdal S, Prasad A, McDonald F. Zinc tolerance test in uremia. *Ann Intern Med.* 1986;104:50-52.

[29] Foote J, Hinks L. Zinc absorption in haemodialysis patients. *Ann Clin Biochem.* 1988;25:398-402.

[30] Antoniou L, Shalhoub R, Elliot S. Zinc tolerance tests in chronic uremia. *Clinical Nephrology.* 1981;16(4):181-187.

[31] Mahajan S, Bowersox E, Rye D, Abu-Hamdan D, Prasad A, McDonald F, Biersack K. Factors underlying abnormal zinc metabolism in uremia. *Kidney International.* 1989;36(27):S269-S273.

[32] Wildish DE. An evidence-based approach for dietitian prescription of multiple vitamins with minerals. *J Am Diet Assoc.* 2004;104:779-786.

[33] Food and Nutrition Board, Institute of Medicine. *Dietary Reference Intakes for Vitamin C, Vitamin E, Selenium and Carotenoids.* Washington, DC: National Academy Press;2000.

[34] Mahan LK, Escott-Stump S. *Krause's Food, Nutrition and Diet Therapy.* 11th ed. Philadelphia: Saunders; 2004:407-454.

[35] Gottschalk P. Vitamin C and kidney stones: challenging tradition. *Practice, Dietitians of Canada.* 2003;22:4.

[36] Henry EB, Carswell A, Wirz A, Fyffe V, McColl KEL. Proton pump inhibitors reduce the bioavailability of dietary vitamin C. *Alimentary Pharmacology & Therapeutics.* 2005;22(6):539-545.

[37] Food and Nutrition Board, Institute of Medicine. *Dietary Reference Intakes for Calcium, Phosphorus, Magnesium, Vitamin D, and Fluoride.* Washington, DC: National Academy Press;1999.

[38] Food and Nutrition Board, Institute of Medicine. *Dietary Reference Intakes for Thiamin, Riboflavin, Niacin, Vitamin B6, Folate, Vitamin B12, Pantothenic Acid, Biotin and Choline.* Washington, DC: National Academy Press;1999.

[39] Food and Nutrition Board, Institute of Medicine. *Dietary Reference Intakes for Vitamin A, Vitamin K, Arsenic, Boron, Chromium, Copper, Iodine, Iron, Manganese, Molybdenum, Nickel, Silicon, Vanadium and Zinc.* Washington, DC: National Academy Press;2001.

[40] Food and Nutrition Board, Institute of Medicine. Using Dietary Reference Intakes for Nutrient Assessment of Individuals. In: *Dietary Reference Intakes: Applications in Dietary Assessment.* Washington, DC: National Academy Press;2000:45-70.

[41] Avenell A, Handoll HHG, Grant AM. Lessons for search strategies from a systematic review, in The Cochrane Library, of nutritional supplementation trials in patients after hip fracture. *Am J Clin Nutr.* 2001;73:505-510.

[42] Cooper M, Ungar W, Zlotkin S. An assessment of inter-rater agreement of the literature filtering process in the development of evidence-based dietary guidelines. *Public Health Nutrition.* 2006;9(4):494-500.

[43] Brown J, Byers T, Thompson K, Eldridge B, Doyle C, Williams AM. American Cancer Society Workgroup on Nutrition and Physical Activity for Cancer Survivors. Nutrition during and after cancer treatment: a guide for informed choices by cancer survivors. *CA Cancer J Clin.* 2001;51:153-187.

[44] Kong Q, Lillehei KO. Antioxidant inhibitors for cancer therapy. *Med Hypotheses.* 1998;51:405-409.

[45] Labriola D, Livingston R. Possible interactions between dietary antioxidants and chemotherapy. *Oncology.* 1999;13:1003-1012.

[46] Lamson DW, Brignall MS. Antioxidants in cancer therapy; their actions and interactions with oncologic therapies. *Altern Med Rev.* 1999;4:304-329.

[47] Prasad KN, Cole WC, Coppes Z. Efficacy of high dose multiple antioxidants as an adjunct to standard cancer therapy. In: Gupta SK, ed. *Pharmacology and Therapeutics in the New Millennium.* New Delhi, India: Narosa Publishing House; 2001:289-312.

[48] Prasad KN, Kumar A, Kochupillai V, Cole WC. High doses of multiple antioxidant vitamins: essential ingredients in improving the efficacy of standard cancer therapy. *J Am Coll Nutr.* 1999;18:13-25.

[49] Pace A, Savarese A, Picardo M, Maresca V, Pacetti U, Del Monte G, Biroccio A, Leonetti G, Jandolo B, Cognetti F, Bove L. Neuroprotective effect of vitamin E supplementation in patients treated with cisplatin chemotherapy. *Journal of Clinical Oncology.* 2003;21:927-931.

[50] Lappe JM, Travers-Gustafson D, Davies KM, Recker RR, Heaney RP. Vitamin D and calcium supplementation reduces cancer risk: results of a randomized trial. *Am J Clin Nutr.* 2007;85:1586-1591.

[51] Bischoff HA, Stahelin HB, Dick W, Akos R, Knecht M, Salis C, Nebiker M, Theiler R, Pfeifer M, Begerow B, Lew RA, Conzelmann M. Effects of vitamin D and calcium supplementation on falls: A randomized controlled trial. *Journal of Bone and Mineral Research.* 2003;18(2):343-351.

[52] Larsen ER, Mosekilde L, Foldspang A. Vitamin D and calcium supplementation prevents osteoporotic fractures in elderly community dwelling residents: A pragmatic population-based 3-year intervention study. *Journal of Bone and Mineral Research.* 2004;19(3):370-378.

[53] Chapuy M-C, Chapuy P, Meunier PJ. Calcium and vitamin D supplements: effects on calcium metabolism in elderly people. *Am J Clin Nutr.* 1987;46(2):324-328.

[54] Dawson-Hughes B, Harris SS, Krall EA, Dallal GE. Effect of withdrawal of calcium and vitamin D supplements on bone mass in elderly men and women. *Am J Clin Nutr.* 2000;72(3):745-750.

[55] Grados F, Brazier M, Kamel S, Mathieu M, Hurtebize N, Maamer M, Garabedian M, Sebert JL, Fardellone P. Prediction of bone mass density variation by bone remodeling markers in postmenopausal women with vitamin D insufficiency treated with calcium and vitamin D supplementation. *The Journal of Clinical Endocrinology & Metabolism.* 2003;88(11):5175-5179.

[56] Grados F, Brazier M, Kamel S, Duver S, Heurtebize N, Mamer M, Mathieu M, Garabedian M, Sebert JL, Fardellone P. Effects on bone mineral density of calcium and vitamin D supplementation in elderly women with vitamin D deficiency. *Joint Bone Spine.* 2003;70(3):203-208.

[57] Harwood RH, Sahota O, Gaynor K, Masud T, Hosking DJ. A randomised, controlled comparison of different calcium and vitamin D supplementation regimens in elderly women after hip fracture: The Nottingham Neck of Femur (NoNOF) Study. *Age and Ageing.* 2004;33(1):45-51.

[58] Honkanen R, Alhava E, Parviainen M, Talasniemi S, Monkkonen R. The necessity and safety of calcium and vitamin D in the elderly. *JAGS.* 1990;38(8):862-866.

[59] Krieg MA, Jacquet AF, Bremgartner M, Cuttelod S, Thiebaud D, Burckhardt P. Effect of supplementation with vitamin D_3 and calcium on quantitative ultrasound of bone in elderly institutionalized women: A longitudinal study. *Osteoporosis International.* 1999;9(6):483-488.

[60] Meier C, Woitge HW, Witte K, Lemmer B, Seibel MJ. Supplementation with oral vitamin D_3 and calcium during winter prevents seasonal bone loss: A randomized

controlled open-label prospective trial. *Journal of Bone and Mineral Research.* 2004;19(8):1221-1230.

[61] Meunier P. Prevention of hip fractures by correcting calcium and vitamin D insufficiencies in elderly people. *Scand J Rheumatol.* 1996;25(103):75-80.

[62] Porthouse J, Cockayne S, King C, Saxon L, Steele E, Aspray T, Baverstock M, Birks Y, Dumville J, Francis RM, Iglesias C, Puffer S, Sutcliffe A, Watt I, Torgerson DJ. Randomised controlled trial of calcium and supplementation with cholecalciferol (vitamin D₃) for prevention of fractures in primary care. *BMJ.* 2005;330(7498):1003.

[63] Johnell O. Review: Vitamin D plus calcium, but not vitamin D alone, prevents osteoporotic fractures in older people. *Evid Based Med.* 2006;11(1):13.

[64] Feskanich D, Weber P, Willett WC, Rockett H, Booth SL, Colditz GA. Vitamin K intake and hip fractures in women: a prospective study. *Am J Clin Nutr.* 1999;69:74-79.

[65] Brown JP, Josse RG. The Scientific Advisory Council of the Osteoporosis Society of Canada. 2002 clinical practice guidelines for the diagnosis and management of osteoporosis in Canada. *CMAJ;* 2002:1-60.

[66] Gottschalk P. Reviewing the safety of vitamin A supplementation in the elderly. Unpublished literature review: Toronto Rehabilitation Institute; 2003.

[67] Stauber PM, Sherry B, VanderJagt D, Bhagavan H, Garry P. A longitudinal study of the relationship between vitamin A supplementation and plasma retinol, retinyl esters and liver enzymes in a healthy elderly population. *Am J Clin Nutr.* 1991;54:878-883.

[68] Krasinski SD, Russell RM, Otradovec CL, Sadowski JA, Hartz SC, Jacob RA, McGandy RB. Relationship of vitamin A and vitamin E intake to fasting plasma retinol, retinol-binding protein, retinyl esters, carotene, alpha-tocopherol, and cholesterol among elderly people and young adults: Increased plasma retinyl esters among vitamin A supplement users. *Am J Clin Nutr.* 1989;49:112-120.

[69] Johnson EJ, Krall EA, Dawson-Hughes B, Dallal GE, Russell RM. Lack of an effect of multivitamins containing vitamin A on serum retinyl esters and liver function tests in healthy women. *J Am Coll Nutr.* 1992;11:682-686.

[70] Tripp F. The use of dietary supplements in the elderly: current issues and recommendations. *J Am Diet Assoc.* 1997;97:S181-S183.

[71] Michäelsson K, Lithell H, Vessby B, Melhus H. Serum retinol levels and the risk of fracture. *N Engl J Med.* 2003;348:287-294.

[72] Cook DJ, Guyatt GH, Laupacis A, Sackett DL. Rules of evidence and clinical recommendations on the use of antithrombotic agents. *Chest.* 1992;102:305S-311S.

[73] Cook DJ, Guyatt GH, Laupacis A, Sackett DL, Goldberg RJ. Clinical recommendations using levels of evidence for antithrombotic agents. *Chest.* 1995;108:227S-230S.

[74] Guyatt G, Rennie D, eds. *Users' Guides to the Medical Literature: A Manual for Evidence-Based Clinical Practice.* Chicago: AMA Press; 2002.

[75] Guyatt G, Rennie D, eds. *Users' Guides to the Medical Literature: Essentials of Evidence-Based Clinical Practice.* Chicago: AMA Press; 2002.

[76] Craig JC, Irwig LM, Stockler MR. Evidence-based medicine: useful tools for decision making. *Med J Aust.* 2001;174:248-253.

[77] MacMahon S, Collins R. Reliable assessment of the effects of treatment on mortality and major morbidity, II: observational studies. *Lancet.* 2001;357:455-462.

[78] Feskanich D, Singh V, Willett WC, Colditz GA. Vitamin A intake and hip fractures among postmenopausal women. *JAMA.* 2002;287:47-54.

[79] Hirano L. Vitamin C and chronic wound healing. Unpublished literature review: Toronto Rehabilitation Institute; 2007.

[80] North G, Booth A. Why appraise the evidence? A case study of vitamin C and the healing of pressure sores. *Journal of Human Nutrition and Dietetics.* 1999;12:237-244.

[81] Taylor TV, Rimmer S, Day B, Butcher J, Dymock IW. Ascorbic acid supplementation in the treatment of pressure-sores. *Lancet.* 1974;2(7880):544-546.

[82] ter Riet G, Kessels AG, Knipschild PG. Randomized clinical trial of ascorbic acid in the treatment of pressure ulcers. *J Clin Epidemiol.* 1995;48:1453-1460.

[83] Committee on Diet and Health, National Research Council. Dietary supplements. In: *Diet and Health: Implications for Reducing Chronic Disease Risk.* Washington, DC: National Academy Press. 1989:509-526.

[84] Earnest C, Cooper KH, Marks A, Mitchell TL. Efficacy of a complex multivitamin supplement. *Nutrition.* 2002;18:738-742.

[85] Shenkin A. Clinical nutrition and metabolism group symposium on nutrition in the severely-injured patient. Part 2. Micronutrients in the severely-injured patient. *Proceedings of the Nutrition Society.* 2000;59:451-456.

[86] Tébi A, Belbraouet S, Chau N, Debry G. Plasma vitamin, beta-carotene, and alpha-tocopherol status according to age and disease in hospitalized elderly. *Nutrition Research.* 2000;20:1395-1408.

[87] Ferreira Da Cunha D, Freire De Carvalho Da Cunha S, Do Rosario Del Lama Unamuno M, Vannucchi H. Serum levels assessment of vitamin A, E, C, B_2 and carotenoids in malnourished and non-malnourished hospitalized elderly patients. *Clinical Nutrition.* 2001;20:167-170.

[88] Position of the American Dietetic Association. Vitamin and mineral supplementation. *J Am Diet Assoc.* 1996;96:73-77.

[89] Troppmann L, Gray-Donald K, Johns T. Supplement use: Is there any nutritional benefit? *J Am Diet Assoc.* 2002;102:818-825.

[90] Holick M. High prevalence of vitamin D inadequacy and implications for health. *Mayo Clin Proc.* 2006;81(3):353-373.

[91] Looker AC. Body fat and vitamin D status in black versus white women. *The Journal of Clinical Endocrinology & Metabolism.* 2005;90(2):635-640.

[92] Nesby-O'Dell S, Scanlon KS, Cogswell ME, Gillespie C, Hollis BW, Looker AC, Allen C, Doughertly C, Gunter EQ, Bowman BA. Hypovitaminosis D prevalence and determinants among African American and white women of reproductive age: third National Health and Nutrition Examination Survey 1988-94. *Am J Clin Nutr.* 2002;76:187-192.

[93] Yadrick MK, Kenney MA, Winterfeldt EA. Iron, copper, and zinc status: response to supplementation with zinc or zinc and iron in adult females. *Am J Clin Nutr.* 1989;49:145-150.

[94] Fischer PWF, Giroux A, L'Abbe MR. Effect of zinc supplementation on copper status in adult man. *Am J Clin Nutr.* 1984;40:743-746.

[95]   Rink L, Gabriel P. Zinc and the immune system. *Proceedings of the Nutrition Society.* 2000;59:541-552.

[96]   Palmer ME, Haller C, McKinney PE, Klein-Schwartz W, Tschirgi A, Smolinske SC, Woolf A, Sprague BM, Ko R, Everson G, Nelson LS, Dodd-Butera T, Bartlett WD, Landzberg BR. Adverse events associated with dietary supplements: An observational study. *Lancet.* 2003;361:101-106.

[97]   Bastian H. Learning from evidence based on mistakes. *BMJ.* 2004;329:1053.

[98]   Sleeper RB, Kennedy SM. Adverse reaction to a dietary supplement in an elderly patient. *Ann Pharmacother.* 2003;37:83-86.

[99]   Mallory MA, Sthapanachai C, Kowdley KV. Iron overload related to excessive vitamin C intake [see comment]. [Case Reports. Letter]. *Ann Intern Med.* 2003;139(6):532-533.

[100] Position of the American Dietetic Association. Food fortification and dietary supplements. *J Am Diet Assoc.* 2001;101(1):115-125.

[101] Makoff R. Vitamin replacement therapy in renal failure patients. *Miner Electrolyte Metab.* 1999;25:349-351.

[102] Makoff R, Gonick H. Renal failure and the concomitant derangement of micronutrient metabolism. *Nutrition in Clinical Practice.* 1999;14(5):238-246.

[103] Munteanu A, Zingg JM, Azzi A. Anti-atherosclerotic effects of vitamin E - myth or reality? *J Cell Mol Med.* 2004;8:59-76.

[104] Singh U, Jialal I. Anti-inflammatory effects of alpha-tocopherol. *Ann N Y Acad Sci.* 2004;1031:195-203.

[105] Kushi LH, Folsom AR, Prineas RJ, Mink PJ, Wu Y, Bostick RM. Dietary antioxident vitamins and death from coronary heart disease in postmenopausal women. *N Engl J Med.* 1996;334(18):1156-1162.

[106] Rimm EB, Stampfer MJ, Ascherio A, Giovannucci E, Colditz GA, Willett WC. Vitamin E consumption and the risk of coronary heart disease in men. *N Engl J Med.* 1993;328(20):1450-1456.

[107] Stampfer MJ, Hennekens CH, Manson JE, Colditz GA, Rosner B, Willett WC. Vitamin E consumption and the risk of coronary disease in women. *N Engl J Med.* 1993;328(20):1444-1449.

[108] Lee IM, Cook NR, Gaziano JM, Gordon D, Ridker PM, Manson JE, Hennekens CH, Buring JE. Vitamin E in the primary prevention of cardiovascular disease and cancer: the Women's Health Study: a randomized controlled trial. *JAMA.* 2005;294(1):56-65.

[109] Ricupero M. Vitamin E and secondary prevention in cardiovascular disease. Unpublished literature review: Toronto Rehabilitation Institute; 2007.

[110] Miller III ER, Pastor-Barriuso R, Dalal D, Riemersma RA, Appel LJ, Guallar E. Meta-analysis: High-dosage vitamin E supplementation may increase all-cause mortality. *Ann Intern Med.* 2005;142(1):37-46.

[111] Lonn E, Bosch J, Yusuf S, Sheridan P, Pogue J, Arnold JM, Ross C, Arnold A, Sleight P, Probstfield J, Dagenais GR. HOPE and HOPE-TOO Trial Investigators. Effects of long-term vitamin E supplementation on cardiovascular events and cancer: a randomized controlled trial. *JAMA.* 2005;293(11):1338-1347.

[112] Greenberg ER. Vitamin E supplements: Good in theory, but is the theory good? *Ann Intern Med.* 2005;142(1):75-76.

[113] Blendon RJ, DesRoches CM, Benson JM, Brodie M, Altman DE. Americans' views on the use and regulation of dietary supplements. *Arch Intern Med.* 2001;161:805-810.

[114] Johnson KA, Bernard MA, Funderburg K. Vitamin nutrition in older adults. *Clin Geriatr Med.* 2002;18:773-799.

[115] Willett WC, Stampfer MJ. What vitamins should I be taking, doctor? *N Engl J Med.* 2001;345:1819-1824.

[116] Trang HM, Cole DE, Rubin LA. Evidence that vitamin D_3 increases serum 25-hydroxyvitamin D more efficiently than does vitamin D_2. *Am J Clin Nutr.* 1998;68(4):854-858.

[117] Health Canada. Information Update: Vitamin D and Health; [cited 2007 18 Jun]. Accessed from: http://www.hc-sc.gc.ca/ahc-asc/media/advisories-avis/2007/2007_72_e.html, 2007.

[118] Health Canada. Section 5: Advice for Different Ages and Stages. *Eating Well with Canada's Food Guide: A Resource for Educators and Communicators*; 2007:38-43.

[119] Calvo MS, Whiting SJ, Barton CN. Vitamin D fortification in the United States and Canada: current status and data needs. *Am J Clin Nutr.* 2004;80:1710S-1716S.

[120] High KP. Nutritional strategies to boost immunity and prevent infection in elderly individuals. *Aging and Infectious Diseases.* 2001;33:1892-1900.

[121] Satia-Abouta J, Kristal AR, Patterson RE, Littman AJ, Stratton KL, White E. Dietary supplement use and medical conditions: The VITAL Study. *Am J Prev Med.* 2003;24:43-51.

[122] Fairfield KM, Fletcher RH. Vitamins for chronic disease prevention in adults. Scientific Review. *JAMA.* 2002;287:3116-3126.

[123] Meydani M. Nutrition interventions in aging and age-associated disease. *Ann N Y Acad Sci.* 2001;928:226-235.

In: Micronutrients and Health Research
Editor: Takumi Yoshida, pp. 207-226

ISBN: 978-1-60456-056-5
© 2008 Nova Science Publishers, Inc.

Chapter VI

EVALUATION OF CHRONIC HEPATIC COPPER ACCUMULATION IN CATTLE

Marta López-Alonso[*]

Universidade de Santiago de Compostela, Departamento de Patoloxía Animal,
Facultade de Veterinaria, 27002 Lugo, Spain.

ABSTRACT

Traditionally cattle were thought to be relatively tolerant of copper (Cu) accumulation, and cattle diets were regularly supplemented with Cu well above physiological needs. In recent years, however, an increasing number of episodes of Cu toxicity have been reported in cattle, in most cases associated with excessive Cu intake in the ration. It has also been reported that dietary supplements leading to Cu accumulation in the liver at concentrations only slightly above normal show negative effects on animal performance, in terms of reduced feed intake and average daily gain (subclinical toxicity). Identification of animals in the silent chronic phase of Cu accumulation is very important to avoid not only economic losses due to subsequent severe disease or death, but also to avoid subclinical disease. Currently available laboratory markers of Cu toxicity are mainly used for diagnostic purposes, i.e. to demonstrate changes associated with clinical manifestations already present. However, there is a clear need to identify markers of early changes, with a capacity to predict risk of Cu accumulation in the liver before actual tissue or functional damage occurs. In this chapter, we evaluate the suitability of some blood parameters as potential markers of hepatic Cu accumulation in cattle during the silent phase as well as the use of *in vivo* biopsies for evaluation of risk of chronic Cu toxicity.

Our results indicate that under moderately high Cu exposure, none of the blood markers currently available accurately predicted hepatic Cu accumulation in cattle and analysis of Cu content in the liver is probably the best diagnostic tool available for assessing the risk of chronic Cu toxicity. However, the limit between safe-adequate Cu

---

[*] Correspondence concerning this article should be addressed to: Marta López-Alonso, Tel: + 34 982 25 23 03; Fax: + 34 982 28 59 40; e-mail: mlalonso@lugo.usc.es.

concentrations and those associated with toxicity is very narrow, and for this reason the total hepatic Cu concentration is not *per se* a good indicator of risk of toxicity in animals with marginal hepatic Cu concentrations. Studies of subcellular hepatic Cu accumulation indicate that the large-granule (lysosomal) fraction has a limited capacity for Cu sequestration and Cu content in this compartment tends to reach a plateau phase at relatively low Cu exposure levels, leading to higher Cu accumulation in the nucleus and cytosol. This pattern of Cu accumulation, as in sheep, may be due to the limited capacity for metallothionein binding of Cu and excretion in bile. Further research into the molecular basis of Cu homeostasis in cattle is essential to better understand the pathogenesis of chronic Cu hepatic accumulation and to validate the use of subcellular Cu parameters as potential markers of the risk of Cu toxicity in cattle.

INTRODUCTION

Copper (Cu) is essential for life processes, as a cofactor for many vital cuproenzymes, yet it is extremely toxic in excess (Horn and Tümer, 1999; Mercer, 2001). Because of this dual role, all living organisms have developed highly specialized homeostatic mechanisms to recruit, deliver and eliminate Cu, and to neutralize its toxic effects. Research in recent years has identified numerous proteins involved in Cu metabolism (notably Cu-binding metallothioneins (MT), and more recently chaperones and Cu ATP-ases), as well as the molecular basis of some human genetic Cu disorders (notably Menkes and Wilson diseases) (Dameron and Harrison, 1998; Harris, 2000, 2001; Mercer, 2001; Mercer and Llanos, 2003), but the mechanisms of Cu homeostasis remain very incompletely understood.

Various animal species show marked variation in their tolerance to increased levels of dietary Cu (Howell and Gooneratne, 1987). Without doubt, sheep are the most susceptible to chronic Cu toxicity, because they do not appear to be able to increase biliary Cu excretion in response to increased Cu intake (Bremner, 1998). In contrast, pigs are very tolerant of Cu, and high concentrations of Cu (250 mg/kg) are used as growth promoters.

Traditionally cattle were thought to be relatively tolerant of Cu exposure (Howell and Gooneratne, 1987; Gooneratne et al., 1989a; Bradley, 1993), and indeed reports of Cu poisoning were, until recently, somewhat rare. In fact, Cu deficiency in cattle is a rather common disorder worldwide, and cattle diets are regularly supplemented with high Cu concentrations (up to 50 mg/kg dry matter), well above physiological requirements (10 mg/kg; NRC, 2000). Such high Cu supplementation has in some cases been justified in view of the interference of Cu with other nutrients, mainly molybdenum and sulphur, but also iron and zinc (Kendall et al., 2001).

In recent years, however, an increasing number of episodes of Cu toxicity have been reported in cattle (Bidewell et al., 2000; VLA, 2001), even at liver Cu concentrations well below those regarded as toxic in the literature (Perrin et al., 1990; Gummow 1996). In most cases, cattle toxicity is associated with excessive Cu intake in the ration, as well as with changes in the type and bioavailability of dietary Cu supplements (Galey et al., 1991; Stefen et al., 1997; Laven et al., 2004) although episodes of chronic Cu toxicity have been also reported in cattle fed Cu concentrations within the normal range (Bradley, 1993). It has also been reported that dietary supplements leading to Cu accumulation in the liver at concentrations only slightly above normal (around 125 mg/kg wet weight) show negative effects on animal performance, in terms of reduced feed intake and average daily gain (Engle and Spears, 2000). Liver Cu concentrations that seemingly could be associated with subclinical chronic Cu toxicity in cattle have been described in many countries where Cu supplements are given well above requirements (Hadrich, 1996; Jilg et al., 1997) or where there is contamination of pastures by mining and/or industrial emissions and waste (especially Cu-enriched pig slurry) (Binnerts, 1986; López-Alonso et al., 2000a,b; Tokarnia et al., 2000).

In addition to the negative effects on animal health, excessive Cu supplementation of cattle diets can lead to high Cu residues in meat products for human consumption, mainly in the liver (the organ that accumulates the highest Cu concentrations). Studies carried out in several countries to monitor metal concentrations in meat and meat products indicate that Cu concentrations are generally high and above the maximum admissible levels established in countries such as Canada or Australia (100 and 150 mg/kg respectively; Langlands et al., 1987; Salisbury et al., 1991). In Europe, although high Cu concentrations have been frequently described in cattle products in countries as Germany (Hadrich, 1996), United Kingdom (Bidewell, 2000) and our own region of Galicia in NW Spain (López-Alonso et al., 2000a), the European Union has not yet established maximum admissible levels in animal products for human consumption. However, the European Food Safety Authority has declared that there is an urgent need to establish these maximum levels, and to identify appropriate levels of mineral supplementation in animal feeds with the goal of minimizing metal residues in meat. Finally, it should be noted that Cu is a significant environmental contaminant. In fact, Cu has become a major environmental problem in countries with high densities of farming, especially intensive pig farms, on which Cu is added at high concentrations to pig diets as a growth promoter (Poole et al, 1990; L'Herroux et al., 1997; Brumm, 1998; Poulsen, 1998).

Identification of animals in the chronic phase of Cu accumulation is very important to avoid not only economic losses due to subsequent severe disease or death, but also to avoid subclinical disease. It is important to adapt Cu supplementation to physiological needs and to reduce it in regions where Cu content in animal feed is already adequate: this will indirectly protect animal health, reduce Cu concentration in meat and meat products for human consumption, and reduce the environmental impact associated with the use of animal slurries on agricultural land.

HEPATIC CHRONIC CU ACCUMULATION

Because of susceptibility of sheep to chronic Cu toxicity and the clinical similarity to Cu disorders in humans, hepatic Cu metabolism in sheep has been widely studied (Corbett et al., 1978; Gooneratne et al., 1979, 1980; Kumaratilake and Howell 1987, 1989; Haywood et al., 2001, 2004; Simpson et al., 2004) and susceptibility is considered to be related to the sheep's inability to accumulate large amounts of Cu as MT in the livers. Although the role of MT in Cu metabolism has not been completely elucidated (Luza and Speisky, 1996; Dameron and Harrison, 1998; Harrison and Dameron, 1999) it is generally accepted to be in the cellular detoxification of the metal. Hepatic subcellular distribution studies in sheep (Corbett et al., 1978; Gooneratne et al., 1979; Saylor and Leach, 1980; Kumaratilake and Howell, 1989) have shown that during the early stages of Cu accumulation, as in most mammals, Cu accumulates mainly in the cytosol bound to MT; however unlike other species, sheep have a limited capacity to accumulate large amounts of Cu-MT in the livers and saturation occurs very soon. As Cu is absorbed from the intestine, it enters the liver where Cu is either utilized in normal hepatocyte metabolism, stored bound to MT or, if Cu balance is positive, excreted into the bile (Bremner, 1991) (Figure 1). MT seems to play a main role in the Cu excretion into the bile, both by a direct route through the hepatocyte cytoplasm or, more importantly, by the hepatolysosomal route, in which Cu-MT are sequestered by the lysosomes for excretion in the bile (Gooneratne et al., 1989b). If there is a large influx of Cu into the liver, the capacity of the MT to bind Cu and the lysosomes to remove Cu from the cytosol can be exceeded, and Cu starts to accumulate at a higher rate in other organelles (mainly in the nucleus), or, at higher Cu accumulations, may even remain as free Cu ions in the cytosol; in both cases Cu is responsible for severe changes in liver structure and function (Bremer, 1991; Bremner, 1998; Cisternas et al., 2005).

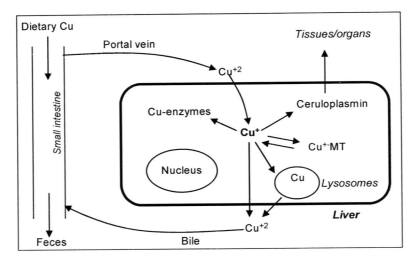

Figure 1. Pathway of Cu in the body. Cu is absorbed by the enterocytes of the small intestine and reaches the liver through the portal circulation. In the liver, Cu is either utilized in normal hepatocyte metabolism, stored bound to MT or, if Cu balance is positive, excreted into the bile. Cu is exported to the tissues as ceruloplasmin.

Once the MT binding sites become saturated the uptake of Cu by the lysosomes is initiated. Lysosomal accumulation is probably linked to Cu-induced autophagy and has generally been assumed to be part of a detoxification process and a prelude to biliary excretion of the metal (although there are also non-lysosomal pathways for biliary Cu excretion; Bremner, 1998). Thus, the sequestration of excess Cu by the proliferating lysosomes may be responsible for the maintenance of a constant concentration of Cu in the cytosol of the liver cells (Kumaratilake and Howell, 1989). At the beginning of this storage lysosomes predominantly increase in number; however, as Cu loading increases, the lysosomal production may be significantly reduced (or may cease at a critical Cu level) and excess Cu accumulated in already present lysosomes, resulting in an increase in their volume (Howell and Gooneratne, 1987). The existing lysosomes may then become saturated and, therefore, the concentration of Cu in the cytosol and nucleus of these cells can no longer be retained and a constant proportion and may rapidly rise to toxic values. Although the mechanisms of liver necrosis in Cu-loaded animals are not completely understood, it has been suggested that the excess of Cu accumulation in the lysosomes leads to rupture of the membrane, resulting in leakage of acid hydrolases into the cytoplasm and destruction of the liver cells (Gooneratne et al., 1980) but it is also possible that the Cu accumulation in the nuclear fraction destabilize DNA and inhibit RNA polymerase activity, leading to a nuclear disorganization and the subsequent death of the cell (Bremner, 1998). The increase of Cu-free ions concentrations in the cytosol may also affect the metabolic activity in microsomes, cause lipid peroxidation of membranes, and lead to degeneration and necrosis of the cells (Kumaratilake and Howell, 1989; Peña et al., 1999; Pinchuk and Lichtenberg, 1999)

Chronic Cu poisoning is a two-stage process (Howell and Gooneratne, 1987). The first stage is the *pre-haemolytic phase*, during which lysosomes are able to sequester Cu and it accumulates in the liver over a period of weeks or months without any signs of liver damage or clinical evidence of disease being manifested. However, once the lysosomes are overloaded, usually following a stressful event of some sort, the storage of excess Cu in the nucleus and cytosol is responsible for the lesions in the liver cells. Cu is then released from the liver, usually causing a haemolytic crisis (*haemolytic phase*). In fact the disease is generally clinically silent and basically undetectable until the haemolytic crisis occurs. In line with this, a recent study notes that in herds with clinical Cu toxicity, the clinical cases represent only a small proportion of the actual cases of Cu poisoning (Laven et al., 2004).

IDENTIFICATION OF ANIMALS IN THE SILENT CHRONIC PHASE OF CU ACCUMULATION

Laboratory findings most commonly associated with a diagnosis of chronic Cu toxicity are associated with the haemolytic phase of the disease and include raised serum bilirubin, the presence of haemoglobin in urine and methaemoglobinaemia. Ante-mortem plasma Cu concentrations slightly increase during the pre-haemolitic phase and plasma Cu concentrations are highest when the haemolytic crisis is imminent. During the clinical phase of Cu poisoning, plasma or serum Cu is usually greater than 3 mg/l. Elevations of serum concentrations of liver enzymes is one of the earliest biochemical changes in the pre-haemolitic phase with increased glutamate dehydrogenase (GLDH) aspartate aminotransferase (AST) and gamma-glutamyl transferase (GGT) concentrations. Diagnosis of chronic Cu toxicity is confirmed by determination of Cu concentrations both in the liver and kidney. In general, it is accepted that Cu concentrations above 150 mg/kg wet weight in the liver (safe-adequate range: 25-100 mg/kg wet weight; Puls., 1994) and 15 mg/kg wet weight in the kidney (reference range: 4-6 mg/kg wet weight) respectively are indicative of toxicity (Bidewell et al., 2000).

On the contrary, identification of animals during the silent chronic phase of Cu accumulation is very difficult because adequate diagnostic markers are not available.

Currently available laboratory markers of Cu toxicity in non-lethal samples (mainly blood), both from humans and animals, are mainly used for diagnostic purposes (i.e. to identify changes associated with clinical manifestations already present; Araya et al., 2003; Ortolani et al., 2003) and the only precise methods for evaluating chronic Cu accumulation in the liver during the silent phase are measurement of Cu concentration in, or histological studies of, *in vivo* liver biopsies. However, there is a clear need to identify markers of early changes, with a capacity to predict risk of Cu accumulation in the liver before actual tissue or functional damage occurs, which could be used in cattle for clinical diagnosis in a routine way. Acquisition of these markers should ideally be non-invasive and should function as a sensitive index of Cu accumulation even in the absence of substantial functional damage.

Development of Potential Blood Markers of Hepatic Cu Accumulation

As indicated, Cu concentration in blood or serum, together with Cu concentrations in liver and kidney in samples obtained at necropsy, are among the most widely clinical tools used for diagnosis of chronic Cu toxicity during the haemolytic phase (Auza et al., 1999; Bidewell et al., 2000); this is because hepatic necrosis leads to a sudden release of Cu into the blood during the terminal stages of Cu poisoning. However, Cu concentrations in blood or serum do not appear to be useful indicators of hepatic chronic Cu accumulation during the silent or pre-haemolitic phase. Several authors have reported that serum/plasma Cu concentration is a poor indicator of Cu loading of the liver (Vermunt and West, 1994; Auza et al., 1999; Minatel and Carfagnini, 2002; Laven and Livesey, 2006); in fact, animals considered to be deficient or in the low-normal part of the reference range on the basis of evaluation of serum Cu concentrations have been found to be at or near a toxic state on the basis of necropsy results or examination of hepatic biopsy specimens (Blakley and Hamilton, 1985). It is only when liver stores reach a critical threshold that acute hepatic necrosis develops, releasing liver Cu stores and causing transient high serum Cu concentrations (Tessman et al., 2001). Our own observations in cattle under moderately high hepatic Cu accumulation indicate that serum Cu concentration was not significantly associated with hepatic Cu concentration (López-Alonso et al., 2006); on the contrary the whole-blood Cu concentration showed a statistically significant association with Cu accumulation in the liver. Whole-blood Cu concentration, although nowadays not commonly used for assessing animals' Cu status (Suttle, 1993), might be a better indicator of Cu accumulation in the liver. In fact a recent study on potential biomarkers of Cu over-exposure has demonstrated that Cu is able to bind with high affinity to some erythrocyte proteins (Speisky et al., 2003); however, further research is still necessary to better characterize these proteins and validate their use as markers of Cu exposure.

In serum or plasma, Cu is present in three major forms, in two pools between which Cu does not appear to be exchangeable: the main pool containing Cu as CP, corresponding to Cu exported from the liver to tissues; and a second pool containing Cu in albumin- and amino-acid- bound forms, mainly corresponding to Cu transported from the intestine to the liver in the portal circulation (Cousins, 1985; Linder et al., 1998). Our own results (López-Alonso et al., 2006), like in other studies (Blakley and Hamilton, 1985; Stoszed et al, 1986), indicate that hepatic Cu and CP activity are not correlated either at normal or high levels of hepatic Cu accumulation. This is because, once the animal reaches adequate Cu status in the liver, CP as well as Cu-dependent enzymes such as superoxide dismutase in erythrocytes attain a maximal activity that is not increased with further hepatic Cu accumulation (Baker et al., 1989; Rock et al., 2000); in addition, CP levels vary with factors such as age and gender (Fisher et al., 1990; Milne, 1994), and increase rapidly in response to factors other than Cu excess, such as exercise and various inflammatory and infection conditions (Harris, 1997; Beshgetoor and Hambidge, 1998).

In an attempt to find potential markers of Cu exposure, and taking into account that CP, the main Cu-containing component in blood, is affected by factors other than Cu exposure, the non-CP fraction (a calculated value) has recently been used as a marker of Cu exposure in humans (Eife et al., 1999; Araya et al., 2003). It has been demonstrated that serum non-CP Cu levels are positively correlated with total serum Cu both in humans receiving high dietary Cu as well as in patients with high Cu load (such as Wilson's disease and other forms of childhood cirrhosis). We also have found that the non-CP Cu fraction was highly correlated with serum Cu in cattle with moderately high hepatic Cu accumulation (López-Alonso et al., 2006), and most importantly both the serum and the whole-blood non-CP fraction were significantly associated with Cu concentration in the liver. However, the strength of these associations, though better than that between whole-blood and hepatic Cu, is still too low for accurate prediction of Cu accumulation in the liver.

Another parameter that has previously been proposed as a marker of Cu deficiency status in ruminants, especially in cases of Cu interactions with molybdenum and iron at high concentrations, is CP/serum-Cu ratio (Mackenzie et al., 1997; Arnhold et al., 1998; Kendall et al., 2001). In cattle with moderately high hepatic Cu accumulation (López-Alonso et al., 2006), CP/serum-Cu ratio was negatively correlated with hepatic Cu level, indicating that as Cu accumulation increases in the liver, proportionally less Cu in serum is bound to CP; however, the strength of this association was low to be considered a suitable marker of chronic hepatic Cu accumulation.

Finally, hepatic enzymes have been also clinical parameters widely used for diagnosis of clinical chronic Cu toxicity (Auza et al., 1999; Bidewell et al., 2000) because hepatic necrosis leads to a sudden release of hepatic enzymes into the blood during the terminal stages of Cu poisoning. Several authors have postulated that hepatic enzymes may also be useful early markers during the long-term subclinical phase of hepatic Cu accumulation (Humann-Ziehank et al., 2001; Laven et al., 2004), based on the fact that during this silent phase some cells undergo necrosis, leading to increases in enzyme activity in the blood. However, in line with our own results in cattle (López Alonso et al., 2006), other authors (Weaver et al.,1990; Sutherland et al., 1992) have found only weak correlations between serum enzyme activity and hepatic Cu levels or clinical manifestations of hepatic insufficiency. During the chronic progressive hepatic Cu accumulation phase only a few hepatocytes undergo necrosis at any specific time (0.45% of liver volume; Gooneratne et al., 1980), so such elevations are transitory, and unless samples are obtained at least once a week, they may not be detected (Howell and Gooneratne, 1987; Ortolani et al., 2003).

Early Functional Markers of Chronic Hepatic Cu Accumulation: Study of Liver Biopsy

As previously mentioned, clinical diagnosis of chronic Cu toxicity is confirmed after measurement of Cu concentrations both in the liver and kidney, Cu concentrations in excess of 150 and 15 mg/kg wet weight in the liver and kidney respectively being indicative of Cu poisoning (Bidewell et al., 2000). However, it is important to consider than only a proportion of cases have a massively elevated liver Cu concentration of more than double the upper limit of the reference range (25-100 mg/kg wet weight; Puls, 1994) and some animals have marginal hepatic Cu concentrations either just or below 150 mg/kg wet weight. In example, in a study in which chronic Cu intoxication was induced experimentally in cattle (Gummow, 1996), clinical signs of Cu toxicity were observed in animals that had a mean ±SD liver Cu concentration of 152±56.6 (range: 69-194) mg/kg wet weight. Furthermore, Perrin et al. (1990) described an episode of chronic Cu toxicity in a dairy herd that resulted from an error in the formulation of the feed; the mean ±SD wet weight Cu concentration in the livers of these animals was 126 ± 17.5 (range: 51-313) mg/kg. In these cases determination of Cu concentrations in the kidney was essential to confirm the clinical diagnosis (Bidewell et al., 2000), the degree of chronic hepatic injury being positively correlated with increasing concentrations of renal Cu (Robinson et al., 1999).

During the pre-haemolitic phase hepatic Cu accumulation, and therefore the animal risk of suffering from chronic Cu toxicity, must be evaluated in small samples obtained by *in vivo* biopsy. However, as indicated, the limit between safe-adequate hepatic Cu concentrations and those associated with chronic toxicity is very narrow, and for this reason the total hepatic Cu concentration *per se* is not, in our opinion, a good indicator of the risk of toxicity. Results of experimental studies in Cu loaded-animals indicate that toxicity appears once the liver capacity to store Cu is overloaded, which depends in great manner on the form in which the Cu is bound, mainly on the concentrations of MTs and the lysosomes capability to sequester the excess of Cu (Lopez-Alonso et al., 2006). Evaluation of MT concentrations and Cu bound to lysosomes could give a better indication of the risk of the animal to Cu toxicity.

DETERMINATION OF HEPATIC MT CONCENTRATIONS

Although initially was though that MT had a main role in detoxification of heavy metals (when discovered in horse kidney in 1957 by Margoshies and Vallee), later research attributed to these proteins a new role on metabolic regulation of Zn and Cu, as well as a radical-scavenging action that is closely regulated to the biological defense mechanism (Nordbeg, 1998).

The marked differences between animal species to Cu toxicity seems to be highly related to their ability to synthesise MT and the accumulation of Cu-MT. Thus, the toxicity of Cu is reduced in the liver of species, such as pig and dog, in which most of the hepatic Cu is bound to MT (Mehra and Bremner, 1984; Bremner and Beattie, 1990) and it is very high in other species, such as sheep, in which only a small proportion of the Cu is bound in this way. In cattle, although it has been suggested that there is limited capacity to accumulate large amounts of Cu as monomeric MT in the liver (Bremner and Marshall, 1974; Bremner, 1980), only a little information is available in the literature on MT concentrations. Understanding of Cu-MT homeostasis in cattle has become increasingly important, as this protein may additionally be involved in the pathogenesis of certain important neurological disorders and prion diseases (Mercer, 2001; Bounias and Purdey, 2002; Hanlon et al., 2002). Henry et al. (1994) found that sheep and cattle have only moderate hepatic MT levels (about 200 mg/kg) compared to pigs and dogs (500-600 mg/kg) and similar results have been observed in cattle exposed to moderately high Cu concentrations (López-Alonso et al., 2005a).

In spite of the assumed role of MT on hepatic Cu excretion this metal is a poor inducer of MT synthesis. Although it has been demonstrated that Cu can induce MT synthesis in laboratory animals, this only happens when administrated in a very large dose, such as by intraperitoneal injections, and variations of dietary Cu have little effect on liver MT expression, until the levels are extremely high (Mercer, 1997). However, most animal species, including ruminants, have a limited capacity to induce MT synthesis in response to increased dietary Cu intake (Saylor et al., 1980; Bremner and Beattie, 1995) even at very high concentrations. On the contrary, MT concentrations in cattle are strongly dependent on the Zn status of the animal (Figure 2) and it has been assumed that the levels of Zn in the liver are extremely important in controlling the synthesis and degradation of MT in most of the animal species (Bremner 1980): MT concentrations in the hepatocyte are very low in Zn-deficient animals and MT synthesis appeared to be stimulated by Zn supplementation of the diet (Saylor et al., 1980; Bremner and Beattie, 1990; Lee et al., 1994; Yu and Beynen, 1994).

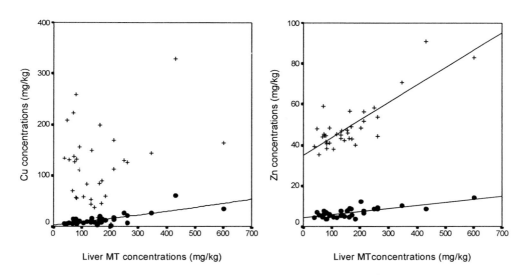

Figure 2. Relationship between MT and Cu and Zn concentrations (mg/kg wet weight) in the liver of cattle under moderately high Cu-exposure (+: total metal; •: bound to MT).

Although Cu is a poor inducer of MT synthesis, Cu can bind to MT by competing with Zn for the binding sites (Figure 2). This is because Cu has a higher avidity to MT than Zn, Cu can compete with and displace Zn from the MT even after Zn has induced its synthesis (Bremner and Beattie, 1995; Bremner, 1998). So, although Zn is essential for inducing MT synthesis, in the presence of Cu, it could be regarded as having a passive binding role to complete the full complement of metals and, thus, maintain the structural integrity of the protein (Bremner and Beattie, 1995). Moreover, the amount of Cu bound to MT will be highly dependent on the Zn status of the animal (López-Alonso et al., 2005a), and Cu-MT can be accurately calculated as a function of the Zn status of the animal. Although there are marked differences between species in the ability of Cu to bind to MT, Zn supplementation in the diet increases the amount of Cu-MT and, on the contrary, no Cu-MT is ever found in the liver of Zn-deficient animals, even in species like the pig in which 80% of liver Cu can be present as MT if the Zn status is normal (Bremner, 1987; Bremner, 1998).

The ability of Cu to displace Zn from the MT binding sites is very variable and depends on factors such as species, route of Cu administration and, especially, on the relative Cu and Zn content in the liver (Bremner and Beattie, 1990). As we have found in cattle during the chronic phase of hepatic Cu accumulation, the proportion of metal binding sites occupied by Cu increases when the ratio Cu:Zn in the liver cell is higher (Figure 3A): as liver Cu concentrations increase in cattle, more MT binding sites are occupied by Cu. Similar results have been obtained in experimental studies in sheep and cattle exposed to very high dietary Cu levels (Bremner and Marshall, 1974; Saylor et al., 1980), Cu being the only metal bound to MT in extreme Cu-loading (Bremner and Beattie, 1995).

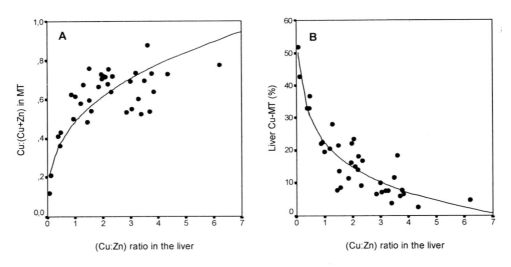

Figure 3. Relationship between (A) the proportion of binding sites of MT occupied by Cu (i.e.: Cu:(Cu+Zn) and (B) the proportion (%) of Cu bound to MT of the total Cu in the liver and the Cu:Zn ratio (by weight) in the liver of cattle under moderately high Cu-exposure.

The proportion of the total hepatic Cu bound to MT in cattle (Figure 3B) as well as in sheep (Saylor et al., 1980; Bremner 1987) is also very variable and has been associated with the relative proportions of Cu and Zn in the liver cell. When the Cu:Zn ratio is very low, which means there is no appreciable Cu accumulation, nearly half of the total hepatic Cu is bound to MT; however, when Cu accumulation increases the percentage of Cu-MT drastically decreases, being very low at high levels of Cu exposure (López-Alonso et al., 2005a). This suggests again that cattle, as with sheep, have a limited capacity to accumulate Cu-thioneins in their livers (Bremner, 1980). If the Cu biliary excretion in cattle is dependent on the Cu bound to MT, as in sheep, these results could indicate that at a high level of Cu exposure, the lysosomes capacity for Cu sequestering and elimination through the bile could be close to saturation (Corbett et al., 1978; Gooneratne et al., 1979) and the animals could be at risk of Cu toxicity.

DETERMINATION OF SUBCELLULAR HEPATIC CU CONCENTRATIONS

Hepatic subcellular distribution studies (Corbett et al., 1978; Gooneratne et al., 1979; Saylor and Leach, 1980; Kumaratilake and Howell, 1989) have shown that during the early stages of hepatic Cu accumulation in sheep, as in most mammals, Cu accumulates mainly in the cytosol bound to MT; however, unlike other species, sheep have a limited capacity to accumulate large amounts of Cu-MT in the liver, and saturation occurs very soon. Once the MT binding sites become saturated, uptake of Cu by lysosomes (in the large-granule fraction) is initiated for subsequent excretion in bile. Lysosomes are essential Cu storage organelles that protect the hepatic cell from the toxic effects of the metal; as long as lysosomes are able to sequester Cu, it can accumulate in the liver for weeks or months, without any clinical signs of liver damage (Howell and Gooneratne, 1987). However, once the lysosomes are overloaded, the storage of excess Cu in the nucleus and cytosol leads to cellular lesions.

In cattle hepatic subcellular Cu distribution has been poorly studied (López-Alonso et al., 2005b). Our own observations indicate that the distribution of Cu among in the different subcellular fractions in cattle (Figure 4) appears to be very similar to that described in sheep, in which the highest proportion of Cu is generally found in the large-granule fraction, followed by the cytosol and the nucleus, while the microsomal fraction contains relatively little Cu (Corbett et al., 1978; Gooneratne et al., 1979; Saylor and Leach, 1980; Kumaratilake and Howell, 1989). By contrast, in most other mammalian species, most Cu in the liver (i.e. 50% or more) is located in the cytosol, whereas the large-granule fraction accounts for only 20% (Evans, 1973; Corbett et al., 1978; Saylor and Leach, 1980). These differences in the intracellular distribution of Cu between sheep and cattle and other species less susceptible to Cu toxicity may be attributable to the limited ability of these ruminant species to synthesize soluble metal-binding proteins (Saylor and Leach, 1980).

In cattle, as in sheep, the capacity of the different subcellular fractions to accumulate Cu change with increasing total liver Cu concentration. The most marked variation was in the large-granule fraction, in which the rate of increase in Cu concentration per unit increase in total liver Cu concentration gradually declined, reaching a plateau at a projected total liver concentration of about 450 mg/kg, 4.5 times the generally accepted safe-adequate liver Cu concentration in this species (López-Alonso et al., 2005b). Subcellular studies in sheep have demonstrated that the large-granule fraction begins to plateau at a hepatic Cu concentration of between 160-180 mg/kg wet weight, less than two times the safe adequate concentration (Corbett et al., 1978; Gooneratne et al., 1979; Saylor and Leach, 1980). In other species less susceptible to Cu toxicity, such as rats, the capacity of the large-granule fraction becomes saturated at hepatic Cu levels of between 210-300 mg/kg wet weight, nearly 100 times the normal hepatic concentration in this species (Lal and Sourkes, 1971; Corbett et al., 1978). This indicates that cattle, although to a lesser extend than sheep, may have a limited capacity to accumulate Cu in the large-granule (i.e. lysosomal) fraction, and thus that saturation of the lysosomal Cu compartment tends to occur at a lower total Cu level than in other animal species. In the opinion of Saylor and Leach (1980), the poor Cu homeostasis in sheep may not reflect an inability of lysosomes to sequester Cu, but rather the lack of adequate soluble metal-binding-protein synthesis in response to increased Cu intake; if this were the case, there would be no increase in the accumulation of Cu in the large-granule fraction, primarily because protein-bound Cu is not available for sequestration. In other animal species in which Cu-MT is an important Cu storage form, the large-granule fraction shows a strong capacity for accumulating Cu, and in Cu-loaded animals Cu content in the large-granule fraction continues to be a linear function of the hepatic Cu concentration (Evans, 1973) until much higher total hepatic Cu concentrations.

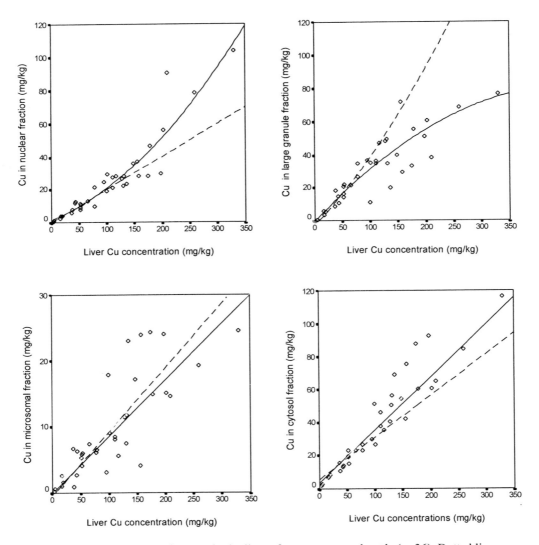

Fig 4. Subcellular distribution of copper in the liver of copper-exposed cattle (n=36). Dotted lines were obtained by regression considering only animals with safe-adequate total Cu levels (< 100 mg/kg, n=18).

Similarly than in sheep, in cattle once large-granule Cu accumulation starts to slow Cu accumulates at a faster rate in the nuclear fraction (see Gooneratne et al., 1979; Saylor and Leach, 1980; Kumaratilake and Howell, 1989). In fact, interpretation of variations in Cu content in the nuclear fraction in Cu-exposed animals is not easy, because during Cu accumulation lysosomes become larger and denser and tend to sediment in the nuclear fraction, so the observed increase in Cu content in this latter fraction is at least partly attributable to the storage of Cu by "dense" lysosomes which sediment with these heavy fractions (Howell and Gooneratne, 1987). Morphometric studies in sheep have demonstrated, however, that lysosomes predominantly increase in number rather than in volume before haemolysis (Gooneratne et al., 1980), and lysosomes do not become heavier and sediment with nuclei until Cu accumulation in the large-granule fraction has reached its plateau (Gooneratne et al., 1979). In cattle (López-Alonso et al., 2005b) the cytosol fraction continued to accumulate Cu after lysosomal Cu sequestration declined, though this Cu was not bound to MT. These findings are in agreement with those of Corbett et al. (1978) and Gooneratne et al. (1979) in sheep; these authors observed an increase in the proportion of Cu in the cytosol fraction with increasing Cu loading. However, these rises in the proportion of Cu in the cytosol were not as marked as those observed in the nucleus in pre-haemolytic animals, and indeed other studies in sheep have found no such rises (Saylor and Leach, 1980; Kumaratilake and Howell, 1989). Finally, the microsomal compartment played only a minor role in Cu accumulation in the cattle studied by us and, as in sheep, Cu tended to accumulate at a lower rate in this compartment as total liver Cu concentration increased (Gooneratne et al., 1979; Saylor and Leach, 1980; Kumaratilake and Howell, 1989).

THE ROLE OF ZINC IN HEPATIC CU ACCUMULATION IN CATTLE

Mutual antagonism between Cu and Zn has been regarded as a prime example of competitive biological interactions between metals with similar chemical and physical properties (Bremner and Beattie, 1995). As indicated, MT concentrations in cattle, as well as the amount of Cu bound to MT, are strongly dependent on the Zn status of the animal (López-Alonso et al., 2005a) and Cu-MT can be accurately calculated as a function of the Zn status of the animal; therefore knowledge of the Zn status of the animal could give valuable information about the risk of suffering chronic Cu toxicity.

In the liver, interactions between the two metals occur mainly in the cytosol, where Cu can compete with and displace Zn from MT binding sites, as we have previously described, in which this displacement is proportional to the total liver Cu concentration. Gooneratne et al. (1979) have demonstrated that in Cu-loaded sheep the proportion of Zn in the cytosol fraction decreases with increasing Cu loading, and that it is increasingly taken up by other subcellular compartments, notably the large-granule fractions (heavy and light mitochondrial fractions). However, Saylor and Leach (1980) did not find any significant effect of Cu exposure on the subcellular distribution of Zn in sheep exposed to different Zn and Cu levels in the diet. Our observations in cattle under to moderately high Cu exposure (López-Alonso et al., 2005b), Cu loading did not have a significant effect on Zn concentration in the cytosol, although liver Cu concentration was positively associated with Zn content in the large-granule fraction; this finding, together with the strong positive association between Cu bound to MT and Zn in the large-granule fraction, could indicate that Zn displaced from the MT is taken up by lysosomes for subsequent excretion. Although it may seem paradoxical to suppose that Cu displaced Zn from cytosolic MT, given that Zn levels in the cytosol were not affected by total liver Cu concentration in that study, this observation can be explained by taking into account that in the cytosol, in addition to MT, Zn is a component of superoxide dismutase and other high-molecular-weight proteins, which represent most of the soluble Zn and hardly vary with hepatic Cu levels (Bremner and Marshall, 1974; Saylor et al., 1980).

CONCLUSION

Under moderately high Cu exposure none of the blood markers currently available accurately predicted hepatic Cu accumulation in cattle and analysis of Cu content in the liver is probably the best diagnostic tool available for assessing the risk of chronic Cu toxicity. At a clinical diagnostic level, study of hepatic *in vivo* biopsy has focused on the measurement of total Cu concentration, whereas Cu intracellular distribution and MT concentrations have been poorly studied. This is possibly due to the fact that liver samples obtained by *in vivo* biopsy are generally too small for this kind of study, and may not be representative of Cu accumulation in the whole organ. In our opinion, the evaluation of intracellular Cu and Zn distribution (and particularly Cu concentration in lysosomes) and MT concentrations (as indicated, also related to neurodegenerative disorders) would give us very relevant information about the risk of suffering the clinical phase of chronic Cu toxicity. Further research into the molecular basis of Cu homeostasis in cattle is essential to better understand the pathogenesis of chronic Cu hepatic accumulation and to validate the use of subcellular Cu parameters as potential markers of the risk of Cu toxicity in cattle in samples obtained by *in vivo* biopsy.

REFERENCES

Araya, M.; Olivares, M.; Pizarro, F.; Gonzalez, M.; Speisky, H. & Uauy, R. (2003). Cu exposure and potential biomarkers of Cu metabolism. *Biometals, 16*, 199-204.

Arnhold, W.; Anke, M.; Glei, M.; Rideout, B.; Stalis, I.; Lowenstine, L.; Edwards, M.; Schüppel, K.F.; Eulenberger, K. & Nötzold, G. (1998). Determination of copper status in ruminants. *Trace Elements and Electrolytes, 15*, 65-69.

Auza, N.J.; Olson, W.G.; Murphy, M.J. & Linn, J.G. (1999). Diagnosis and treatment of Cu toxicosis in ruminants. *Journal of the American Veterinary Medicine Association, 214*, 1624-1628.

Baker, A.; Turkey, E.; Bonham, M.P.; O'Connor, J.M.; Strain, J.J.; Flynn, A. & Cashman, K.D. (1999). No effect of copper supplementation on biochemical markers of bone metabolism in healthy adults. *British Journal of Nutrition, 82*, 283-290.

Beshgetoor, D. & Hambidge, M. (1998). Clinical conditions altering copper metabolism in humans. *American Journal of Clinical Nutrition, 67*, 1017S-1021S.

Bidewell, C.A.; David, G.P. & Livesey, C.T. (2000). Copper toxicity in cattle. *The Veterinary Record, 147*, 399-400.

Binnerts, W.T. (1986). The copper status of cattle in the Netherlands. *Tijdchr Diergeneeskd, 111*, 321-324.

Blakley, B.R. & Hamilton, D.L. (1985). Ceruloplasmin as an indicator of copper status in cattle and sheep. *Canadian Journal Comparative Medicine, 49*, 405-408.

Bounias, M. & Purdey, M. (2002). Transmissible spongiform encephalopathies: a family of etiologically complex diseases. A review. *The Science of the Total Environment, 297*, 1-19.

Bradley, C.H. (1993). Copper poisoning in a dairy herd fed a mineral supplement. *Canadian Veterinary Journal, 34*, 287-292.

Bremner, I. (1980). Absorption, transport and distribution of copper. *Excerpta Medica (Ciba Foundation Symposium 79)*, 23-48.

Bremner, I. (1987). Interactions between metallothionein and trace elements. *Progress in Food an Nutrition Science, 11*, 1-37.

Bremner, I. (1991). Nutritional and physiological significance of metallothionein. *Methods in Enzimology, 205*, 25-35.

Bremner, I. (1998). Manifestations of copper excess. *American Journal of Clinical Nutrition, 67*,1069S-1073S.

Bremner, I. & Marshall, R.B. (1974). Hepatic copper-and zinc-binding proteins in ruminants. 2. Relationship between Cu and Zn concentrations and the occurrence of a metallothionein-like fraction. *British Journal of Nutrition, 32*, 293-299.

Bremner, I. & Beattie, J.H. (1990). Metallothionein and trace minerals. *Annual Reviews of Nutrition, 10*, 63-83.

Bremner, I. & Beattie, J.H. (1995). Copper and zinc metabolism in health and disease: Speciation and interactions. *Proceedings of the Nutrition Society, 54*, 489-499.

Brumm, M.C. (1998). Sources of manure: Swine. In: J.L. Hatfield & B.A. Stewart (Eds.), *Animal waste utilization: Effective use of manure as a soil resource (49-64)*. Michigan: Ann Arbor Press.

Charmley, L.L. & Symonds, H.W. (1985). A comparison of the ability of cattle and pigs to clear excess copper from the plasma and excrete it in bile. TEMA 5. *Commonwealth Agriculture Bureau Scotland, 5*, 339-341.

Cisternas, F.A.; Tapia, G. & Arredondo, M. (2005). Early histological and functional effects if chronic Cu exposure in rat liver. *BioMetals, 18*, 541-551.

Corbett, W.S.; Saylor W.W.; Long, T.A. & Leach, R.M. (1978). Intracellular distribution of hepatic copper in normal and copper-loaded sheep. *Journal of Animal Science, 47*, 1174-1179.

Cousins, R.J. (1985). Absorption, transport, and hepatic metabolism of copper and zinc: special reference to metallothionein and ceruloplasmin. *Physiological Reviews, 65*, 238-309.

Dameron, C.T. & Harrison, M.D. (1998). Mechanisms for protection against copper toxicity. *American Journal of Clinical Nutrition, 67*, 1091S-1097S.

Eife, R.; Weiss, M.; Müller-Hocker, J.; Lang, T.; Barros, V.; Sigmund, B.; Thanner, F.; Welling, P.; Lange, H.; Wolf, W.; Podeck, B.; Kittel, J.; Schramel, P. & Reiter, K. (1999). Chronic poisoning by Cu in tap water: II. Cu intoxication with predominantly systemic symptoms. *European Journal of Medical Research, 4*, 224-228.

Engle, T.E. & Spears, J.W. (2000). Effects of dietary copper concentration and source on performance and copper status of growing and finishing steers. *Journal of Animal Science, 78*, 2446-2451.

Evans, G.W. (1973). Copper homeostasis in the mammalian system. *Physiological Reviews, 53*, 535-570.

Fisher, P.W.F.; Lábbé, M.R. & Giroux, A. (1990). Effects of age, smoking, drinking, exercise and estrogen use on indices of copper status in healthy adults. *Nutrition Research, 10*, 1081-1090.

Galey, F.D.; Maas, J.; Tronstad, R.J.; Woods, L.W.; Jonson, B.J.; Litlefield, E.S.; Wallstrum, R. & Dorius, L.C. (1991). Copper toxicosis in two herds of beef calves following injection with copper disodium edetate. *Journal of Veterinary Diagnostic and Investigation, 3*, 260-263.

Gooneratne, S.R.; Buckey W.T. & Christensen, D.A. (1989a). Review of copper deficiency and metabolism in ruminants. *Canadian Journal of Animal Science, 69*, 819-845.

Gooneratne, S.R.; Laarveld, B.; Chaplin, R.K. & Christensen, D.A. (1989b). Profiles of [67]Cu in blood, bile, urine and faeces from [67]Cu-primed lambs: effect of [99]Mo-labelled tetrathiomolybdate on the metabolism of recently stored tissue [67]Cu. *British Journal of Nutrition, 61,* 355-371.

Gooneratne, S.R.; Howell, J.McC. & Cook, R.D. (1980). An ultrastructural and morphometric study of the liver of normal and copper-poisoned sheep. *American Journal of Pathology, 99*, 429-450.

Gooneratne, S.R.; Howell, J.McC. & Gawthorne, J. (1979). Intracellular distribution of copper in the liver of normal and copper loaded sheep. Research in Veterinary Science, 27, 30-37.

Gummow, B. (1996). Experimentally induced chronic copper toxicity in cattle. *Onderstepoort Journal of Veterinary Research, 63*, 277-288.

Hadrich, J. (1996). High amounts of Cu in calf's livers. Recent data and estimation of potential health hazards. *Deutsche Lebensmittel-Rundschau, 92*, 103-113.

Hanlon, J.; Monks, E.; Hughes, C.; Weavers, E. & Rogers, M. (2002). Metallothionein in bovine spongiform encephalopathy. *Journal of Comparative Pathology, 127*, 290-299.

Harris, E.D. (1997). Copper. In: R.A. O'Dell & B.L. Sunde (Eds.), *Handbook of Nutritionally Essential Mineral Elements (231-273)*. New York: Marcel Decker.

Harris, E.D. (2000). Cellular copper transport and metabolism. *Annual Review of Nutrition, 20*, 291-310.

Harris, E.D. (2001). Copper homeostasis: The role of cellular transporters. *Nutrition Reviews, 59*, 281-285.

Harrison, M.D. & Dameron, C.T. (1999). Molecular mechanism of copper metabolism and the role of the Menkes disease protein. *Journal of Biochemical and Molecular Toxicology, 13*, 93-105.

Haywood, S.; Muller, T.; Muller, W.; Heinz-Erian, R.; Tanner, M.S. & Ross, G. (2001). Copper-associated liver disease in North Ronaldsay sheep, A possible animal model for non-Wilsoniam hepatic copper toxicosis of infancy and childhood. *Journal of Pathology, 195*, 264-269.

Haywood, S.; Muller, T.; Mackenzie, A.M.; Muller, W.; Tanner, M.S.; Heinz-Erian, R.; Willians, C.L. & Loughran,M.J. (2004). Copper-induced hepatotoxicosis withhepatic stellate cell activation and severe fibrosis in North Ronaldsay lambs:a model for non-Wilsoniam hepatic copper toxicosis in infants. *Journal of Pathology, 130*, 266-277.

Henry, R.B.; Liu, J.; Choudhuri, S. & Klaassen C.D. (1994). Species variation in hepatic metallothionein. *Toxicology Letters, 74*, 23-33.

Horn, N. & Tümer, Z. (1999). Molecular genetics of intracellular copper transport. *Journal of Trace Elements in Experimental Medicine, 12*, 297-313.

Howell, J.McC. & Gooneratne, R.S. (1987). The pathology of copper toxicity in animals. In: J. McC. Howell & J.M. Gawthorne (Eds.) *Copper in Animals and Man, Vol. II.* (53-78) Florida: CRC Press.

Humann-Ziehank, E.; Coenen, M.; Ganter, M. & Bickhardt, K. (2001). Long-term observation of subclinical chronic Cu poisoning in two sheep breeds. *Journal of Veterinary Medicine Series A-Physiology Pathology Clinical Medicine, 48*, 429-439.

Jilg, T.; Unglaub, W. & Eckstein, B. (1997). Influence of Cu supplementation in milk replacers on the Cu concentration of calf livers. *Fleischwirtschaft, 77*, 559-562.

Kendall, N.R.; Illingworth, D.V. & Telfer, S.B. (2001). Cu responsive infertility in British Cattle: the use of a blood caeruloplasmin to Cu ratio in determining a requirement for Cu supplementation. In: M. G. Diskin (Ed.) *Fertility in the high producing dairy cow. Occasional Publication No 26 British Society of Animal Science (429-432)* Edinburgh.

Kumaratilake, J.S. & Howell, J.McC. (1987). Histochemical study of the accumulation of copper in the liver of sheep. *Research in Veterinary Science, 42*, 73-81.

Kumaratilake, J.S.& Howell, J.McC. (1989). Intracellular distribution of copper in the liver of copper-loaded sheep –a subcellular fractionation study. *Journal of Comparative Pathology, 101*, 161-176.

L'Herroux, L. L.; Le Roux, S.; Appriou, P. & Martinez, J. (1997). Behaviour of metals following intensive pig slurry applications to a natural field treatment process in Brittany (France). *Environmental Pollution, 97*, 119-130.

Langlands, J.P.; Donald, G.E. & Smith, A.J. (1987). Analysis of data collected in a residue survey: Cu and zinc concentratiosn in liver, kidney and muscle in Australian sheep and cattle. *Australian Journal of Experimental Agriculture, 27*, 485-491.

Laven, R.A.; Livesey, C.T.; Offer, N.W. & Fountain, D. (2004). Apparent subclinical hepatopathy due to excess copper intake in lactating Holstein cattle. *Veterinary Record, 155*, 120-121.

Laven, R.A. & Livesey, C.T. (2006). An evaluationof the effect od clotting and processing of blood sampleson the recovery of copper from bovine blood. *The Veterinary Journal, 171*, 295-300.

Lee, J.; Treloar, B.P. & Harris, P.M. (1994). Metallothionein and trace element metabolism in sheep tissues in response to high and sustained zinc dosages. I. Characterization and turnover of metallothionein isoforms. *Australian Journal of Agricultural Research, 45,* 303-320.

Linder, M.C.; Wooten, L.; Cerveza,P.; Cotton, S.; Shulze R. & Lomeli, N. (1998). Copper transport. *American Journal of Clinical Nutrition, 67,* 965S-971S.

Livesey, C.T. (2002). Investigation of copper poisoning in adult cows by veterinary laboratories agency. *Cattle Practice, 10,* 289-294.

López-Alonso, M.; Crespo, A.; Miranda, M.; Castillo, C.; Hernández, J. & Benedito, J.L. (2006). Assesement of some blood parameters as potential markers of hepatic copper accumulation in cattle. *Journal of Veterinary Diagnostic and Investigation, 18,* 71-75.

López-Alonso, M.; Prieto Montaña, F.; Miranda, M.; Castillo, C.; Hernández, J. & Benedito, J.L. (2005a). The role of metallothionein and zinc in hepatic Cu accumulation in cattle. The Veterinay Journal, 169, 262-267.

López-Alonso, M.; Montaña, F.P.; Miranda, M.; Castillo, C.; Hernández , J.; Benedito, J.L., (2005b). Intracellular distribution of copper and zinc in the liver of copper-exposed cattle from northwest Spain. *The Veterinary Journal, 170,* 332-338.

López-Alonso, M.; Benedito, J.L.; Miranda, M.; Castillo, C.; Hernández , J. & Shore, R.F., (2000b). Arsenic, cadmium, lead, copper and zinc in cattle from Galicia, NW Spain. *The Science of the Total Environment, 246,* 237-248.

López-Alonso, M.; Benedito, J.L.; Miranda, M.; Castillo, C.; Hernández, J. & Shore, R.F. (2000a) The effect of pig farming on copper and zinc accumulation in cattle in Galicia (North-Western Spain). *The Veterinary Journal 160,* 259-266

Luza, S.C. & Speisky, H.C. (1996). Liver copper storage during development, Implications for cytotoxicity. *American Journal of Clinical Nutrition, 63,* S812-820.

Mackenzie, A.M.; Allinworth, D.V.; Jackson, D.W. & Teifer, S.B. (1997). A comparison of methods of assessing copper status in cattle. In: P.W.F. Fischer; M.R. L'Abbé; K. A. Cackell & R.S. Gibson (Eds.) *Trace Elements in Man and Animals*, TEMA 9. (301-302) Alberta: NRC Research Press. Banff.

Margoshes, M. & Vallee, B.L. (1957). A cadmium protein from equine kidney cortex. *Journal of the American Chemical Society, 79,* 4813-4814.

Mehra, R.K. & Bremner, I. (1984). Species differences in the occurrence of copper-metallothionein in the particulate fractions of the liver of copper-loaded animals. *Biochemical Journal, 219,* 539-546.

Mercer, J.F.B. (2001). The molecular basis of Cu-transport diseases. *Trends in Molecular Medicine, 7,* 64-69.

Mercer, J.F.B. (1997). Gene regulation by copper and the basis for copper homeostasis. *Nutrition, 13,* 48-49.

Mercer, J.F.B. & Llanos, R.M. (2003). Molecular and cellular aspects of copper transport in developing mammals. *Journal of Nutrition, 133,* 1481S-1484S.

Milne, D.B. (1994). Assessment of copper status. *Clinical Chemistry, 40,* 1479-1484.

Minatel,L. & Carfagnini, J.C. (2002). Evaluation of the diagnosis value of plasma copper levels in cattle. *Preventive Veterinary Medicine, 53,* 1-5.

Nordberg, M. (1998). Metallothioneins, historical review and state of knowledge. *Talanta, 46,* 243-254.

NRC (2000). *Nutrient requirements of Beef Cattle.* (7th ed). Washington, DC.: National Academy Press.

Ortolani, E.L.; Machado, C.H. & Araripe; M.C. (2003). Assessment of some clinical and laboratory variables for early diagnosis of cumulative copper posioning in sheep. *Veterinary and Human Toxicology, 45*, 289-293.

Peña, M.O.O.; Lee, J. & Thiele, D.J. (1999). A delicate Balance: Homeostatic control of copper uptake and distribution. *Journal of Nutrition, 129*, 1251-1260.

Perrin, D.J.; Schiefer, B. & Blakley, B.R. (1990). Chronic copper toxicity in a dairy herd. *Canadian Veterinary Journal, 31*, 629-632.

Pinchuk, I. & Lichtenberg, D. (1999). Copper-induced LDL peroxitation: interrelated dependencies of the kinetics on the concentrations of copper, hydroperoxides and tocopherol. *FEBS Letters, 450*, 186-190.

Poole, D.B.R.; Mcgrath, D.; Fleming, G.A. & Moore, W. (1990). Effects of applying copper-rich pig slurry to grassland. *Irish Journal of Agricultural Research, 29*, 34-40.

Poulsen, H.D. (1998). Zinc and copper as feed additives, growth factors or unwanted environmental factors. *Journal of Animal and Feed Sciences, 7*, 135-142.

Puls, R. (1994). *Mineral levels in animal health.* Clearbrook, Sherpa International.

Robinson, F.R.; Sullivan, J.M.; Brelage, D.R.; Sommers, R.L. & Everson, R.J. (1999). Comparison of hepatic lesions in veal calves with concentrations of copper, iron and zinc in liver and kidney. *Veterinary and Human Toxicology, 41*, 171-174.

Rock, E.; Mazur, A.; O'Connor, J.M.; Bonham, M.P.; Rayssiguier, Y. & Strain, J.J. (2000). The effect of copper supplementation on red blood cell oxidizability and plasma antioxidants in middle-aged healthy volunteers. *Free Radical Biology and Medicine, 28*, 324-329.

Salisbury, C.D.C.; Chan, W. & Saschenbrecker, P. (1991). Multielement concentrations in liver and kidney tissues from five pecies of Canadian slaughter animals. *Journal of AOAC International, 74*, 587-591.

Saylor, W.W. & Leach, R.M. (1980). Intracellular distribution of copper and zinc in sheep, effect of age and dietary levels of the metals. *Journal of Nutrition, 110*, 448-459.

Saylor, W.W.; Morrow, F.D. & Leach, R.M. (1980). Copper- and zinc-binding proteins in sheep liver and intestine, Effects of dietary levels of the metals. *Journal of Nutrition, 110*, 460-468.

Simpson, D.M.; Beynon, R.J.; Robertson, D.H.L.; Loughran, M.J. & Haywood, S. (2004). Copper-associated liver disease: A proteomics study of copper challenge in a sheep model. *Proteomics, 4*, 524-536.

Speisky, H.; Navarro, P.; Cherian, M.G. & Jimenez, I. (2003). Copper-binding proteins in human erythrocytes, Searching for potential biomarkers of copper over-exposure. *Biometals, 16*, 113-123.

Steffen, D.J.; Carlson, M.P. & Casper, H.H. (1997). Copper toxicosis in suckling beef calves associated with improper administration of copper oxide boluses. *Journal of Veterinary Diagnostic and Investigation, 9*, 443-446.

Stoszed, M.J.; Mika, P.G.; Oldfield, J.L. & Weswig, P.H. (1986). Influence of copper supplementation on blood and liver copper in cattle fed tall fescue or quackgrass. *Journal of Animal Science, 62*, 263-271.

Sutherland, R.J.; Deol, H.S. & Hood, P.J. (1992). Changes in plasma bile acids, plasma amino acids, and hepatic enzymes pols as indices of functional impairment in liver-damaged sheep. *Veterinary Clinical Pathology, 21*, 51-56.

Suttle, N. (1993). Overestimation of copper deficiency. *Veterinary Record, 133*, 123-124.

Tessman, R.K.; Lakritz, J.; Tyler, J.W.; Casteel, S.W.; Willians, J.E. & Dew, R.K. (2001). Sensitivity and specifity of serum copper determination for detection of copper deficiency in feeder calves. *Journal of the American Veterinary Medicine Association, 218*, 756-760.

Tokarnia, C.H.; Dobereiner, J.; Peixoto, P.V. & Moraes, S.S. (2000). Outbreak of copper poisoning in cattle fed poultry litter. *Veterinary and Human Toxicology, 42*, 92-95.

Vermunt, J.J. & West, D.M. (1994). Predicting copper status in beef cattle using serum copper concentrations. *New Zealand Veterinary Journal, 42*, 194-195.

VLA Surveillance Report (2001). July sees an increased incidence of copper poisoning in cattle. *The Veterinary Record, 149*, 257-260.

Weaver, D.M.; Tyler, J.W.; Marion, R.S.; Castell, S.W.; Loiacono, C.M. & Turk, J.R. (1999). Subclinical copper accumulation in llamas. *Canadian Veterinary Journal, 40*, 422-424.

Wikse, S.E.; Herd, D.; Field, R. & Holland, P. (1992). Diagnosis of copper deficiency in cattle. *Journal of the American Veterinary Medicine Association, 200*, 1625-1629.

Yu, S. & Beynen, A.C. (1994). High zinc intake reduces biliary copper excretion in rats. *Journal of Animal Physiology and Animal Nutrition, 72*, 169-175.

In: Micronutrients and Health Research
Editor: Takumi Yoshida, pp. 227-247

ISBN: 978-1-60456-056-5
© 2008 Nova Science Publishers, Inc.

Chapter VII

ZINC, COPPER, MANGANESE AND MAGNESIUM IN LIVER CIRRHOSIS

Dario Rahelic[1], Milan Kujundzic[2] and Velimir Bozikov[1]

[1]Division of Endocrinology, Diabetology and Metabolic Disorders,
[2]Division of Gastoenterology,
Dubrava University Hospital, Zagreb, Croatia.

ABSTRACT

The role of trace elements in the pathogenesis of liver cirrhosis and its complications is still not clearly understood.

Zinc, copper, manganese and magnesium are essential trace elements whose role in liver cirrhosis and its complications is still a matter of research.

Zinc is associated with more than 300 enzymatic systems. Zinc is structured part of Cu-Zn superoxide dismutase, important antioxidative enzyme. Zinc acts as an antioxidant, a membrane and cytosceletal stabilizator, an anti-apoptotic agent, an important co-factor in DNA synthesis, an anti-inflammatory agent, etc. Copper is an essential trace element which participates in many enzymatic reactions. Its most important role is in redox processes. Reactive copper can participate in liver damage directly or indirectly, through Kupffer cell's stimulation. Scientists agree that copper's toxic effects are related to oxidative stress. Manganese is a structural part of arginase, which is an important enzyme in the urea metabolism. Manganese acts as an activator of numerous enzymes in Krebs cycle, particularly in the decarboxilation process.

Magnesium is important for the protein synthesis, enzyme activation, oxidative phosphorilation, renal potassium and hydrogen exchange etc.

Since zinc, copper, manganese and magnesium have a possible role in the pathogenesis of liver cirrhosis and cirrhotic complications, the aim of our study was to investigate the serum concentrations of mentioned trace elements in patients with liver cirrhosis and compare them with concentrations in controls.

Serum concentrations of zinc, copper, manganese and magnesium were determined in 105 patients with alcoholic liver cirrhosis and 50 healthy subjects by means of plasma sequential spectrophotometer. Serum concentrations of zinc were significantly lower (median 0.82 vs. 11.22 µmol/L, p<0.001) in patients with liver cirrhosis in comparison to controls. Serum concentrations of copper were significantly higher in patients with liver cirrhosis (median 21.56 vs. 13.09 µmol/L, p<0.001) as well as manganese (2.50 vs. 0.02 µmol/L, p<0.001). The concentration of magnesium was not significantly different between patients with liver cirrhosis and controls (0.94 vs. 0.88 mmol/L, p=0.132). There were no differences in the concentrations of zinc, copper, manganese and magnesium between male and female patients with liver cirrhosis. Only manganese concentration was significantly different between Child-Pugh groups (p=0.036). Zinc concentration was significantly lower in patients with hepatic encephalopathy in comparison to cirrhotic patients without encephalopathy (0.54 vs. 0.96 µmol/L, p=0.002). The correction of trace elements concentrations might have a beneficial effect on complications and maybe progression of liver cirrhosis. It would be recommendable to provide analysis of trace elements in patients with liver cirrhosis as a routine.

Keywords: Zinc, Copper, Manganese, Magnesium, Liver cirrhosis, Trace elements.

1. LIVER CIRRHOSIS

1.1. Epidemiology

According to data from the World Health Organization (WHO) chronic liver disease causes more than 1.4 million death outcomes per year. Liver cirrhosis mortality rates vary across the countries. A cirrhosis mortality rate in Great Britain is now among the highest in Europe (28.9 per 100.000 in man and 12.8 in women). Between 1987-1991 and 1997-2001, cirrhosis mortality in man in Scotland doubled more than once (112% increase) and in women increase almost by two-thirds (67%) (Leon et al., 2006 a,b). On the contrary, in Sweden decrease in liver cirrhosis mortality has been observed. In the last fifteen years an age standardized mortality rate of liver cirrhosis was about 4 per 100.000 deaths per year (Stokkeland et al., 2006).

The regional differences in cirrhosis mortality rates follow a north-south gradient, with the lowest rates in Northern and the highest in Southern Europe. In 1995 cirrhosis mortality rates in Northern Europe for men were about 12.2 per 100.000 and for women 4.8. On the contrary, in Southern Europe cirrhosis mortality rates were about 33.7 for men and 12.1 for women. Some exceptions were noticed in order to obtain general pattern. France has substantially higher death rates than other southern European countries like Greece, Spain and Italy (Ramstedt, 2002).

Taking into account that liver cirrhosis has important impact on overall mortality, even small progress in explaining the liver cirrhosis pathogenesis could have positive influence on disease progression.

1.2. Definition

Liver cirrhosis is, according to the WHO, a diffuse process characterized by fibrosis and conversion of normal liver architecture to structural abnormal nodules without normal lobular organization.

1.3. Etiology

There are numerous causes of liver cirrhosis. Alcohol is the most common cause in the Western countries but viral infection is the most common cause world-wide. Other causes, like hereditary hemochromatosis, Wilson's disease, α1-antitrypsin deficiency, galactosemia, autoimune disease, Budd-Chiari syndrome, secondary biliary cirrhosis, hepatic venous congestion, thrombosis of portal vein, infection, sarcoidosis, drugs, etc. are less common.

1.4. Alcoholic Liver Disease

Ethanol is metabolized in the liver through three pathways, by alcohol dehydrogenase / aldehyde dehydrogenase (ADH), microsomal ethanol oxidative system (MEOS) and by catalase.

More than 80% of ethanol is metabolized through first pathway. Consequently, an increase in the NADH/NAD ratio occurs, what inhibits many NAD+ dependent enzymes.

Liver changes caused by alcohol consumption include fatty liver, alcoholic hepatitis and alcoholic (Laenec's) liver cirrhosis. Fatty liver is initial, reversible phase of alcoholic liver disease characterized by the development of fatty vacuole in hepatocytes due to the impaired fatty acid metabolism.

Alcoholic hepatitis is characterized by hepatocyte necrosis, infiltration of polymorphonuclear leucocytes mainly in zone 3, then by dense cytoplasmic inclusions called Mallory bodies and by hiatal sclerosis (Jensen et al, 1994 a,b). Mallory bodies are not specific for alcoholic liver disease, because they can be found also in Wilson's disease and primary biliary cirrhosis.

Liver cirrhosis is pathohystological term characterized by necrosis of liver parenchyma, fibrosis and development of regeneratory lobules. According to the lobular size, liver cirrhosis can be divided on micronodular, macronodular and mixed cirrhosis. Micrinodular cirrhosis is characterized by lobules smaller than 3 mm in diameter and macronodular by lobules above 3 mm in diameter.

Alcoholic liver cirrhosis is usually micronodular, but during the time can transform to macronodular cirrhosis.

1.5. Pathogenesis of Alcoholic Liver Disease

Alcoholic liver cirrhosis is caused by toxic effects of alcohol on the liver, lipid peroxidation and immunologic alterations. After absorption, alcohol is transformed to acetaldehyde. Accumulation of acetaldehyde alters hepatocyte function. Also, the product of alcohol metabolism is reduced nicotinamide-adenine dinucleotide (NADH) which accumulates in the cytosol and mitochondria of hepatocytes. That results in inhibition of many NAD+ dependent enzymes like the enzymes of β-oxidation. All that cause decreased oxidation of fatty acids with increased export of very low density lipoprotein (VLDL) and hypertriglyceridemia which are commonly associated with alcohol use (Crabb & Estonius, 1998). Consequently, fat deposition occurs within the liver what cause so called *fatty liver*. Acetaldechide can also modify liver proteins and DNA forming neoantigens which can be recognized by the immune system and cause immunological reaction. Acetaldechyde stimulates collagen synthesis by stellate cells. Acetaldechyde reduces mitochondrial glutathione concentration. Alcohol by itself causes increased oxygen consumption with consequent centrilobular hypoxia.

In the condition of low blood and tissue alcohol concentration, ADH has a key role in the metabolism of alcohol. When tissue concentration increases above 10 mmol/L MEOS starts to metabolize alcohol. MEOS is situated in microsomes of smooth endoplasmic reticulum. Chronic alcohol consumption causes an increase in MEOS activity 5 to 10 times. Main role in MEOS has isoenzyme CYP2E1 from cytochrom P450 family. CYP2E1 metabolizes ethanol but also acetaldechyde and many other drugs what explains the increased toxicity of therapeutic doses of some drugs in alcoholics (Vucelic et al., 2002).

Chronic alcohol consumption leads to the induction of CYP2E1 with generation of oxygen radicals and lipid peroxidation. Also, alcohol sensitizes Kupffer cells and stellate cells and probably inhibits regeneration of injured hepatocytes (Crabb & Estonius, 1998). Reactive oxygen species cause hepatocyte injury by lipid peroxidation.

In pathogenesis of liver cirrhosis important occurrences are necrosis of hepatocytes, hepatocellular regeneration, fibrosis and destruction of lobular structure with forming pseudolobules.

In fibrogenesis, necrosis of hepatocytes occurs first. In the early phase, as mentioned above, products of cell inflammation, like proteinases and free oxygen radicals, cause necrosis of hepatocytes with consequent release of numerous cytokines. Changes of extracellular matrix occur in further phase. Those changes include non-proportional increase in a concentration of some extracelular matrix molecules, changes on molecules and their transposition within the matrix.

There is a multiple increase in concentration of extracellular matrix molecules like collagen, glycoproteins and proteoglycans. Chronic alcohol intake also stimulates production and releasing of numerous cytokines by stimulated Kupffer cells. One of the most important cytokine in fibrogenesis is certainly transforming growth factor β (TGF-β). Released cytokines stimulate stellate cells on proliferation and collagen synthesis.

On the other hand, degradation of protein matrix has also important role in fibrogenesis (Sherlock et al., 2002). Matrix degradation is regulated by metalloproteinase (Arthur & Iredale, 1994; Arthur, 2000). The most important metalloproteinases are collagenases (MMP-

1 and MMP-13, which disolve type I, II and III collagen), gelatinase (MMP-2 and MMP-9, which disolve type IV collagen) and stromelisins (MMP-3 and MMP-10, which disolve proteoglycans, laminin, fibronectin, etc.) (Takahara et al., 1995). All these enzymes are synthesized by Kupffer cells and activated stellate cells. Metalloproteinases are inhibited by tissue metalloproteinase inhibitors (TIMP). Activated stellate cells synthesize TIMP-1. Therefore, stellate cells have important role in degradation and synthesis of connective tissue (Iredale et al., 1992).

Fibrosis alters the liver structure and obstructs biliary and vascular pathways with clinical consequences.

1.6. Clinical Manifestations of Liver Cirrhosis

Fatty infiltration causes nonspecific symptoms or abnormal laboratory results of liver function. The liver is usually enlarged. In advanced alcoholic liver disease common symptoms are loss of appetite, weight loss, nausea, jaundice, abdominal pain and edema. Liver cirrhosis is characterized by an enlarged liver in the beginning and small, fibrous liver in advanced stages, enlarged spleen, portal hypertension with esophageal varices, hepatic encephalopathy, anemia, etc.

1.7. Treatment of Patients with Liver Cirrhosis

Treatment of liver cirrhosis is mostly symptomatically. Usually, the main problem in patients with liver cirrhosis is the treatment of complications like hepatic encephalopathy, hepatorenal syndrome and bleeding from esophageal varices.

Numerous studies have tried to focus on prevention of alcoholic liver cirrhosis and progression of alcoholic liver disease to liver cirrhosis. There were also numerous studies which have tried to slow down progression of liver disease and prevent complications. As the oxidative stress has important role in pathogenesis of liver cirrhosis, trace elements have become important substrate for investigations of pathogenesis of liver cirrhosis and its complications.

Trace elements certainly have important role in pathogenesis of liver cirrhosis and its complications.

2. TRACE ELEMENTS

2.1. Definition

Trace elements are present in human body in very small concentration *(ppm - pars per million)*.

Development of new laboratory methods has allowed better quality and quantity determination of trace elements, as well as better understanding of their role in numerous metabolic processes.

There are essential and nonessential trace elements. Essential trace elements are those necessary for life and normal body function. According to Cotzias (Cotzias, 1967), essential trace elements are iron (Fe), zinc (Zn), copper (Cu), manganese (Mn), cobalt (Co), iodine (J), molybdenum (Mo), selenium (Se) and chromium (Cr). There is an additional division of trace elements on incontestable essential trace elements and »probably essential trace elements for humans«. Incontestably essential trace elements are iron (Fe), zinc (Zn), copper (Cu), chromium (Cr), iodine (I), cobalt (Co), molybdenum (Mo) and selenium (Se). Probably essential trace elements are manganese (Mn), tin (Sn), nickel (Ni), fluor (F), silicon (Si), vanadium (Va), calcium (Ca) and magnesium (Mg).

Trace elements entry includes ingestion by food and water. Normal nutrition satisfies requirements of human body for trace elements.

Concentration of trace elements is different in different drinking waters. Food processing, especially industrial, influences (mostly decrease) concentration of trace elements. There is also a question of trace element supplementation in patients with long-term parenteral nutrition.

All above mentioned suggests that an intake of trace elements in human body by food or by drink water varies.

Trace elements form moderately stable complexes with enzymes, nucleic acids and other ligands, changing and controlling their function, while other form compact static complexes and become integral functional components of enzymes (Speech et al., 2001). Therefore, it is obvious that some trace elements participate in numerous biochemical reactions which are necessary for life, like oxygen transport and release, redox processes, etc.

Optimal concentration of trace elements is within narrow range between their deficiency and toxicity.

Deficiency of trace elements is usually caused by the inadequate intake or other factors, like an increased loss caused by diarrhea, malabsorption after surgical resection of small intestine, by forming metal complexes with food ingredients which do not allow absorption, increase urinary losses, increase losses caused by pancreatic juices or other exocrine secretions, etc. The deficiency can as well be caused by the antagonistic actions of some trace elements on absorption or transportation of other trace elements, for example, in the case of intake of zinc and copper or copper and molibden. The intake of one trace element can also cause the deficiency of the other trace elements.

Toxic effects of trace elements depend on chemical shape, way of entry in the body, biological ligands, tissue distribution, concentration and velocity of elimination.

Toxicity mechanisms include enzyme inhibition by binding to essential amino-acid residuum, changing both function and structure of nucleic acids, inhibition of synthesis, influence on membrane permeability, inhibition of phosphorilation, etc (Kasper et al., 2005).

As it would be difficult to present role of all trace elements in liver cirrhosis we choose to present only zinc, copper, manganese and magnesium according to data from our research.

2.2. Zinc, Copper, Manganese and Magnesium in Liver Cirrhosis

The role of trace elements in pathogenesis of liver cirrhosis and its complications is still not clearly understood. In fibrogenesis the initial occurrence is hepato-cellular necrosis. In the early phase, inflammation cell products, proteinases and reactive oxygen radicals, may initiate hepato-cellular necrosis with consecutive releasing of numerous cytokines. Following hepatic injury, there is an increase in extracellular matrix, the activation of stellate cells, the increase in rough endoplasmatic reticulum and expression of smooth muscle specific α-actin (Friedman, 1993).

Activated stellate cells are influenced by numerous cytokines. Some of them have proliferative effect on stellate cells while others stimulate fibrogenesis (Pinzani, 1995).

Zinc, copper, manganese and magnesium are essential trace elements whose role in liver cirrhosis and its complications is still a matter of research. There are contrary reports about their serum concentrations in patients with liver cirrhosis.

2.2.1. Zinc

Zinc is incontestably essential trace element in humans. In nature zinc is especially present in sea food, cereals, vegetable, milk, walnuts etc. Average daily intake is approximately 12-15 mg. From oral intake, only 20-30% will be absorbed. In the enteric cell zinc induces synthesis of metalothionein, low molecular weight protein and when this process ends further absorption of zinc decreases. About two thirds of absorbed zinc is bounded on albumin and other is bounded on ß-2 microglobulin. Normal plasma concentration of zinc is 0.85-1.10 µg/mL.

In adult people renal excretion is approximately 300-600 µg per day. Renal tubular absorption decreases with tiazid diuretics administration (Prasad et al., 1996). Increased urinary losses are common in nephrotic syndrome, liver cirrhosis and other hypoalbuminic states, during penicillamine administration, catabolic states after burning, trauma, surgery, hemolytic anemia, etc. Decreased serum concentration of zinc is common in patient with acute myocardial infarction, infection, hepatitis, etc. (Kasper et al., 2005).

Lower serum concentration of zinc is common in patients with liver cirrhosis due to decreased intake, decreased absorption, decreased bioavailability and increased losses due to malabsorption, diarrhea or increased urinary losses.

There is a reduced liver protein synthesis in patients with liver cirrhosis with consequently decreased zinc bioavailability.

Zinc participates in more than 300 enzymatic systems (Christianson, 1991). Zinc is involved in synthesis of nucleic acid, protein synthesis, testosterone secretion, cerebral function etc. Zinc presents natural defense from reactive oxygen radicals through antioxidative enzyme, Cu-Zn superokside dysmutase (Speich et al., 2001). Its role in storage and release of hormones, neurotransmision, visual processes and cognitive processes were also described (Truong-Tran et al., 2000; Vallee et al., 1993).

Zinc acts as an antioxidant, membrane and cytoskeletal stabilizator, anti-apoptotic agent, important cofactor in DNA synthesis, anti-inflamatory agent etc. (Truong-Tran et al., 2001).

In the last decade role of zinc in apoptosis was considered intensively (Truong-Tran et al., 2000; Zalewski et al., 1993; Sunderman, 1995; Wyllie, 1997). Apoptosis is important in early embryonic development, what has been found in investigations with zinc deficient rats (Record et al., 1985).

Ethanol consumption induces apoptosis in liver and lymphoid tissue as well as many other. According to the published data it seems that zinc has influence on apoptosis of blood mononuclear cells by inhibiting the mitochondrial pathway of cell death. It was suggested that mitochondrial pathway of ethanol-related immune cell death may be inhibited by zinc supplementation (Szuster-Ciesielska et al., 2005).

On the other hand, it seems that zinc at pharmacologic concentrations stimulates cytokine expression and induces apoptosis of peripheral blood mononuclear cells (Chang et al., 2006).

The role of zinc in Alzheimer disease has also been investigated (Anderson et al., 1996).

Zinc has also role in glucose metabolism. Decreased secretion of insulin and impaired glucose tolerance were found in zinc deficient patients (Marchesini et al., 1998). Zinc is also integral part of insulin molecule and crucial for the synthesis, storage and secretion of insulin in pancreatic islet cells (Grungreiff et al., 2005; Chausmer, 1998; Blostein-Fuji et al., 1997). There has been hypothesed that zinc deficiency could be a link between liver cirrhosis and "liver" diabetes mellitus (Grungreiff et al., 2005). Zinc supplementation increases glucose disposal due to the increased non-insulin-mediated glucose uptake, without any systematic effect on insulin secretion and sensitivity (Marchesini et al., 1998).

Zinc has an important role in fibrogenesis. Some of zinc metalloenzymes, like DNA and RNA polymerases, have a great impact on regeneration of liver parenchyma. In fibrogenesis, zinc acts antagonistically to copper (Arakawa et al., 2003).

Zinc inhibits the cross-linking of covalent bonds in collagen through lysyl oxidase (Sato et al., 2005).

Zinc is a structure part of collagenasis. On the other hand, zinc is the inhibitor of prolyl hydroxilase, which is important enzyme in collagen synthesis (Camps et al., 1992).

In some studies, in the early phase a positive correlation between liver regeneration and zinc tissue concentration was found (Milin et al., 2005). In regenerated liver translocation of metallothionein to the nuclei is noticed where zinc participate in cell cycle processes (Tsujikawa et al., 1994).

Zinc is an activator of ornithin transcarbomoilase which participates in ammonia metabolism.

Zinc also participates in amino-acid metabolism, therefore its role in portal encephalopathy was investigated. Studies have showed that long-term oral zinc supplementation in patients with liver cirrhosis improve urea synthesis from ammonia and amino-acids with consequently decrease in concentration of ammonia and improvement clinical features of liver cirrhosis (Marchesini et al., 1996).

According to the results from clinical trials, zinc has a positive effect on the oxydative stress. Zinc supplementation in protein deficient rats resulted in increased activity of catalase, glutathion peroxidase, glutathion reductase and glutathion-S-transferase (Sidhu et al., 2005).

Zinc supplementation in those patients leads to significant increase in reduced glutathion concentration (GSH) and increased superoxide dismutase (SOD) activity in comparison to control group. By zinc supplementation in mentioned research serum concentration of copper, iron and selenium were normalized.

The results suggested possible influence of zinc on antioxidative enzymes activity and its possible effect on concentration of other trace elements.

The research on animal models showed that zinc supplementation has a protective effect on ethanol induced liver damage.

Zinc supplementation decreases ethanol induced zinc depletion and decrease in cytochrom P450 2E1 (CYP2E1) activity. Also, zinc supplementation increases activity of alcohol dehydrogenase in liver. That partially can explain zinc influence on the oxidative stress.

Zinc has also the important role in preserving of intestinal integrity as well as in prevention of endotoxemia with consequent inhibition of TNF-α synthesis induced by endotoxine (Kang et al., 2005).

Mentioned effects of zinc are independent from metallothioneine. Zinc supplementation has protective effect on ethanol induced decreasing of glutathione concentration, decreasing glutathione peroxidase activity and increasing glutathione reductase activity in liver (Zhou et al., 2005).

Zinc inhibits free oxygen radicals generation and increases antioxidative pathways activity.

According to Camps (Camps et al., 1992) zinc supplementation leads to decreased lipid peroxidation, collagen deposition, inhibition of prolyl-hydroxilase and increased collagenase activity.

Zinc induces synthesis of metallothionein. Metallothionein is effective cytoprotective agent against ethanol induced liver damage. Its protective effect can be explained by its influence on oxidative stress (Zhou et al., 2002).

Also, ZNF 267 (*zinc finger protein* 267) mRNA expression is increased in stellate cells of patients with liver cirrhosis. ZNF 267 is binding for MMP-10 and presents negative regulator of transcription MMP-10 and indirectly enhances fibrogenesis in the liver (Schnabl et al., 2005). The role of MMP-10 was mentioned above. All mentioned suggests the important role of zinc in fibrogenesis and pathogenesis of liver cirrhosis and its complications.

2.2.2. Copper

Copper is an essential trace element which participates in many enzymatic reactions. Copper has the most important role in redox processes, where presents donator of electron on mitochondrial level.

Copper absorbed in duodenum, binds for ceruloplasmin, albumin and transcuprein. More than 90% of copper in plasma binds for ceruloplasmin, and the rest binds for albumin and transcuprein (Luza et al., 1996).

In hepatocite copper is incorporated into ceruloplasmin and metallothionein, cistein rich protein, which binds also other heavy metals, like cadmium and mercury. Metallothionein acts as a factor of detoxicaton in gastrointestinal mucosa, but also prevents copper induced cytotoxicity (Luza et al., 1996; Sato et al., 2005). Copper enters into the cell by two copper transporting enzymes, ATP-ase ATP7A i ATP7B, products of genes for Menkel and Wilson's disease. Copper elimination is mainly through hepatobiliary tract, and around 4% by urinary tract.

Copper participates in gene expression. Copper is a cofactor of many enzymes, like superoxide dismutase, important antioxidative enzyme, furthermore enzyme tirosinase, which is necessary for melanin synthesis in human body, as well as many other enzymes. Copper influences on metabolism of iron, its absorption, incorporation in hemoglobin, etc.

Toxic effect of copper was focus of interest of many scientists. One of proposed model was that metallothionein saturated with copper entry to lysosomes, where is incompletely demolished and polymerized, forming insoluble material containing reactive copper which, together with iron, run lisosomal lipid peroxidation. That consequently causes hepatocyte necrosis.

Reactive copper participates in liver damage directly or indirectly, through stimulation of Kupffer and other cells (Klein et al., 1998). Toxic effect of copper is explained through its role in production of oxygen radicals (Bremner, 1998). Oxygen radicals can cause destruction of cell lipids, nucleic acids, proteins and carbohydrates, what results in the impairment of cell function and cell integrity.

Copper is also very important in fibrogenesis. Copper is the cofactor of lysil oxidase, which is involved in the formation of molecular bridges in collagen. An excessive accumulation of copper in the liver and an increase in the copper concentration promote hepatic fibrosis (Arakawa and Suzuki, 1993; Sato et al., 2005).

2.2.3. Manganese

Manganese is an essential trace element discovered in 1774. Manganese entries the human body by ingestion. Only 3-4% of ingested manganese is absorbed. Proportion of absorbed manganese can increase in specific states, like hypochromic anemia. In plasma manganese is transported by transmanganin (Kasper et al., 2005). In the body manganese is accumulated in mitochondria. The highest concentration of manganese is in enteric system, liver, pancreas, kidney, lungs and muscles. It passes hemato-encephalic barrier and can be accumulated in the brain in the state of prolonged exposition. Mainly, manganese is excreted through hepatobiliary system. Partly is reabsorbed in small intestine and the rest is excreted by feces.

Ingestion of manganese substances can cause destruction of gastrointestinal mucosa with bleeding. Chronic intoxication with manganese leads to degenerative changes in basal ganglia, especially in globus pallidus and corpus striatum (Spahr et al., 1996; Rose et al., 1999). Decreased synthesis of dopamine and decreased conversion causes decreased concentration of dopamine in corpus striatum. Possible explanation could be decreased activity of tyrosine kinase and other oxidative enzymes situated in mitochondria, where manganese is especially accumulated. Gradually, in three phases, symptoms like those in Parkinson disease develop in patients intoxicated with manganese.

Manganese is a structural part of arginase, which is an important enzyme in the urea metabolism. Manganese acts as an activator of numerous enzymes in Krebs cycle, particularly in the decarboxilation process.

Glutamine synthesis is also manganese metalloenzyme what confirms the role of manganese in antioxidative system. Manganese influences on skeletal growth, synthesis of nucleic acids, proteins, hemoglobin, lipid and carbohydrates metabolism, etc.

According to the results of the studies, there is a common increased serum concentration of manganese in patients with hepatic encephalopathy. There are opinions that toxicity of manganese contributes to occurrence of hepatic encephalopathy. Prevention of manganese accumulation and decrease in serum manganese concentration could have beneficial effect on mental status of patients with liver cirrhosis (Hauser et al., 1996).

Several studies have showed accumulation of manganese in basal ganglia in patients with liver cirrhosis. Extrapyramidal symptoms could be explained as a result of copper toxicity on dopaminergic function of basal ganglia (Spahr et al., 1996; Rose et al., 1999).

2.2.4. Magnesium

Magnesium is the fourth frequent cation in human body. It occurs in soft tissues and bones. Only 1-5% of magnesium is situated extracellularly. The main part of magnesium originates from ingested food. About 1/3 of ingested magnesium will be absorbed. Mostly, magnesium will be excreted through urinary system. Around 30% is bounded to serum proteins, 15% is in complexes and around 50% is available in ionized form. Magnesium bounded to serum proteins is mainly (75%) bounded to albumins, α-1 and α-2 globulins. Parathyroid hormone is important regulator of magnesium concentration acting through regulation of renal tubular reabsorption.

Magnesium is important in protein synthesis, activation of enzymes, oxidative phosphorilation, etc.

Magnesium also has an important role on the level of neuromuscular connection where slows down neuromuscular impulse inhibiting acetylcholine. That is the main reason why disturbance in magnesium equilibrium causes neuromuscular symptoms.

Magnesium deficiency is usually caused by kidney disease, chronic alcoholism, excessive diuresis, malabsorption, sever diarrhea, etc. Magnesium deficiency causes increased muscular excitability due to the increased acetylcholine activity, with consequent muscular tremor. Mental disorders include confusion and hallucinations. Magnesium influences on heart conductive system and magnesium deficiency can cause arrhythmia. Magnesium intoxication usually caused by acute or chronic renal insufficiency, cause hyporeflexity, cardiac arrhythmia, respiratory depression and coma.

According to the results of published studies, there is a decreased serum concentration of magnesium in patients with liver cirrhosis (Rocchi et al., 1994). Study of Stergiou has showed that spironolactone decreases magnesium excretion by decreasing furosemide-induced renal excretion of potassium and magnesium (Stergiou et al., 1993).

Since zinc, copper, manganese and magnesium have the possible role in the pathogenesis of liver cirrhosis and cirrhotic complications, the aim of our study was to investigate the serum concentrations of mentioned trace elements in patients with liver cirrhosis and compared them with concentrations in controls.

3. MATERIAL AND METHODS

3.1. Subjects

The study included 105 patients with diagnosed liver cirrhosis of ethylic etiology who were hospitalized from 2000 to 2005 in the Division of Gastroenterology at Dubrava University Hospital, with median age 55 years. Seventy eight (74%) of them were male and twenty seven (26%) were female. According to the Child-Pugh classification patients with liver cirrhosis were divided in Child-Pugh A, B and C group. There were 35 subjects in every Child-Pugh group.

Inclusion criteria were alcoholic liver cirrhosis (diagnosed by anamnestic data of alcohol consumption, laboratory and pathohistological findings, negative markers of viral hepatitis and normal values of ceruloplasmine), ability to sign the Informed consent and age 18 to 70.

Exclusion criteria were vegetarianism, Wilson's disease, malign disease, acute liver failure, impaired renal function (creatinine clearance <60 ml/min), multiorganic failure and inability to sign the Informed consent.

The control group consisted of 50 healthy subjects (median age 52 years) who were performed laboratory analysis as part of systematic medical examinations. There were 35 (70%) males and 15 (30%) females.

The Informed consent was obtained from all study subjects. The study protocol was approved by the Ethics Committee of Dubrava University Hospital. The protocol was carried out in accordance with the ethics guidelines of the Helsinki Declaration.

3.2. Methods

Blood samples were collected without anticoagulans and serum was stored in a freezer on -20°C until processing. In processing 1 ml of serum was taken, 1.5 ml of concentrated nitric acid and 0.5 ml 30% H_2O_2 were added on account of the digestion. After the digestion the sample was cooling for 20 minutes. The solution was transferred into a 10 ml container and was supplemented with ultra clean water. The concentrations of trace elements were determined by means of plasma sequential spectrophotometer TraceScan (Thermo Jarrell Ash, USA). Data were presented with median and 5-95 percentile range and compared using Wilcoxon and Kruskal-Wallis non-parametric tests. Statistics was done using MedCalc software (MedCalc Software, Mariakerke, Belgium). Only $p < 0.05$ was considered significant.

4. RESULTS

The serum concentrations of zinc, copper, manganese and magnesium in patients with liver cirrhosis and controls are presented in Table 1. The serum concentration of zinc was significantly lower in patients with liver cirrhosis in comparison to the controls (0.82 µmol/L vs. 11.22 µmol/L, $p < 0.001$). The serum concentration of copper was significantly higher in patients with liver cirrhosis in comparison to the controls (21.56 µmol/L vs. 13.09 µmol/L, p<0.001) as well as manganese concentration (2.50 μmol/L vs. 0.02 μmol/L, p<0.001). The concentration of magnesium was not significantly different between patients with liver cirrhosis and controls (Table 1, p=0.132). There were no differences in the concentrations of zinc, copper, manganese and magnesium between male and female patients with liver cirrhosis (Table 2).

The data in Table 3 show that the serum levels of manganese were significantly different between Child-Pugh groups (H=9.21, p=0.036). An additional analysis showed that the serum levels of manganese were significantly higher in patients with Child-Pugh C liver cirrhosis (6.30 μmol/L) in comparison to patients with Child-Pugh A (2.00 μmol/L , z=-3.09, p=0.002) and B liver cirrhosis (2.10 μmol/L, z=-2.06, p=0.039). The concentrations of zinc, copper, and magnesium did not differ significantly between Child-Pugh groups (Table 3).

The serum concentrations of zinc, copper, manganese and magnesium in cirrhotic patients with and without hepatic encephalopathy are represented in Table 4. The concentration of zinc was significantly lower in patients with hepatic encephalopathy in comparison to cirrhotic patients without encephalopathy (0.54 μmol/L vs. 0.96 μmol/L, p=0.002). There were no differences in serum concentrations of other trace elements between patients with or without encephalopathy. The serum concentrations of zinc, copper, manganese and magnesium in cirrhotic patients with and without ascites are represented in Table 5. Only manganese concentration was significantly different between patients with and without ascites. Namely, serum manganese concentration was higher in cirrhotic patients with ascites in comparison to the cirrhotic patients without ascites (4.10 μmol/L vs. 1.80 μmol/L, p<0.001).

Table 1. Serum concentrations of zinc, copper, manganese and magnesium in patients with liver cirrhosis and controls

Trace elements	Subjects (N=105) median and 5 - 95 percentiles	Controls (N=50) median and 5 - 95 percentiles	Statistics z	p
Zinc (μmol/L)	0.82 (0.24–1.74)	11.22 (9.23–15.10)	10.05	<0.001
Copper (μmol/L)	21.56 (11.17–30.60)	13.09 (11.17–19.95)	-7,66	<0.001
Manganese (μmol/L)	2.50 (0.01–29.65)	0.02 (0.01–0.40)	-8,21	).001
Magnesium (mmol/L)	0.94 (0.63–1.36)	0.88 (0.56–1.12)	-1.51	132

Table 2. Serum concentrations of zinc, copper, manganese and magnesium in male and female patients with liver cirrhosis

Trace elements	Male (N=78) median and 5 - 95 percentiles	Female (N=27) median and 5 - 95 percentiles	Statistics z	p
Zinc (μmol/L)	0.84 (0.25–1.70)	0.74 (0.20–1.99)	-0.32	0.750
Copper (μmol/L)	21.18 (9.86–30.07)	23.56 (15.49–32.12)	1.58	0.113
Manganese (μmol/L)	2.10 (0.01–31.20)	3.70 (0.08–29.55)	1.45	0.146
Magnesium (mmol/L)	0.96 (0.58–1.40)	0.88 (0.71–1.36)	-1.05	0.293

Table 3. Serum concentrations of trace elements in Child-Pugh groups

Trace elements	Child-Pugh A (N=35) median and 5 - 95 percentiles	Child-Pugh B (N=35) median and 5 - 95 percentiles	Child-Pugh C (N=35) median and 5 - 95 percentiles	Statistics	
				H	p
Zinc(μmol/L)	1.06 (0.38–1.49)	0.78 (0.26–1.94)	0.54 (0.14–1.45)	19.24	0.053
Copper (μmol/L)	19.98 (13.75–29.84)	22.30 (10.51–31.65)	23.20 (9.75–29.76)	1.00	0.608
Manganese (μmol/L)	2.00 (0.12–9.42)	2.10 (0.01–27.62)	6.30 (0.01–35.75)	9.21	0.036
Magnesium (mmol/L)	0.93 (0.65–1.18)	0.96 (0.65–1.38)	0.88 (0.40–1.53)	5.34	0.084

5. DISCUSSION

Mechanisms linked on ethanol metabolism, especially oxidative stress, redox potentials and acetaldehyde, participate in the emergence of liver damage. Trace elements play an important role in oxidative stress and redox potentials. A possible role of zinc, copper, manganese and magnesium in pathogenesis of liver cirrhosis and its complications is still subject of researches.

In our research the serum levels of zinc were significantly lower in patients with liver cirrhosis in comparison to controls (Table 1, median 0.82 μmol/L in patient with liver cirrhosis and 11.22 μmol/L in controls, p<0.001). The results confirm Kugelmans' research (Kugelmas et al., 2000), which explained low zinc levels with low ingestion due to protein reluctance, increased loss in gastroenterological system due to diarrhea or intestinal malabsorption and increased urinary losses. The assumption is also based on the research of McClain (McClain et al., 1991) and Extremera (Extremera et al., 1990). Protein deficiency occurs frequently due to the poor dietary intake. Our results confirm findings of decreased serum concentrations of zinc in patients with liver cirrhosis. Possible explanations for the decreased zinc levels in cirrhotic patients are mentioned above.

In Celik's research (Celik et al., 2002) the decrease in both serum and ascites zinc content was found in patients with liver cirrhosis. The interaction between zinc and copper in their intestinal absorption and their competition for binding sites on the carrier proteins and cellular uptake may be regulators of their homeostasis. Maybe this can explain inverse concentrations of zinc and copper. Zinc binds on albumin, transferrin and metalloproteins in the cell, so relative concentrations of these proteins might regulate the serum concentration of zinc (Celik et al., 2002; Mertz, 1981).

The serum copper content was found significantly increased in patients with liver cirrhosis in comparison to the control group (Table 1, median 21.56 μmol/L in patient with liver cirrhosis and 13.09 μmol/L in controls, p<0.001). It could be explained with copper's role in the redox process. Redox cycling between Cu^{2+} and Cu^{1+} can catalyze the production of toxic hydroxyl radicals (Askwith et al., 1998; Harrison et al., 2000). It is a well known fact that redox processes and oxidative stress play an important role in the pathogenesis of liver cirrhosis.

Serum concentrations of manganese were significantly higher in cirrhotic patients in comparison to the controls (Table 1, median 2.50 μmol/L in cirrhotic patients and 0.02 μmol/L in controls, p<0.001). Higher serum levels of manganese in Krieger's research (Krieger et al., 1995) as well as in research of Layrargues and co. (Layrargues et al., 1998) were also found in cirrhotic patients.

Moscarella did not find any significant difference in the concentrations of manganese between the cirrhotic patients and the controls (Moscarella et al., 1994). After all, it seems that serum levels of manganese are higher in patients with liver cirrhosis than in healthy people. Manganese is secreted in bile so the concentration of manganese increases in cholestatic liver disease, which could be one of the possible explanations why manganese accumulation is common in liver cirrhosis (Krieger et al., 1995).

It has been suggested that a possible mechanism responsible for manganese accumulation in the pallidum of patients include a decrease in biliary excretion and increased systemic availability due to the portosystemic shunting.

Intrahepatic shunting or portosystemic shunting also have an additional effect on manganese accumulation. In the study of Rose and co. (Rose et al., 1999) pallidal manganese concentrations were the highest in shunted rats, which confirms that shunting is a major determinant of manganese accumulation in the brain. Manganese accumulation in the brain was confirmed by several clinical studies (Krieger et al., 1995; Rose et al., 1999; Hauser et al., 1996, Spahr et al., 1996).

The difference between serum concentrations of magnesium in cirrhotic patients and controls was not significant (Table 1, median 0.94 mmol/L in cirrhotic patients and 0.88 mmol/L in controls, p= 0.132). Results are opposite to Kosch's research (Kosch et al., 2000). In that research serum levels of magnesium were lower in patients with liver cirrhosis in comparison to patients with liver steatosis and controls. In addition, the research of Rocchi (Rocchi et al., 1994) and Suzuki (Suzuki et al., 1996) confirmed the same. Our research did not confirm lower concentrations of magnesium in patients with liver cirrhosis. That partially could be explained with influence of spironolactone on magnesium levels. Namely, in Stergiou's research (Stergiou et al., 1993) spironolactone in health subjects decreased urine excretion of magnesium and in cirrhotic patients antagonized magnesiuric effect of furosemide. Our patients with liver cirrhosis mostly have spironolactone in their standard therapy. However, there were no differences in serum concentration of magnesium between patients who were taking spironolactone and those who were not taking spironolactone.

There was a slight decrease in serum zinc concentrations in patients with more severe clinical state of liver cirrhosis according to Child-Pugh classification but these differences in our research were not significant.

As zinc is bound to albumin in the serum, it has been thought that the serum zinc concentration would decrease with advancing grades of hepatic fibrosis (Hatano et al., 2000). Yoshida found that patients with decompensated liver cirrhosis have lower levels of zinc than patients with compensated cirrhosis (Yoshida et al., 2001). However, in Hatano's research

(Hatano et al., 2000) serum zinc levels did not differ significantly between grades of hepatic fibrosis.

Copper levels in our research were similar in all three Child-Pugh groups (Table 3), as well as in Hatano's research.

Serum levels of manganese were higher in patients with Child-Pugh C liver cirrhosis in comparison to those in Child-Pugh A and B cirrhosis. Our results are contrary to Spahr's research (Spahr et al., 1996) who found similar concentrations of manganese in all three Child-Pugh groups. It seems that manganese concentrations are higher in patients with severe liver cirrhosis possible due to the advanced intrahepatic and portosystemic shunting.

In our study magnesium levels were similar in all Child-Pugh groups. Moscarella's research (Moscarella et al., 1994) also confirms similar levels in compensated and decompensated liver cirrhosis. However, Wang found that magnesium deficiency occurs more frequently in severe liver disease (Wang et al., 2004). Significantly lower zinc levels were found in cirrhotic patients with hepatic encephalopathy

(Table 4, median 0.54 μmol/L in patients with encephalopathy and 0.96 μmol/L without encephalopathy, p= 0.002), which was confirmed in other studies (Grungreiff et al., 2000; Riggio et al. 1992). There are some findings that zinc supplementation can cause increased releasing of glutamine from skeletal muscle and also activate glutamine synthetasis, which can decrease the level of ammonia and improve hepatic encephalopathy (Grungreiff et al., 2000). That can be explained with the fact that zinc supplementation increases the hepatic activity of ornithine transcarbamoylase, key enzyme of the urea cycle, which consecutively increases urea formation and decreases ammonia levels (Riggio et al., 1992). The rationale for use of zinc is also its ability to induce intestinal and hepatic metallothionein synthesis. Zinc decreases copper absorption by increasing the formation of Cu-metallothionein in intestinal epithelial cells (Friedman, 2004). However, Riggio found that short-term zinc supplementation has no influence on hepatic encephalopathy (Riggio et al., 1991).

Table 4. Serum concentrations of trace elements in cirrhotic patients with and without hepatic encephalopathy

Trace elements	Without encephalopathy (N=83) median and 5 - 95 percentiles	With encephalopathy (N=22) median and 5 - 95 percentiles	Statistics	
			z	p
Zinc (μmol/L)	0.96 (0.25–1.77)	0.54 (0.19–1.11)	-3.07	0.002
Copper (μmol/L)	21.56 (13.07–31.43)	21.31 (9.85–29.31)	-1.21	0.227
Manganese (μmol/L)	2.20 (0.01–31.38)	4.90 (0.01–26.94)	0.66	0.506
Magnesium (mmol/L)	0.95 (0.63–1.36)	0.90 (0.53–1.37)	-1.72	0.086

Considering all, zinc supplementation could have a positive influence on hepatic encephalopathy but before the implementation of this result in the treatment, further researches are necessary.

The levels of manganese were not significantly different between patients with liver cirrhosis and hepatic encephalopathy and patients without encephalopathy (Table 4, p=0.506), which is opposite to the researches of Hauser (Hauser et al., 1996) and Krieger (Krieger et al., 1995). They found increased concentrations of manganese and suggested a beneficial effect of prevention of accumulation or decreasing manganese concentration in patients with liver cirrhosis. Rose and Layrargues found increased concentrations of manganese in basal ganglia of cirrhotic patients in comparison to the controls (Rose et al., 1999; Layrargues et al., 1998).

Manganese concentrations were significantly higher in cirrhotic patients with ascites in comparison to those without ascites (Table 5, median 4.10 µmol/L in patients with ascites and 1.80 µmol/L in patients without ascites, p<0.001). The levels of zinc, copper and magnesium were within reference range. Our results are contrary to the research of Pasqualetti and co. who found significantly lower magnesium concentrations in patients with ascites (Pasqualetti et al., 1987). Therefore, it is necessary to research the possible role of manganese in emergence of ascites in patients with liver cirrhosis.

Finally, decreased serum concentrations of zinc and increased levels of manganese in patients with liver cirrhosis could have an important role in the pathogenesis of liver cirrhosis and its complications, especially in hepatic encephalopathy. The supplementation of zinc could improve hepatic encephalopathy. The decrease in manganese levels could also have a beneficial effect on the neurological status in patients with liver cirrhosis and hepatic encephalopathy. Increased concentrations of manganese in cirrhotic patients with ascites inspire further researches about a possible role of manganese in the pathogenesis of ascites in patients with liver cirrhosis. Maybe, decreasing of manganese levels might also have beneficial effect on prevention or volume of ascites.

Table 5. Serum concentrations of trace elements in cirrhotic patients with and without ascites

Trace elements	Without ascites (N=45) median and 5 - 95 percentiles	With ascites (N=60) median and 5 - 95 percentiles	Statistics	
			z	p
Zinc (µmol/L)	0.97 (0.36–1.57)	0.69 (0.18–1.78)	1.77	0.077
Copper (µmol/L)	20.25 (11.84–30.47)	22.42 (10.74–30.82)	-0.28	0.778
Manganese (µmol/L)	1.80 (0.01–11.20)	4.10 (0.01–31.80)	-3.43	< 0.001
Magnesium (mmol/L)	0.92 (0.64–1.13)	0.94 (0.54–1.46)	-0.58	0.564

6. CONCLUSION

Considering all that, the correction of serum trace elements concentrations would have a beneficial effect on some complications of liver cirrhosis and maybe on progression of the disease, so it would be recommendable to provide laboratory analysis of trace elements in patients with liver cirrhosis as a routine.

REFERENCES

Anderson, AJ; Su, JH; Cotman, CW. DNA damage and apoptosis in Alzheimer's disease: colocalization with c-Jun immunoreactivity, relationship to brain area, and effect of postmortem delay. *J. Neurosci*, 1996, 16, 1710-16.

Arakawa, Y; Suzuki, I. Hepatic disease and trace elements. *The Journal of Therapy*, 1993, 75, 894-905.

Arthur, MJP; Iredale, JP. Hepatic lipocytes, TIMP-1 and liver fibrosis. *J.Roy.Coll.Phys.*, 1994, 28, 200.

Arthur, MJP. Fibrogenesis II. Metalloproteinases and their inhibitors in liver fibrosis. *Am J Physiol Gastrointest Liver Physiol*, 2000, 279 (2), 245-9.

Askwith, CC; Kaplan, J. Iron and copper transport in yeast and its relevance to human disease. TIBS, 1998, 23, 135-8.

Blostein-Fuji, A; DiSilvestro, RA; Frid, D; Katz, C; Malarkey, W. Short-term zinc supplementation in women with non-insulin-dependent diabetes mellitus effects on plasma 5' nucleotididase activity, insulin-like growth factor-1 concentrations and lipoprotein oxidation rates in vitro. *Am J Clin Nutr*, 1997, 66, 639-42.

Bremner, I. Manifestation of copper excess. *Am J Clin Nutr*, 1998, 67 (5), 1069s-1073s.

Camps, J; Bargallo, T; Gimenez, A; Alie, S; Caballeria, J; Pares, A; Joven, J; Masana, L; Rodes, J. Relationship between hepatic lipid peroxidation and fibrogenesis in carbon tetrachloride-treated rats: effect of zinc administration. *Clin Sci.*, 1992, 83(6), 695-700.

Celik, HA; Aydin, HH; Ozsaran, A; Kilincsoy, N; Batur, Y; Ersoz, B. Trace elements analysis of ascitic fluid in benign and malignant disease. *Clin Biochem*, 2002, 35(6), 477-81.

Chang, KL; Hung, TC; Hsieh, BS; Chen, YH; Chen, TF; Cheng, HL. Zinc at pharmacologic concentrations affects cytokine expression and induces apoptosis of human peripheral blood mononuclear cells. *Nutrition,* 2006, 22(5), 465-74.

Chausmer, AB. Zinc, insulin and diabetes. *J Am Coll Nutr*, 1998, 17, 109-15.

Christianson, DW. The structure biology of zinc. *Adv. Prot. Chem.*, 1991, 42, 281-335.

Cotzias, GC. Trace Substances. Eviron Health-Proc, *Univ. Mo. Annu Conf,* 1967, 5.

Crabb, DW; Estonius M. Alcoholic Liver Disease and Nonalcoholic Steatohepatitis. In: Stein JH. *Internal Medicine*. St. Louis: Mosby; 1998; 2194-99.

Extremera, B; Maldonado, MA; Martinez, MR; Hinojosa, JC; Ruiz, AD; Moreno, R. Zinc and liver cirrhosis. *Acta Gastroenterologica Belgica*, 1990, 53 (3), 292-8.

Friedman, SL. The cellular basis of hepatic fibrosis: mechanisms and treatment strategies. *N Engl J Med*, 1993, 328, 1828-35.

Friedman, SL; Keeffe EB. *Handbook of liver disease*. Second edition. Philadelphia: Churchill Livingstone, Sabre Zagreb; 2004.

Grungreiff, K; Grungreiff, S; Reinhold, D; Zinc deficiency and hepatic encephalopathy: Results of long-term follow-up on zinc supplementation. *Journal of Trace Elements in Experimental Medicine*, 2000, 13 (1), 21-31.

Grungreiff, K; Reinhold, D. Liver cirrhosis and "liver" diabetes mellitus are linked by zinc deficiency. *Medical hypothesis*, 2005, 64, 316-7.

Harrison, MD; Jones, CE; Solioz, M; Dameron, CT. Intracellular copper routing: the role of copper chaperones. *TIBS*, 2000, 25, 29-32.

Hatano, R; Ebara, M; Fukuda, H; Yoshikawa, M; Sugiura, N; Kondo, F; Yukawa, M; Saisho, H. Accumulation of copper in the liver and hepatic injury in chronic hepatitis C. *Journal of Gastroenterology & Hepatology*, 2000, 15 (7), 786-91.

Hauser, RA; Zesiewich, TA; Martinez, C; Rosemurgy, AS; Olanow, CW. Blood manganese correlates with brain magnetic resonance imaging changes in patients with liver disease. *Can J Neur Sci.*, 1996, 23 (2), 95-8.

Iredale, JP; Murphy, G; Hembry, RM et al. Human hepatic hepatocytes synthesise tissue inhibitor of metalloproteinases-1 (TIMP-1): implications for regulation of matrix degradation in liver. *J.Clin.Invest.* 1992, 90, 282.

Jensen, K (a); Gluud, C. Mallory body: morphological, clinical and experimental studies (part 1 of a literature survey). *Hepatology*, 1994, 20, 1061.

Jensen, K (b); Gluud, C. Mallory body: theories on development and pathological significance (part 2 of a literature survey). *Hepatology*, 1994, 20, 1330.

Kang, YJ; Zhou, Z. Zinc prevention and treatment of alcoholic liver disease. *Mol Aspects Med.* 2005, 26(4-5), 391-404.

Kasper, DL; Braumwald, E; Fauci, A; Hauser, S; Longo, D; Janeson, JL. *Harrison's Principles of Internal Medicine.* 16th edition. New York: McGraw-Hill; 2005.

Klein, D; Lichtmannegger, J; Heinzmann, U; Muller-Hocker, J; Michaelsen, S; Summer, KH. Association of copper to metallothionein in hepatic lysosomes of Long-Evans cinnamon (LEC) rats during the development of hepatitis. *Eur J Clin Invest*, 1998, 28 (4), 302-10.

Kosch, MA; Nguyen, SQ; Tokmak, F; Schodjaian, K; Hausberg, M; Rahn, KH; Kisters, K. Zinc and magnesium status in patients with liver disease due to chronic alcoholism. *Journal of Trace & Microprobe Techniques*, 2000, 18 (4), 529-33.

Krieger, D; Krieger, S; Jansen, O; Gass, P; Theilmann, L; Lichtnecker, H. Manganese and chronic hepatic encephalopathy. *Lancet*, 1995, 346, 270-4.

Kugelmas, M. Preliminary Observation: Oral Zinc Sulfate Replacement is effective in Treating Muscle Cramps in Cirrhotic Patients. *J Am Coll Nutr*, 2000, 19 (1), 13-15.

Layrargues, GP; Rose, C; Spahr, L; Zayed, J; Normandin, L; Butterworth, RF. Role of manganese in pathogenesis of portal-systemic encephalopathy. *Metabolic Brain Disease*, 1998, 13 (4), 311-7.

Leon, DA (a); McCambridge. J. Liver cirrhosis mortality rates in Britain from 1950 to 2002: an analysis of routine data. *Lancet*, 2006, 367, 52-6.

Leon, DA (b); McCambridge. J. Liver cirrhosis mortality rates in Britain, 1950 to 2002. *Lancet*, 2006, 367, 645.

Luza, SC; Speisky, HC. Liver copper storage and transport during development: implication for cytotoxicity. *Am J Clin Nutr*, 1996, 63 (5), 812s-20s.

Marchesini, G; Fabri, A; Bianchi, G; Brizi, M; Zoli, M. Zinc Supplementation and Amino Acid-Nitrogen Metabolism in Patients With Advanced Cirrhosis. *Hepatology*, 1996, 23, 1084-92.

Marchesini, G; Bugianesi, E; Ronchi, M; Flamia, R; Thomaseth, K; Pacini, G. Zinc Supplementation Improves Glucose Disposal in Patients With Cirrhosis. *Metabolism*, 1998, 47 (7), 792-8.

McClain, CJ; Marsano, L; Burk, RF; Bacon, B. Trace elements in liver disease. *Semin Liver Dis.*, 1991, 11, 321-39.

Mertz, W. Essential trace elements. *Science*, 1981, 213 (4514), 1332-8.

Milin, C; Tota, M; Domitrovic, R; Giacometti, J; Pantovic, R; Cuk, M; Mrakovcic-Sutic, I: Jakovac, H; Radosevic-Stasic, B. Metal Tissue Kinetics in Regenerating Liver, Thymus, Spleen and Submandibular Gland After Partial Hepatectomy in Mice. *Biol Trace Elem Res*, 2005, 108, 225-43.

Moscarella, S; Duchini, A; Buzzelli, G. Eur. J. Gastroenterol. *Hepatol.*, 1994, 6 (7), 633.

Pasqualetti, P; Casale, R; Colantonio, D; Di Lauro, G; Festuccia, V; Natali, L; Natali, G. Serum levels of magnesium in hepatic cirrhosis. *Quad Sclavo Diag*, 1987, 23 (1), 12-7.

Pinzani, M. Hepatic stellate (Ito) cells: expanding roles for a liver-specific pericyte. *J Hepatol.*, 1995, 22, 700.

Prasad, R; Kaur, G; Nath, R; Walia, BN. Molecular basis of pathophysiology of Indian childhood cirrhosis: role of nuclear copper accumulation in liver. *Molecular & Cellular Biochemistry*, 1996, 156 (1), 25-30.

Ramstedt, M. Alcohol-Related Mortality in 15 European Countries in the Postwar Period. *Eur J Popul*, 2002, 18, 307-23.

Record, IR; Tulsi, RS; Dreosti, IE; Fraser, FJ. Cellular necrosis in zinc-deficient rat embryos. *Teratology*, 1985, 32, 397-405.

Riggio, O; Ariosto, F; Merli, M; Caschera, M; Zullo, A; Balducci, G; Ziparo, V. et al. Short-term oral zinc supplementation does not improve chronic hepatic encephalopaty. Results of a double-blind crossover trial. *Dig Dis Sci*, 1991, 36, 1204-8.

Riggio, O; Merli, M; Capocaccia, L; Caschera, M; Zullo, A; Pinto, G; Gaudio, E. et al. Zinc supplementation reduces blood ammonia and increase liver ornithine trancarbamylase activity in experimental cirrhosis. *Hepatology*, 1992, 16, 785-9.

Rocchi, E; Borella, P; Borghi, A; Paolillo, F; Pradelli, M; Farina, F; Casalgrandi, G. Zinc and magnesium in liver cirrhosis. *Eur J Clin Invest*, 1994, 24 (3), 149-55.

Rose, C; Butterworth, RF; Zayed, J; Normandin, L; Todd, K; Michalak, A; Spahr, L; Huet, PM; Pomier-Layrargues, G. Manganese Deposition in Basal Ganglia Structures Results From Both Portal-Systemic Shunting and Liver Dysfunction. *Gastroenterology*, 1999, 117, 640-4.

Sato, C; Koyama, H; Satoh, H; Hayashi, Y; Chiba, T; Ohi, R. Concentrations of Copper and Zinc in Liver and Serum Samples in Biliary Atresia Patients at Different Stages of Traditional Surgeries. *Tohoku J. Exp. Med.*, 2005, 207, 271-7.

Schnabl, B; Hu, K; Muhlbauer, M; Hellerbrand, C; Stefanovic, B; Brenner, DA; Scholmerich, J. Zinc finger protein 267 is up-regulated during the activation process of human hepatic stellate cells and functions as a negative transcriptional regulator of MMP-10. *Biochem Biophys Res Commun*, 2005, 335(1), 87-96.

Sherlock, S; Dooley, J. *Disease of the liver and biliary system.* 11th edition. Oxford: Blackwell Science Ltd.; 2002.

Sidhu, P; Garg, ML; Dhawan, DK. Protective effects of zinc on oxidative stress enzymes in liver of protein-deficient rats. *Drug Chem Toxicol*, 2005, 28(2), 211-30.

Spahr, L; Butterworth, RF; Fontaine, S; Bui, L; Therrien, G; Milette, PC; Lebrun, LH; Zayed, J; Leblanc, A; Pomier-Layrargues, G. Increased Blood manganese in Cirrhotic Patients:

Relationship to Pallidal Magnetic Resonance Signal Hyperintensity and Neurological Symptoms. *Hepatology*, 1996, 24, 1116-20.

Speich, M; Pineau, A; Ballereau, F. Minerals, trace elements and related biological variables in athlets and during physical activity.*Clin Chim Acta*, 2001, 321(1-2), 1-11.

Stergiou, GS; Mayopoulousymvoulidou, D; Mountokalakis, TD. Attenuation by spironolactone of the magnesiuric effect of acute fursemid administration in patients with liver cirrhosis and ascites. *Mineral & Electrolyte Metabolism*, 1993, 19 (2), 86-90.

Stokkeland, K; Brandt, L; Ekbom, A; Ösby, U; Hultcrantz, R. Morbidity and mortality in liver cirrhosis in Sweden 1969-2001 in relation to alcohol consumption. *Scand J Gastroenterol*, 2006, 41, 463-8.

Sunderman, FW. The influence of zinc on apoptosis. *Ann. Clin. Lab. Sci.*, 1995, 25, 134-42.

Suzuki, K; Oyama, R; Hayashi, E; Arakawa, Y. Liver disease and essential trace elements. Nippon Rinsho. *Japanese Journal of clinical medicine*, 1996, 54 (1), 85-92.

Szuster-Ciesielska, A; Daniluk, J; Bojarska-Junak, A. Apoptosis of blood mononuclear cells in alcoholic liver cirrhosis. The influence of in vitro ethanol treatment and zinc supplementation. *Toxicology*, 2005, 212, 124-34.

Takahara, T; Furui, K; Funaki, J; Nakayama, Y; Itoh, H; Miyabayashi, C. Increased expression of matrix metalloproteinase-II in experimental liver fibrosis in rats. *Hepatology*, 1995, 21, 787-95.

Truong-Tran, AQ; Ho, LH; Chai, F; Zalewski, PD. Celular zinc fluxes and the regulation of apoptosis / gene-directed cell death. *J.Nutr.*, 2000, 130 (Suppl.), 1459 S - 66 S.

Troung-Tran, AQ; Carter, J; Ruffin, R; Zalewski PD. New insights into the role of zinc in the respiratory epithelium. *Immunol Cell Biol*, 2001, 79, 170-7.

Tsujikawa, K; Suzuki, N; Sagawa, K. Induction and subcellular localization of metallothionein in regenerating rat liver. *Eur J Cell Biol*, 1994, 63, 240-6.

Vallee, BL; Falchuk; KH. The biochemical basis of zinc physiology. *Physiol. Rev.*, 1993, 73, 79-118.

Vucelic, B; Hrstic, I. Ciroza jetre. In: Vucelic B. et al. *Gastroenterologija i hepatologija*. Zagreb: Medicinska naknada; 2002; 1269-80.

Wang, F; Cao, J; Ma, L; Jin, Z. Study on cellular and serum concentration of calcium and magnesium in periferal blood cells of cirrhosis. *Chin J Hepatol*, 2004, 12 (3), 144-7.

Wyllie, AH. Apoptosis: an overview. *Br. Med. Bull.*, 1997, 53, 451-65.

Yoshida, Y; Higashi, T; Nouso, K; Nakatsukasa, H; Nakamura, S; Watanabe, A; Tsuji, T. Effects of zinc deficiency/zinc supplementation on ammonia metabolism in patients with decompensated liver cirrhosis. *Acta Medica Okayama*, 2001, 55 (6), 349-55.

Zalewski, PD; Forbes, IJ; Betts, WH. Correlation of apoptosis with change in intracellular labile Zn using Zinquin a new specific fluoroscent probe for zinc. *Biochem. J.*, 1993, 296, 403-8.

Zhou, Z; Sun, X; Kang, J. Metallothionein Protection against Alcoholic Liver Injury through Inhibition of Oxidative stress. *Experiment. Biol. Med.*, 2002, 227, 214-22.

Zhou, Z; Wang, L; Song, Z; Saari, JT; McClain, CJ; Kang, YJ. Zinc supplementation prevents alcoholic liver injury in mice through attenuation of oxidative stress. *Am J Pathol*, 2005, 166(6), 1681-90.

In: Micronutrients and Health Research
Editor: Takumi Yoshida, pp. 249-261

ISBN: 978-1-60456-056-5
© 2008 Nova Science Publishers, Inc.

Chapter VIII

DIACYLGLYCEROL OIL: ITS EFFICACY AND MECHANISMS

Shinichiro Saito, Koichi Yasunaga, Masao Takeshita,
Hideto Takase, Shinichi Meguro, Yoshihisa Katsuragi,
Noboru Matsuo and Ichiro Tokimitsu
Health Care Food Research Laboratories, Kao Corporation, Tokyo, Japan.

ABSTRACT

Diacylglycerol (DAG), which consists mainly of 1,3-DAG, is a naturally occurring oil present in low concentrations in vegetable oils that has a long history of use as food. Compared with conventional triacylglycerol (TAG) oil, DAG has beneficial effects in humans and rodents, with no adverse effects.

Long-term ingestion of DAG prevents body fat accumulation compared to TAG ingestion in humans and rodents. DAG and TAG with a similar fatty acid composition have similar energy values and are absorbed similarly in rats, suggesting that these properties are not associated with the anti-obesity effect of DAG. DAG stimulates β-oxidation gene expression in the liver, small intestine, and skeletal muscle, and decreases the postprandial respiratory quotient, suggesting that dietary DAG induces fat oxidation postprandially and chronically, which might be one of the mechanisms underlying the anti-obesity effect of DAG. Additionally, DAG protects against the development of glucose intolerance and impaired insulin resistance in animal models of metabolic abnormalities, suggesting that DAG helps to maintain appropriate carbohydrate metabolism in addition to appropriate fat metabolism.

A single oral administration of DAG decreases postprandial plasma triglyceride (TG) levels compared with those after TAG administration. A potential explanation for this difference was generated by studies in which the lymphatic transport of chylomicrons after 1,3-DAG ingestion was significantly delayed and reduced, presumably as a result of poor reesterification of fatty acids onto 1-monoacylglycerol (MAG) in the intestinal mucosa. Another mechanism was suggested by the results of a recent study in which DAG administration decreased TG levels, but increased MAG and

1,3-DAG levels in secreted chylomicrons compared with TAG administration, thus leading to a more rapid clearance of DAG-chylomicrons by lipoprotein lipase-mediated lipolysis than that of TAG-chylomicrons.

Plant sterols (PS) are cholesterol-lowering agents. A review of previous human studies indicates that the effective dose of PS is 0.4 g/day when dissolved in DAG, whereas that of PS dissolved in TAG is estimated to be at least 0.8 g/day. PS at 0.5 g/day dissolved in DAG oil, but not in TAG oil, has cholesterol-lowering effects, suggesting that PS act synergistically with DAG, or that DAG enhances the actions of PS. Further studies are needed, however, to clarify the mechanism.

In conclusion, DAG and PS/DAG are useful for the prevention of metabolic abnormalities, and are expected to decrease risk factors for disease when incorporated into human daily dietary habits.

INTRODUCTION

The global epidemic of obesity over the last two decades is driving the large increase in health risks for chronic disease such as heart disease, hypertension, cancer, and diabetes [1], and setting the scene for an impending wave of cardiovascular morbidity and mortality [2,3]. The accumulation of fat in the abdomen, liver, and muscle is thought to be closely related to obesity-related insulin resistance [4,5] and metabolic syndrome [6,7]. Several factors are proposed to be involved in the pathophysiology of metabolic syndrome, particularly obesity and insulin resistance, which are lifestyle-related factors [8]. Therefore, changes in lifestyle, especially dietary habits, might be one of the most effective ways to prevent the development of metabolic syndrome.

Table 1. Relative contribution of mono-, di-, and triacylglycerols in selected edible oils

	MAG	DAG	TAG	Others
Soybean	--	1.0	97.9	1.1
Cottonseed	0.2	9.5	87.0	3.3
Palm	--	5.8	93.1	1.1
Corn	--	2.8	95.8	1.4
Safflower	--	2.1	96.0	1.9
Olive	0.2	5.5	93.3	2.3
Rapeseed	0.1	0.8	96.8	2.3
Lard	--	1.3	97.9	0.8

Source: Ref. 1.

Diacylglycerol (DAG) is a naturally occurring oil present at levels of 0.8 to 9.5 % in vegetable oils (Table 1) [9], and has a long history of human consumption. Cottonseed and olive oil contain greater amounts of DAG than other commonly used edible oils. DAG is used as a food additive in small amounts, but the 1,3-specific lipase-catalyzed reverse reaction currently allows for large-scale production of DAG, which is commercially available in the United States and Japan as cooking oil, and in processed oil and fat products. DAG occurs in two isoforms, 1,2 (or 2,3)-diacyl-sn-glycerol (1,2-DAG) and 1,3-diacyl-sn-glycerol (1,3-DAG) (Figure 1) [10]. 1,2-DAG can exist as 1,2-sn-DAG or 2,3-sn-DAG, but the difference between these enantiomers has no effect on the fat and oil chemistry or dietetics [10]. In most natural edible oils and manufactured DAG oil, ~70 % (w/w) of the DAG is present as the 1,3-isoform [11]. DAG and conventional triacylglycerol (TAG) oil have a similar fatty acid composition as well as similar taste, appearance, stability against oxidation and heating, and cooking properties [12,13]. DAG can be easily incorporated into food products such as mayonnaise, spreads, and salad dressing.

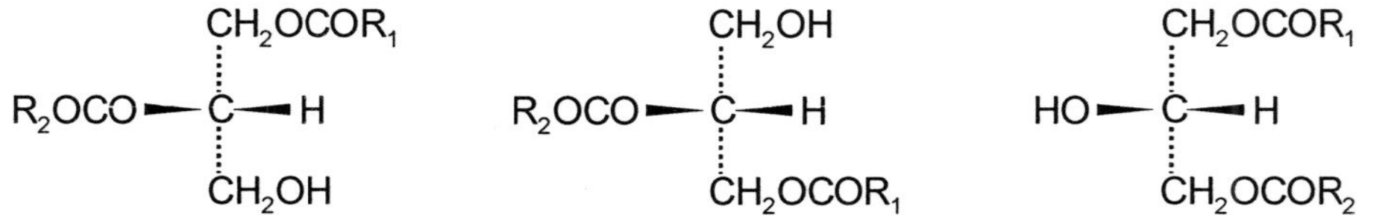

1,2 -diacyl-sn-glycerol 2,3 -diacyl-sn-glycerol 1,3 -diacyl-sn-glycerol

Figure 1. Structure of diacylglycerol. Stereospecific numbering system is represented as "sn".

DAG has beneficial effects compared with TAG in humans and rodents and does not have severe adverse effects in humans [14,15]. Therefore, DAG is approved as a "generally recognized as safe" food ingredient by Food and Drug Administration in the United States [12,14,16] and as a "food for specific health use" by the Ministry of Health, Labor, and Welfare in Japan [11,12,14].

Foods containing DAG consisting of mainly 1,3-DAG 1) prevent the accumulation of body fat, 2) protect against the development of glucose intolerance and impaired insulin resistance, 3) lower postprandial plasma triglyceride (TG) levels, and 4) work synergistically with plant sterols (PS) against hypercholesterolemia in comparison with foods containing TAG. The present review summarizes the results of recent DAG studies with a focus on the efficacy and potential mechanisms of action.

1.1. Preventive Effect on Body Fat Accumulation

The long-term ingestion of DAG consisting of mainly 1,3-DAG prevents body fat accumulation in humans and rodents, in comparison to TAG with a similar fatty acid composition. In a low-fat diet feeding study, Watanabe et al. reported that daily ingestion of a 10 % (w/w) DAG diet for 4 weeks reduced the body fat ratio in Sprague-Dawley (SD) rats compared with a 10 % (w/w) TAG diet [17]. Conversely, however, Sugimoto et al. reported that body weight, and epididymal and perirenal adipose tissue weights were not significantly different between young (7 weeks of age) and old (8 months of age) Wistar rats ingesting a 10 % DAG or 10 % TAG diet (w/w) feeding for 1, 4, 8, or 12 weeks [18]. The contradiction between these two reports suggests that there are variations in the ant-obesity effects of relatively low-dose DAG ingestion that are dependent upon study conditions such as animal age, feeding duration, breeding circumstances, etc. On the other hand, relatively high-fat (15

% - 30 %) DAG diet (w/w) suppressed body weight gain and body fat accumulation compared with a diet with same percentage of TAG. Murase et al. reported that ingesting a 15 % (w/w) DAG diet concomitant with 5 % (w/w) lard for 8 months suppressed body weight gain and the accumulation of white adipose tissue compared with a 15 % (w/w) TAG diet concomitant with 5% (w/w) lard in C57BL/6J mice [19]. They also reported that the white adipose tissue weight and liver TG content after 5 months ingestion of a 30 % (w/w) DAG diet were significantly lower than after ingestion of a 30 % (w/w) TAG diet in C57BL/6J mice [20]. Consistently, Taguchi et al. reported that the increase in hepatic TG was significantly lower after ingesting a 30 % (w/w) DAG diet than after a 30 % (w/w) TAG diet in high-fat fed SD rats [21]. Moreover, Meng et al. reported that body weight, abdominal adipose tissue weight, and liver TG content were lower in SD rats fed a 20 % (w/w) DAG diet compared with those fed a 20 % (w/w) TAG diet [22]. These data suggest that the favorable effects of DAG are more likely to be observed under conditions of excessive energy intake with high fat.

In humans, Nagao et al. conducted a long-term comparative study of DAG and TAG oil consumption in 38 mildly overweight Japanese men (mean±standard error [SE] of body mass index [BMI]; 24.1 ± 0.4 kg/m^2) [23]. In this double-blind parallel study, 10 g of the 50 g oil in the daily diet was replaced with the test oil for a period of 16 weeks, and there was a significant decrease in body weight, visceral and subcutaneous fat, and waist circumference in the DAG consumption group compared with the TAG consumption group. Similarly, in United States populations, Maki et al. reported that body weight and body fat were significantly reduced in the DAG group compared with the TAG group in 127 overweight obese men (mean±standard deviation of BMI; 34.5 ± 3.7 kg/m^2) during 6-month consumption of 8 to 9 g test oils under a mild hypo-calorie condition [24]. On the other hand, in non-overweight healthy subjects (BMI<23 kg/m^2), 12-week consumption of DAG did not affect body weight [14,25], indicating that DAG does not induce unnecessary weight loss in lean subjects.

Overall, many studies in humans and rodents suggest that DAG is beneficial for maintaining appropriate weight when incorporated into daily dietary habits, and the anti-obesity effect is strongly associated with the suppression of body fat accumulation, suggesting that DAG ingestion contributes to reduce health risk factors such as insulin resistance and dyslipidemia associated with obesity. It is possible that the loss of fat mass after DAG consumption is a result of enhanced postprandial or even chronic fat utilization, as described below.

1.2. Mechanisms Underlying the Anti-Obesity Effect

DAG and TAG with a similar fatty acid composition have similar energy values and undergo similar absorption in rats [26], suggesting that these properties are not associated with the anti-obesity effect of DAG. In studies with C57BL/6J mice, Murase et al. reported that long-term ingestion of DAG stimulated β-oxidation gene expression in the liver [20] and small intestine [19] together with the suppression of body fat accumulation, compared with TAG. Consistent with these reports, Murata et al. reported that dietary DAG compared with

TAG decreased the activities of enzymes involved in the fatty acid oxidation pathway in rat liver [27]. These observations suggest that the stimulation of fatty acid oxidation in the liver and small intestine is partially responsible for the beneficial effects of DAG.

There are two reports suggesting that there is a postprandial increase in fat oxidation after the consumption of a diet containing DAG in humans. Kamphuis et al. reported that fat oxidation was significantly higher after DAG ingestion of than after TAG ingestion in a 24-hour respiratory chamber study [28]. In their study, 33.0 ± 2.3 g of DAG oil was incorporated into each breakfast, lunch, dinner, and snacks during the stay in a respiratory chamber, but there were no differences in postprandial energy expenditure. Saito et al. reported that postprandial energy expenditure tended to be higher ($p<0.1$) and the respiratory quotient was significantly lower after 30 g of DAG ingestion with a single meal than after TAG ingestion [29]. These observations suggest that a DAG diet induces postprandial fat oxidation possibly together with increased energy expenditure, as supported by a couple of animal studies [17,30]. Watanabe et al. reported that postprandial oxygen consumption was higher in the DAG group than in the TAG group in SD rats [17]. Kimura et al. demonstrated increased oxygen consumption, fat oxidation, and decreased respiratory quotient after a single oral ingestion of a DAG emulsion compared with a TAG emulsion in Wistar rats [30] Thus, dietary DAG enhances postprandial and chronic fat oxidation (possibly energy expenditure), and this might be one of the mechanisms underlying the anti-obesity effect of DAG.

2. PROTECTION AGAINST IMPAIRED GLUCOSE TOLERANCE AND INSULIN RESISTANCE

Impaired glucose tolerance and insulin resistance are accompanied by the accumulation of body fat [31,32]. Because DAG has anti-obesity effects in humans and rodents, DAG might have preventive effects against impaired glucose tolerance and insulin resistance. Indeed, Murase et al. reported that the long-term ingestion of DAG oil decreased fasting serum glucose and insulin levels in obese and diabetes-prone mice (C57BL/6J) fed a high-fat diet [19]. Moreover, DAG ameliorates glucose intolerance and prevents the development of impaired glucose tolerance in Otsuka Long-Evans Tokushima Fatty rats [33] and sucrose-fed Wistar rats [34], respectively. These studies suggest that the ingestion of DAG not only prevents the accumulation of body fat but also suppresses the development of abnormal carbohydrate metabolism. In one study, however, glucose intolerance was induced by DAG compared with TAG in genetically obese Wistar rats [35], suggesting that further studies are needed to clarify the effect of DAG on glucose metabolism.

To gain more insight into the effects of DAG on glucose metabolism and molecular changes in metabolic abnormalities, Saito et al. conducted a long-term DAG-diet feeding study in mice lacking brown adipose tissue (BATless mice), which become severely obese and insulin resistant on high fat diets [36]. In that study, a 15-week consumption of a DAG diet reduced weight gain and the accumulation of body fat observed with a TAG-diet, and these effects of DAG were associated with the maintenance of normal insulin sensitivity. Fatty acid oxidation gene expression in skeletal muscle (and possibly the liver and intestine), together with the suppression of hepatic gluconeogenesis gene expression, were stimulated;

nevertheless, whether these molecular changes are causally related to the reduced weight gain could not be determined. Moreover, Saito and colleagues observed a reduction in the expression of tumor necrosis factor (TNF) alpha in white adipose tissue; adipose tissue TNF-alpha expression is closely linked to obesity-induced insulin resistance [37,38]. Because weight loss is associated with decreases in TNF-alpha [39,40], they were unable to determine whether the lower TNF-alpha expression levels in white adipose tissue that they observed in the DAG group was a direct effect of DAG or the result of DAG-induced weight loss.

Overall, although the mechanisms remain unknown and the contradictory results leave the conclusion in dispute, these studies suggest that dietary DAG protects against impaired insulin sensitivity associated with the development of obesity, but further studies are required.

3. LOWERING EFFECT ON PLASMA TG LEVELS

Postprandial lipemia is a characteristic abnormality in obese and insulin -resistant individuals, and contributes to the risk for cardiovascular disease [41,42]. Therefore, it would be helpful to find diet alternatives to improve postprandial lipemia. Recent studies suggest that oral ingestion of DAG, specifically 1,3-DAG, results in lower postprandial plasma TG levels as compared to levels after the ingestion of TAG with a similar fatty acid composition in healthy humans [43,44,45], insulin resistant humans [46], and humans with type II diabetes mellitus [47]. Taguchi et al. reported that the magnitude of postprandial lipemia in 17 healthy subjects ingesting a DAG emulsion was significantly lower (23 %) than that when they ingested a TAG emulsion of 44 g test oil, and the difference was reproducible even with low fat doses (10 and 20 g) [43]. Similarly, Tada et al. demonstrated that serum TG levels at 2, 3, and 8 hours after DAG oil loading (30 g/m^2 body surface area) were significantly lower than those after TAG oil loading, and postprandial serum remnant like particle (RLP)-cholesterol and RLP-TG levels in the DAG group were also significantly lower than those in the TAG group [44]. Tomonobu et al. verified the effect of DAG in a typical meal on postprandial changes in serum TG and RLP-cholesterol compared with TAG, and showed that the area under the curve (0-6 hours) for serum TG and RLP-cholesterol levels after the DAG meal was significantly smaller than that after the TAG meal in 29 healthy subjects with fasting serum TG levels of at least 1.13 mmol/L (100 mg/dL) [45]. In a study in non-diabetic subjects with insulin resistance, Takase et al. reported that the maximum increase in postprandial serum TG levels from baseline positively correlated with the insulin resistance index (homeostasis model assessment) after oral TAG ingestion, but not after DAG ingestion, suggesting that the lowering effect of DAG on postprandial lipemia is closely associated with insulin resistance, and they concluded that DAG would be preferable for individuals with insulin resistance [46]. Consistent with the study in subjects with insulin resistance, the mean increase in area under the curve for serum TG, RLP-cholesterol, and RLP-TG after DAG ingestion is significantly lower when compared with that after TAG ingestion in type II diabetic patients [47].

A potential explanation for the effect of DAG on postprandial lipemia was provided by studies in which the lymphatic transport of chylomicrons was significantly delayed and reduced after 1,3-DAG ingestion [48], presumably as a result of poor reesterification of fatty acids onto 1-monoacylglycerol (MAG) in the intestinal mucosa [19,49,50]. A novel mechanism was suggested in a recent study showing less TG, but more MAG and 1,3-DAG, in secreted chylomicrons after DAG administration in comparison with TAG administration [51]. This difference led to more rapid clearance of DAG-chylomicrons by lipoprotein lipase-mediated lipolysis than of TAG-chylomicrons. It should be noted, however, that a recent study in which DAG consumption appeared to reduce plasma TG levels in a patient homozygous for lipoprotein lipase deficiency [52], leaves the door open to other possible mechanisms by which DAG is associated with reduced postprandial TG concentrations.

Furthermore, in addition to the effect on postprandial plasma TG levels, two studies reported the effects of DAG on fasting serum lipid levels after long-term ingestion of DAG in type II diabetes mellitus [53,54]. Because hypertriglyceridemia is commonly observed in patients with type II diabetes [55], and moderate hypertriglyceridemia persists even after satisfactory blood glucose control in diabetes [56], DAG might be valuable for dietary therapeutic management in diabetes with hypertriglyceridemia.

4. SYNERGISTIC ACTIONS WITH PLANT STEROLS ON HYPERCHOLESTEROL

Plant sterols (PS) are present in all foods of plant origin, such as vegetable oils, fruits, and cereals [57]. In plants, these sterols function as structural components of the cell membrane. PS are structurally similar to cholesterol, but have a slight modification of the aliphatic side chain, and are thought to act primarily in the intestinal lumen [58]. As cholesterol analogs, they compete with cholesterol for absorptive micelles resulting in reduced cholesterol solubility [58]. The affinity of PS for micelles is greater than that of cholesterol [59]. In spite of these properties, the reduction in cholesterol absorption by PS is incomplete, with only 30 % to 40 % decreased absorption efficiency being reported, even with high PS doses [60,61]. Therefore, a daily intake of 2 g PS leads to only a 9 % to 14 % reduction in plasma low density lipoprotein (LDL)-cholesterol concentrations with no effects on plasma high density lipoprotein (HDL)-cholesterol or TG [62]. Although PS are generally safe and have a long history of human consumption [63], several recent studies have reported negative effects of PS on serum fat-soluble (pro)vitamin levels such as carotenoids and tocopherol (vitamin E) [64]. Because of this negative effect, it would be worthwhile to estimate the minimum effective dose of PS and to avoid excessive intake. According to a meta-analysis review of previous human studies, the effective dose of PS in a variety of foods is estimated to be at least 0.8 g/day [63]. In a more recent human study with PS, however, Saito et al. reported that DAG-containing PS (PS/DAG) decreased serum total cholesterol levels at a dose of 0.4 g PS and LDL-cholesterol at a dose of 0.3 g PS in healthy and mildly hypercholesterolemic subjects [65], suggesting that serum cholesterol levels are decreased when PS are dissolved in DAG oil compared to TAG oil despite the lower dose of PS. Indeed, in a comparison of 0.5 g/day PS dissolved in DAG and TAG, the cholesterol-lowering effect of the PS was observed only when it was dissolved in DAG oil [66], suggesting that PS act synergistically with DAG, or that DAG enhances PS actions. On the other hand, in a study on the safety aspects of PS/DAG, serum retinol, alpha-tocopherol, and beta-carotene levels were not altered by a 2-week consumption of excessive doses of PS/DAG (1.2 g PS/30 g DAG oil) [67], suggesting that PS/DAG does not affect serum fat soluble (pro)vitamin levels, even when ingested at three times the effective dose.

Takeshita et al. investigated the usability of PS/DAG for therapeutic management of hypercholesterolemia accompanied by menopause [68] or in patients treated with a cholesterol biosynthesis inhibitor [69]. After 4 weeks ingestion of PS/DAG oil (0.563 g PS intake with DAG oil each day), reductions in serum total (10.2 %), LDL- (12.1 %) cholesterol, apolipoprotein B (9.7 %), and lipoprotein (a) (18.6 %) were induced compared with standard DAG oil (0.050 g PS intake with DAG oil in each day) in postmenopausal women with mild to moderate hypercholesterolemia presumably accompanied by decreased female hormones [68]. These results indicated that PS/DAG might be a useful adjunct to first-line therapy for the management of atherogenic lipoproteins in women after menopause. Additionally, it was reported that PS/DAG reinforced the cholesterol-lowering effect of low-dose pravastatin treatment (10 mg/day) in hypercholesterolemic patients [69], indicating that the practical use of dietary PS/DAG oil in conjunction with pravastatin as a low-dose combined therapy, is beneficial for further reducing blood cholesterol.

CONCLUSION

As reported in several studies of humans and rodents and in reviews of the physiologic properties of DAG [11,12,70-79], DAG might be useful for 1) preventing body fat accumulation, 2) protecting against impaired glucose tolerance and insulin resistance, 3) decreasing postprandial plasma TG levels, and 4) preventing hypercholesterolemia via synergistic actions with PS. Although further studies are required to clarify more detailed mechanisms, DAG and PS/DAG might protect against metabolic abnormalities and decrease the risk factors for chronic diseases when incorporated into human daily dietary habits.

REFERENCES

[1]   Zimmet, P; Alberti, KG; Shaw, J. (2001) Global and societal implications of the diabetes epidemic. *Nature, 13*, 782-787.

[2]   Nigro, J; Osman, N; Dart, AM; Little, PJ. (2006) Insulin resistance and Atherosclerosis. *Endocr Rev, 27*, 242-259.

[3]   Behn, A; Ur, E. (2006) The obesity epidemic and its cardiovascular consequences. *Curr Opin Cardiol, 21*, 353-360.

[4]   Hartz, AJ; Rupley DCJr; Kalkhoff RD; Rimm AA. (1983) Relationship of obesity to diabetes: Influence of obesity level and body fat distribution. *Prev Med, 12*, 351-357.

[5]   Younis, N; Soran H; Farook S. (2004) The prevention of Type 2 diabetes mellitus: Recent advances. *QJM, 97*, 451-455.

[6]   Reaven, GM. (1998) Role of insulin resistance in human disease. *Diabetes, 37*, 1595-1607.

[7] Anonymous expert panel on detection, evaluation, and treatment of high blood cholesterol in adults. (2001) Executive summary of the third report of the NCEP expert panel on detection, evaluation, and treatment of high cholesterol in adults (adult treatment panel III). *JAMA, 285-258*, 2486-2497 (Abstract).

[8] Eckel, RH; Grundy, SM; Zimmet, PZ. (2005) The metabolic syndrome. *Lancet, 365*, 1415-1428.

[9] Flickinger, BD; Matsuo, N. (2003) Nutritional characteristics of DAG oil. *Lipids, 38*, 129-132.

[10] Nakajima, Y; Fukasawa, J; Shimada, A. Physicochemical properties of diacylglycerol (Chapter 18). In: Katsuragi Y; Yasukawa T; Matsuo N; Flickinger BD; Tokimitsu, I; Matlock MG, editors. *Diacylglycerol Oil*. New York: AOCS press; 2004; 182-196.

[11] Yasukawa, T; Katsuragi, Y. Diacylglycerols (Chapter 1). In: Katsuragi Y; Yasukawa T; Matsuo N; Flickinger BD; Tokimitsu, I; Matlock MG, editors. *Diacylglycerol Oil*. New York: AOCS press; 2004; 1-15.

[12] Rudkowska, I; Roynette, CE; Demonty, I; Vanstone, CA; Jew, S; Jones, PJH. (2005) Diacylglycerol: Efficacy and metabolism of action of an anti-obesity agent. *Obes Res, 13*, 1864-1876.

[13] Nishide, T; Shimizu, M; Tiffany, TR; Ogawa, H. Cooking oil: Cooking properties and sensory evaluation (Chapter 19). In: Katsuragi Y; Yasukawa T; Matsuo N; Flickinger BD; Tokimitsu, I; Matlock MG, editors. *Diacylglycerol Oil*. New York: AOCS press; 2004; 182-196.

[14] Yasunaga, K; Glinsmann, WH; Seo, Y; Katsuragi, Y; Kobayashi, S; Flickinger, B; Kennepohl, E; Yasukawa, T; Borzelleca, JF. (2004) Safety aspects regarding the consumption of high-dose dietary diacylglycerol oil in men and women in a double-blind controlled trial in comparison with consumption of a triacylglycerol control oil. *Food Chem Toxicol, 42*, 1419-1429.

[15] Borzelleca, JF; Glinsmann, W; Kennepohl, E. Safety aspects of diacylglycerol oil (Chapter 17). In: Katsuragi Y; Yasukawa T; Matsuo N; Flickinger BD; Tokimitsu, I; Matlock MG, editors. *Diacylglycerol Oil*. New York: AOCS press; 2004; 182-196.

[16] Empie, MW. Regulatory status of diacylglycerol oil in North America, the European Union, Latin America, Australia/New Zealand, and Japan (Chapter 16). In: Katsuragi Y; Yasukawa T; Matsuo N; Flickinger BD; Tokimitsu, I; Matlock MG, editors. *Diacylglycerol Oil*. New York: AOCS press; 2004; 182-196.

[17] Watanabe, H; Onizawa, K; Taguchi, H; Kobori, M; Chiba, H; Naito, S; Matsuo, N; Yasukawa, T; Hattori, M; Shimasaki, N. (1997) Nutritional characterization of diacylglycerol in rats. *J Jpn Oil Chem Soc, 46*, 301-307.

[18] Sugimoto, T; Kimura, T; Fukuda, H; Iritani, N. (2003) Comparisons of glucose and lipid metabolism in rats fed diacylglycerol and triacylglycerol oil. *J Nutr Sci Vitaminol, 49*, 47-55.

[19] Murase, T; Aoki, M; Wakisaka, T; Hase, T; Tokimitsu, I. (2002) Anti-obesity effect of dietary diacylglycerol in C57BL/6J mice: dietary diacylglycerol stimulates intestinal lipid metabolism. *J Lipid Res, 43*: 1312-1319

[20] Murase, T; Mizuno, T; Omachi, T; Onizawa, K; Komine, Y; Kondo H; Hase, T; Tokimitsu, I. (2001) Dietary diacylglycerol suppresses high fat and high sucrose diet-induced body fat accumulation in C57BL/6J mice. *J Lipid Res, 42*, 372-378.

[21] Taguchi, H; Omachi, T; Nagao, T; Matsuo, N; Tokimitus, I; Itakura, H. (2002) Dietary diacylglycerol suppress high fat diet-induced hepatic fat accumulation and microsomal triacylglycerol transfer protein activity in rats. *J Nutr Biochem, 13*, 678-683.

[22] Meng X; Zou, D; Shi, Z; Duan, Z; Mao, Z. (2004) Dietary diacylglycerol prevents high-fat diet-induced lipid accumulation in rat liver and abdominal adipose tissue. *Lipids, 39*, 37-41.

[23] Nagao, T; Watanabe, H; Goto, N; Onizawa, K; Taguchi, H; Matsuo, N; Yasukawa, T; Tsushima, R; Shimasaki, H; Itakura, H. (2000) Dietary diacylglycerol suppresses accumulation of body fat compared to triacylglycerol in men in a double-blind controlled trial. *J Nutr, 130*, 792-797.

[24] Maki, KC; Dacidson, MH; Tsushima, R; Matsuo, N; Tokimitsu, I; Umporowicz, DM; Dicklin, MR; Foster, GS; Ingram, KA; Anderson, BD; Frost, SD; Bell, M. (2002) Consumption of diacylglycerol oil as part of a reduced-energy diet enhances loss of body weight and fat in comparison with consumption of a triacylglycerol control oil. *Am J Clin Nutr, 76*, 1230-1236.

[25] Watanabe, H; Onizawa, K; Naito, S; Taguchi, H; Goto, N; Nagao, T; Matsuo, N; Tokimitsu, I; Yasukawa, T; Tsushima, R; Shimasaki, H; Itakura, H. (2001) Fat-solbule vitamin status in not affected by diacylglycerol consumption. *Ann Nutr Metab, 45*, 259-264.

[26] Taguchi, H; Nagao, T; Watanabe, H; Onizawa, K; Matsuo, N; Tokimitsu, I; Itakura, H. (2001) Energy value and digestibility of dietary oil containing mainly 1,3-diacylglycerol are similar to those of triacylglycerol. *Lipids, 36*, 379-382.

[27] Murata, M; Ide, T; Hara, K. (1997) Reciprocal responses to dietary diacylglycerol of hepatic enzymes of fatty acid synthesis and oxidation in the rat. *Br J Nutr, 77*, 107-121.

[28] Kamphuis, MMJW; Mela, DJ; Westerterp-Plantenga, MS. (2003) Diacylglycerols affect substrate oxidation and appetite in humans. *Am J Clin Nutr, 77*, 1133-1139.

[29] Saito, S; Tomonobu, K; Hase, T; Tokimitsu, I. (2006) Effects of diacylglycerol on postprandial energy expenditure and respiratory quotient in healthy subjects. *Nutrition, 22*, 30-35.

[30] Kimura, S; Tsuchiya, H; Inage, H; Meguro, S; Matsuo, N; Tokimitsu, I. (2006) Effects of dietary diacylglycerol on the energy metabolism. *Int J Vitam Nutr Res, 76*, 75-79.

[31] Bjorntorp, P. (1988) Abdominal obesity and the development of non-insulin-dependent diabetes mellitus. *Diabetes Metab Rev, 4*, 615-622.

[32] Matsuzawa, Y; Shimomura, I; Nakamura, T; Keno, Y; Kotani, K; Tokunaga, K. (1995) Pathophysiology and pathogenesis of visceral fat obesity. *Obes Res, 2 (suppl)*, 187S-194S.

[33] Mori, Y; Nakagiri, H; Kondo, H; Murase, T; Tokimitsu, I; Tajima, N. (2005) Dietary diacylglycerol reduces postprandial hyperlipidemia and ameliorates glucose intolerance in Otsuka Long-Evans Tokushima Fatty (OLETF) rats. *Nutrition, 21*, 933-939.

[34] Meguro, S; Osaki, N; Matsuo, N; Tokimitsu, I. (2006) Effect of diacylglycerol on the development of impaired glucose tolerance in sucrose-fed rats. *Lipids, 41*, 347-355.

[35] Sugimoto, T; Fukuda, H; Kimura, T; Iritani, N. (2003) Dietary diacylglycerol-rich oil stimulation of glucose intolerance in genetically obese rats. *J Nutr Sci Vitaminol, 49*, 139-144.

[36] Saito, S; Hernandez-Ono, A; Ginsberg HN. (2007) Dietary 1,3-diacylglycerol protects against diet-Induced obesity and insulin resistance. *Metabolism*, 56, 1566-1575.

[37] Hotamisligil, GS; Arner, P; Caro, JF; Atkinson, RL; Spiegelman, BM. (1995) Increased adipose expression of tumor necrosis factor-☐ in human obesity and insulin resistance. *J Clin Invest, 95*, 2409-2415.

[38] Hotamisligil, GS. (2003) Inflammatory pathways and insulin action. *Int J Obes Relat Metab Disord, 27*, S53-S55.

[39] Kern, PA; Saghizadeh, M; Ong, JM; Bosch, RJ; Deem, R; Simsolo, RB. (1995) The expression of tumor necrosis factor in human adipose tissue. Regulation by obesity, weight loss, and relationship to lipoprotein lipase. *J Clin Invest, 95*, 2111-2119.

[40] Jellema, A; Plat, J; Mensink, RP. (2004) Weight reduction, but not a moderate intake of fish oil, lowers concentrations of inflammatory markers and PAI-1 antigen in obese men during the fasting and postprandial state. *Eur J Clin Invest, 34*,766-773.

[41] Howard, BV. (1999) Insulin resistance and lipid metabolism. *Am J Cardiol, 84 (1A)*, 28J-32J.

[42] Castro Cabezas, M; Halkes, CJ; Erkelens, DW. (2001) Obesity and free fatty acids: double trouble. *Nutr Metab Cardiovasc Dis, 11*, 134-142.

[43] Taguchi, H; Watanabe, H; Onizawa, K; Nagao, T; Gotoh, N; Yasukawa, T; Tsushima, R; Shimasaki, H; Itakura, H. (2000) Double-blind controlled study on the effects of dietary diacylglycerol on postprandial serum and chylomicron triacylglycerol responses in healthy humans. *J Am Coll Nutr, 19*, 789-796.

[44] Tada, N; Watanabe, H; Matsuo, N; Tokimitsu, I; Okazaki, M. (2001) Dynamics of postprandial remnant-like lipoprotein particles in serum after loading of diacylglycerols. *Clinica Chimica Acta, 311*, 109-117.

[45] Tomonobu, K; Hase, T; Tokimitsu, I. (2006) Dietary diacylglycerol in a typical meal suppresses postprandial increases in serum lipid levels compared with dietary triacylglycerol. *Nutrition, 22*, 128-135.

[46] Takase, H; Shoji, K; Hase, T; Tokimitsu, I. (2005) Effect of diacylglycerol on postprandial lipid metabolism in non-diabetic subjects with and without insulin resistance. *Atherosclerosis, 180*, 197-204.

[47] Tada, N; Shoji, K; Takeshita, M; Watanabe, H; Yoshida, H; Hase, T; Matsuo, N; Tokimitsu, I. (2005) Effects of diacylglycerol ingestion on postprandial hyperlipidemia in diabetes. *Clin Chim Acta, 353*, 87-94.

[48] Yangagita, T; Ikeda, I; Wang, Y; Nakagiri, H. (2004) Comparison of the lymphatic transport of radiolabeled 1,3-dioleoylglycerol and trioleoylglycerol in rats. *Lipids, 39*, 827-832.

[49] Kondo, H; Hase, T; Murase, T; Tokimitsu, I. (2003) Digestion and assimilation features of dietary DAG in the rat small intestine. *Lipids, 38*, 25-30.

[50] Osaki, N; Meguro, S; Yajima, N; Matsuo, N; Tokimitsu, I; Shimasaki, H. (2005) Metabolism of dietary triacylglycerol and diacylglycerol during the digestion process in rats. *Lipids, 40*, 281-286.

[51] Yasunaga, K; Saito, S; Zhang, YL; Hernandez-Ono, A; Ginsberg, HN. (2007) Effects of triacylglycerol and diacylglycerol oils on blood clearance, tissue uptake, and hepatic apolipoprotein B secretion in mice. *J Lipid Res, 48*, 1108-1121.

[52] Yamamoto, K; Asakawa, H; Tokunaga, K; Meguro, S; Watanabe, H; Tokimitsu, I; Yagi, N. (2005) Effects of diacylglycerol administration on serum triacylglycerol in a patient homozygous for complete lipoprotein lipase deletion. *Metabolism, 54*, 67-71.

[53] Yamamoto, K; Asakawa, H; Tokunaga, K; Watanabe, H; Matsuo, N; Tokimitsu, I; Yagi, N. (2001) Long-term ingestion of dietary diacylglycerol lowers serum triacylglycerol in type II diabetic patients with hypertriglyceridemia. *J Nutr, 131*, 3204-3207.

[54] Yamamoto, K; Takeshita, M; Tokimitsu, I; Watanabe, H; Mizuno, T; Asakawa, H; Tokunaga, K; Tatsumi, T; Okazaki, M; Yagi, N. (2006) Diacylglycerol oil ingestion in type 2 diabetic patients with hypertriglyceridemia. *Nutrition, 22*, 23-29.

[55] Kissebah, AH; Alfarsi S; Evans, DJ; Adams, PW. (1982) Integrated regulation of very low density lipoprotein triglyceride and apolipoprotein-B kinetics in non-insulin-dependent diabetes mellitus. *Diabetes, 31*, 217-225.

[56] Stern, MP; Mitchell, BD; Haffner, SM; Hazuda, HP. (1992) Does glycemic control of type II diabetes suffice to control diabetic dyslipidemia? A community perspective. *Diabetes Care, 15*, 638-644.

[57] Ellegard, LH; Andersson, SW; Normen AL. (2007) Dietary plant sterols and cholesterol metabolism. *Nutr Rev, 65*, 39-45.

[58] Ostlund, RE, Jr. (2007) Phytosterols, cholesterol absorption and healthy diets. *Lipids, 42*, 41-45.

[59] Armstrong, MJ; Carey, MC. (1987) Thermodynamic and molecular determinants of sterol solubilities in bile salt micelles. *J Lipid Res, 28*, 1144-1155.

[60] Ostlund, RE, Jr; Spilburg, CA; Stenson, WF. (1999) Sitostanol administered in lecithin micelles potently reduces cholesterol absorption in humans. *Am J Clin Nutr, 70*, 826-831.

[61] Lees, AM; Mok, HYI; Lees, RS; McCluskey, MA; Grundy, SM. (1977) Plant sterols as cholesterol-lowering agents: clinical trials in patients with hypercholesterolemia and studies of sterol balance. *Atherosclerosis, 28*, 325-338.

[62] Plat, J; Kerckhoffs, DAJM; Mensink, RP. (2000) Therapeutic potential of plant sterols and stanols. *Curr Opin Lipidol, 11*, 571-576.

[63] Department of Health and Human Services (Food and Drug Administration). (2000) Food labeling: Health claims; Plant sterol / stanol esters and coronary heart disease; Interim final rule. In: *Federal Register, Vol 65*, 21 CFR Part 101.

[64] Plat, J; Kerckhoff, DAJM; Mensink, RP. (2000) Therapeutic potential of plant sterols and stanols. *Curr Opin Lipidol, 11*, 571-576.

[65] Saito, S; Takeshita, M; Tomonobu, K; Kudo, N; Shiiba, D; Hase, T; Tokimitsu, I; Yasukawa, T. (2006) Dose-dependent cholesterol-lowering effect of a mayonnaise-type product with a main component of diacylglycerol-containing plant sterol esters. *Nutrition, 22*, 174-178.

[66] Meguro, S; Higashi, K; Hase, T; Honda, Y; Otsuka, A; Tokimitsu, I; Itakura, H. (2001) Solubilization of phytosterols in diacylglycerol versus triacylglycerol improves the serum cholesterol-lowering effect. *Eur J Clin Nutr, 55*, 513-517.

[67] Saito, S; Tomonobu, K; Kudo, N; Shiiba, D; Hase, T; Tokimitsu, I. (2006) Serum retinol, alpha-tocopherol, and beta-carotene levels are not altered by excess ingestion of diacylglycerol-containing plant sterol esters. *Ann Nutr Metab, 50*, 372-379.

[68] Takeshita, M; Saito, S; Katsuragi, Y; Yasunaga, K; Matsuo, N; Tokimitsu, I; Yasukawa, T; Nakamura, H. (2007) Combination of plant sterols and diacylglycerol oil lowers serum cholesterol and lipoprotein (a) concentrations in postmenopausal women with mild to moderate hypercholesterolemia. *Eur J Clin Nutri Metab, 2*, 4-11.

[69] Takeshita, M; Katsuragi, Y; Kusuhara, M; Higashi, K; Miyajima, E; Mizuno, K; Mori, K; Obata, T; Ohmori, R; Ohsuzu, F; Onodera, Y; Sano, J; Sawada, S; Tabata, S; Tokimitsu, I; Tomonobu, K; Yamashita, T; Yasukawa, T; Yonemura, A; Nakamura, H. Phytosterols dissolved in diacylglycerol oil reinforce the cholesterol-lowering effect of low-dose pravastatin treatment. *Nutr Metab Cardiovasc Dis, in press.*

[70] Yasukawa, T; Yasunaga, K. (2001) Nutritional function of dietary diacyglycerols. *J Oleo Sci, 50*, 427-432.

[71] Matsuo, N. (2001) Diacylglycerol oil: an edible oil with less accumulation of body fat. *Lipid Tech, 13*, 129-133.

[72] Matsuo, N; Tokimitsu, I. (2001) Metabolic characteristics of diacylglycerol. An edible oil that is less likely to become body fat. *Biochem, 12*, 1098-1102.

[73] Nagao, T; Matsuo, N; Tokimitsu, I. (2002) Diacylglycerol, an edible oil with less body fat accumulation. *Recent Res Devel Nutrition, 5*, 179-187.

[74] Flickinger, BD; Matsuo, N. (2003) Nutrition characteristics of DAG oil. *Lipids, 38*, 129-132.

[75] Tada, N; Yoshida, H. (2003) Diacylglycerol on lipid metabolism. *Curr Opin Lipidol, 12*, 29-33.

[76] St-Onge, M-P. (2005) Dietary fats, teas, dairy, and nuts: potential functional foods for weight control? *Am J Clin Nutr, 81*, 7-15.

[77] Rudkowska, I; Roynette, CE; Demonty, I; Vastone, CA; Jew, S; Jones, PJH. (2005) Diacylglycerol: Efficacy and mechanism of action of an anti-obesity agent. *Obes Res, 13*, 1864-1876.

[78] Kovacs, EMR; Mela, DJ. (2006) Metabolically active functional food ingredients for weight control. *Obes Rev, 7*, 59-78.

[79] Takase, H. (2007) Metabolism of diacylglycerol in humans. *Asia Pac J Clin Nutr, 16* (Suppl 1), 398-403.

In: Micronutrients and Health Research
Editor: Takumi Yoshida, pp. 263-277

ISBN: 978-1-60456-056-5
© 2008 Nova Science Publishers, Inc.

Chapter IX

VITAMINS: DOING DOUBLE DUTY[a]

Franklyn F. Bolander[*]

Department of Biological Sciences, University of South Carolina,
Columbia, SC 29208, USA.

ABSTRACT

Vitamins are organic molecules which are required in small amounts to sustain life but which cannot be made by the organism. Most vitamins are coenzymes, molecules that facilitate the chemical reactions catalyzed by enzymes, while two are hormone precursors, which bind and activate transcription factors. However, both types of vitamins share some of the functions exhibited by the other: vitamin K_2, a coenzyme in γ-carboxylation, can also bind and activate the steroid and xenobiotic receptor (SXR); lipoic acid, a coenzyme in oxidative decarboxylation, can bind and activate the insulin receptor; and nicotinic acid, a component of NAD^+ which is involved with redox reactions, can signal through a G protein-coupled receptor. On the other hand, the active forms of vitamin D and vitamin A, which bind nuclear receptors (VDR and RAR, respectively), can have nongenomic effects by binding and activating enzymes through their receptors. For example, the VDR can bind and stimulate the phosphoinositide 3-kinase, while the RAR can bind and activate protein kinase Cδ. This review explores several of these multifunctional compounds and tries to provide a possible explanation for this double duty from an evolutionary perspective.

---

[a] This review is based, in part, on a shorter review published earlier [1].
[*] Correspondence concerning this article should be addressed to: Franklyn F. Bolander, Department of Biological Sciences University of South Carolina, Columbia, SC 29208. (803) 777-7656 (office); (803) 777-4002 (fax); Bolander@sc.edu.

INTRODUCTION

All known vitamins are divided into two major functional classes. The majority of vitamins are coenzymes that facilitate the chemical reactions catalyzed by enzymes. Two vitamins, vitamins A and D are hormone precursors whose final products, retinoic acid and 1,25-dihydroxycholecalciferol (DHCC), bind and activate a group of ligand-regulated transcription factors, known as the nuclear receptors. As more is learned about these molecules, it is apparent that they have more overlapping functions than was initially appreciated: many of the coenzymes have hormone-like activity that is mediated through receptors, while retinoic acid and DHCC can nongenomically activate a number of enzymes. Such multifunctionality is becoming increasingly common in proteins. This review will examine the "atypical" activity of these vitamins and provide a possible explanation and mechanism for the diversification of their functions.

METABOLIC SYNERGY

Hormones are intercellular messengers that usually have no intrinsic function; rather, their "activity" resides entirely in how a cell responds to their presence. As such, the same hormone can elicit different reactions in different cells or even in the same cell at different stages of development or metabolic states. The recruitment of a molecule as a hormone appears to be fortuitous (chapter 18 in reference [2]): for example, the first chemoreceptors in primitive eukaryotes were probably designed to detect potential food sources, especially amino acids. When multicellularity developed, these receptors and their ligands were internalized to become the first hormones. Amino acids and their derivatives are still among the most abundant chemical messengers in animals. However, some hormones do have enzymatic activity and appear to have been appropriated into the endocrine system because their enzymatic activity provided an important signal. For example, thrombin is a protease activated in blood coagulation. As such, its activity is an indication of tissue damage and it can act as a stress hormone via interaction with a membrane receptor.

Similarly, coenzymes are critical components in many chemical reactions; as such, they can provide the cell with important information about the status of certain metabolic cycles. For example, coenzymes involved with redox reactions are often allosteric regulators of enzymes in the tricarboxylic acid cycle. It would seem perfectly natural for them to be recruited as hormones for more widespread signaling and coordination. Similar linkages have occurred with coenzymes involved with osteogenesis and lipogenesis.

Nicotinic Acid

Nicotinic acid (also called niacin) is 3-pyridinecarboxylic acid. In the body it is coupled to adenine via a ribophosphate bridge to form NAD^+ and $NADP^+$; NAD^+ acts as a hydrogen/electron carrier in catabolic redox reactions, while $NADP^+$ serves the same function in anabolic reactions (chapter 15 in reference [3]). However, nicotinic acid also has independent effects on the cardiovascular system and lipid metabolism; for example, it can dilate blood vessels and lower blood cholesterol, triglycerides, and free fatty acids. As coenzymes, NAD^+ and $NADP^+$ are involved with the cellular metabolism of lipids; as a hormone, nicotinic acid helps to coordinate lipid metabolism throughout the organism.

The antilipolytic effects of nicotinic acid arise from its ability to lower cAMP levels [4]. Traditionally, cAMP is regulated by GTP binding proteins (G proteins), which are molecular switches: when bound to GDP, they are "off"; but when bound to GTP, they are "on". These switches are usually controlled by G protein-coupled receptors (GPCRs). These membrane proteins have seven transmembrane α-helices that are kinked and clustered together to form a ligand binding pocket. The intracellular loops between these helices bind to the G protein. Interhelical bonds stabilize the inactive state; ligand binding disrupts these bonds and the helices rotate to form new bonds with the ligand. The ensuing movement of the loops pries open the nucleotide binding cleft in the G protein to allow GTP to displace the GDP and turn the switch on. This very simple mechanism allows for the rapid evolutionary accommodation of new ligands; indeed, such evolution of GPCRs has been demonstrated in vitro [5]. During evolution, GPCRs have developed binding sites for a number of metabolites, including fatty acids, succinate, α-ketoglutamate, ketone bodies, and bile acids (Table 1) [6]. Therefore, the adaptation of a binding site for coenzymes would not be unreasonable; indeed, GPR109A has been proposed to be the GPCR for nicotinic acid.

Table 1. Examples of receptors for intermediary metabolites

Receptor	Metabolite ligand	Function
GPCRs[a]:		
BG37	Bile acids	Elevates cAMP
GPR40	Medium and long chain fatty acids	Stimulates insulin secretion
GPR41, -43	Short chain fatty acids	Stimulates leptin release and adipogenesis
GPR84	Medium chain fatty acids	Regulates cytokine production
GPR91	Succinate	Hypertension
GPR99	α-Ketoglutamate	Hypertension
GPR109A	Ketone bodies; nicotinic acid(?)	Elevates calcium and arachidonic acid; lowers cAMP
GPR120	Long chain fatty acids	Stimulates MAP kinase and PKB; stimulates GLP-1 release
NRs:		
FXR	Bile acids; lanosterol	Bile acid and cholesterol metabolism
HNF4α	Fatty acyl CoAs	Lipid and carbohydrate metabolism
LXR	Oxysterols	Cholesterol metabolism
PPARα	Polyunsaturated fatty acids	Fatty acid metabolism
PPARγ	Polyunsaturated fatty acids	Adipogenesis
RORα	Cholesterol	Cholesterol homeostasis

[a]All GPCRs except BG37 are coupled to G_i and G_q.

This coenzyme has another link with the endocrine system: cells store triiodothyronine (T_3) in their cytoplasm by binding it to a protein, called μ-crystallin [7]. This reservoir is essential for maintaining adequate cellular T_3 levels, although it also sequesters T_3 and inhibits its transcriptional activity. T_3 binding to μ-crystallin has an absolute requirement for NADPH. Since T_3 mobilizes fatty acids and stimulates their oxidation, sequestration of T_3 by NADPH-activated μ-crystallin might partially explain some of the noncoenzymatic effects of nicotinic acid.

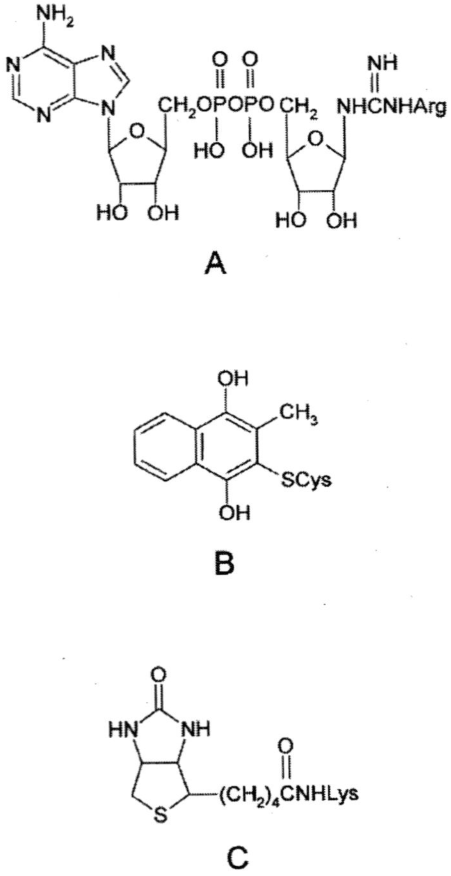

Figure 1. Structure of some vitamins covalently attached to proteins. (A) Mono(ADP-ribosyl)ated arginine, (B) vitamin K_3 bound to cysteine, and (C) biotinylated lysine.

Finally, NAD^+ can be used as a substrate for mono- and poly(ADP-ribosyl) polymerases, which remove the nicotinic acid and attach the remaining moiety to proteins (Figure 1A; chapters 9 and 14 in reference [2]). Although this might be considered an unusal mechanism for hormone action, several hormones can covalently react with their targets: nitric oxide (NO) can S-nitrosylate cysteines in proteins to regulate their activity; insulin can form a disulfide bond with its receptor to affect receptor kinetics; and prostaglandin J_2 can react with a cysteine in NF-κB to inhibit its transcriptional activity. Poly(ADP-ribosyl)ation of histones and some transcription factors has been shown to affect transcription; but the effect of nicotinic acid on blood vessels and lipid metabolism occur too quickly to be explained by gene induction. Alternatively, the G protein, G_s, can be mono(ADP-ribosyl)ated. G_s

stimulates cAMP production by the adenylate cyclase, and mono(ADP-ribosyl)ation enhances this activity. However, nicotinic acid activates G_i to lower cAMP levels. Therefore, the activation of a GPCR is the most likely mechanism for the noncoenzymatic activities of nicotinic acid, while effects on T_3 metabolism may play an ancillary role.

Vitamin K

Vitamin K refers to a group of closely related chemicals known as the 3-methyl-1,4-naphthoquinones (chapter 15 in reference [3]): K_1 (phylloquinone), K_2 (the menaquinones), and K_3 (menadione). All three molecules have the same nucleus. Vitamin K_1 is derived from plants consumed in the diet and has a phytyl side chain. The bacterial flora in the gastrointestinal tract is another source of this nutrient; this form (vitamin K_2) possesses a polyprenyl side chain having from two to nine monomers. However, these side chains are not required for the biological activity of the vitamin and merely make its synthesis more difficult and costly. Therefore, the synthetic version (vitamin K_3) does not have any side chain. Vitamin K is required by enzymes that incorporate an additional carboxy group into the side chain of glutamic acid. The resulting γ-carboxyglutamic acid (Gla) is an excellent chelator of calcium and is found in proteins involved with coagulation and bone formation.

As with nicotinic acid, vitamin K can also act as a hormone to complement its coenzymatic function. However, instead of a GPCR, vitamin K_2 can bind and activate a ligand-regulated transcription factor known as the steroid and xenobiotic receptor (SXR). This nuclear receptor is involved with the metabolism and elimination of endogenously generated toxins and exogenous chemicals by the induction of cytochrome P450, conjugating enzymes, and drug transporters. Interestingly, SXR can also activate several genes related to bone formation and metabolism. Such genes include alkaline phosphatase, which plays a role in bone mineralization; matrix Gla protein, a mineralization inhibitor; and tsukushi, an inhibitor of bone morphogenic protein [8]. As such, both the transcriptional activity of vitamin K_2 and its coenzymatic function facilitate bone formation.

The carboxyterminal domain of nuclear receptors (NR) has a globular structure consisting of a three-tiered stack of α-helices (chapter 6 in reference [2]). Ligand binding within a hydrophobic cavity in this domain triggers a conformational change that creates a coactivator binding groove. The resulting formation of a signaling complex eventually leads to the initiation of transcription. Evolutionarily, ligand binding was an acquired characteristic: that is, although NRs first appeared in the metazoans, only isolated incidences of hormone binding can be documented below the vertebrates [9]. NRs were initially regulated in some other manner: for example, by phosphorylation. The first ligands to appear were probably hydrophobic metabolites, such as fatty acids and cholesterol derivatives (Table 1). In vertebrates, the binding pocket has been modified to accommodate a wide range of hormone structures; and further adaptations to bind coenzymes would not be difficult.

Like nicotinic acid, vitamin K_3 can form protein derivatives (Figure 1B) [10]. For example, tyrosine kinases stimulate a phosphorylation cascade leading to the activation of the mitogen-activated protein kinases (MAPKs). Protein tyrosine phosphatases reverse this effect by dephosphorylation. However, these phosphatases have in their catalytic site a critical cysteine that can react with vitamin K_3. This modification inhibits the phosphatases, which, in turn, prolongs the activation of the MAPKs. Since the susceptibility of cysteine to modification is sensitive to the redox potential of cells, derivatization by vitamin K_3 may be used as a sensor for oxygen stress. Cysteine-110 in histone H3 is another known target for vitamin K_3 modification. This reaction has the potential to effect gene induction, since it only occurs in transcriptionally active regions where this residue is exposed. However, there is no evidence, as yet, that this modification does effect transcription.

Lipoic Acid

Lipoic acid is a fatty acid with a terminal disulfide loop; chemically, it is 6,8-epidithiooctanoic acid, which is also known as thioctic acid (chapter 15 in reference [3]). Although it can be synthesized by humans and, therefore, is not a vitamin in this species, there are other organisms that do require lipoic acid in their diet. It is used as a coenzyme in the glycine cleavage complex that converts two glycines into serine, which in turn is degraded into pyruvate. It is also a coenzyme for pyruvate dehydrogenase, which converts pyruvate into acetate for fatty acid synthesis. The major hormone stimulating lipogenesis is insulin; and it would be evolutionarily advantageous for lipoic acid, which supplies acetate for fatty acid synthesis, to coordinate its activity with that of insulin. In fact, it has been recently discovered that lipoic acid binds the insulin receptor [11]. It appears that its binding to the catalytic site stabilizes the ATP binding loop and activates the receptor tyrosine kinase. Once again the hormone-like activity of a coenzyme complements its enzymatic function.

Biotin

Biotin has an oxothienoimidazole nucleus with a pentanoic side chain that is used to form an amide bond with a lysine in carboxylases. The 1' nitrogen can react with bicarbonate which is then donated to substrates in carboxylation reactions (chapter 14 in reference [3]). Biotin is a coenzyme for four carboxylases: propionyl-CoA carboxylase, which is involved in the catabolism of odd-chain fatty acids and some amino acids; pyruvate carboxylase, which is involved with gluconeogenesis; methylcrotonyl-CoA carboxylase, which is involved with the catabolism of some amino acids; and acetyl-CoA carboxylase, which is the initial step in fatty acid synthesis. In addition to its role in enzymatic carboxylation, biotin is important in the development of the epidermal layer of the skin and its appendages, like nails, hooves, and mammary glands [12]. For example, biotin is necessary for the adequate production of keratin, which is a major component of hoof horn tissue [13], and enhances milk yields and milk protein content in dairy cows [14,15]. Indeed, biotin supplementation has been used to treat hoof lesions in cattle and brittle fingernails in humans. Biotin can also activate genes involved with glucose and lipid metabolism [16]. For example, biotin induces the genes for insulin, its receptor, and glucokinase, which phosphorylates glucose. At the same time, it represses the gene for phosphoenolpyruvate carboxykinase, which is involved with gluconeogenesis. These activities complement at least one of the reactions for which biotin is a coenzyme: acetyl-CoA carboxylase is the rate-limiting step in fatty acid synthesis, which insulin stimulates.

The transcriptional effects of biotin in fibroblasts, hepatocytes [17,18], and mammary epithelium (Bolander, unpublished observations) appear to be mediated by cGMP. First, inhibitors of the soluble guanylate cyclase (sGC), which generates cGMP, and inhibitors of protein kinase G (PKG), a cGMP-activated protein kinase, both block the effects of biotin. Second, cGMP analogs can reproduce the effects of biotin in these tissues. These effects are not related to carboxylation, since cGMP is not involved in carboxylase activity. There are two possible mechanisms by which biotin could activate the sGC: first, NO is a physiological activator of the sGC and NO synthetase can be activated by elevated calcium. Therefore, hormones that use cGMP often bind receptors that are coupled to calcium as a second messenger.

The second potential mechanism for the activation of the sGC is evident from the structure of this molecule. sGC is a dimer composed of two homologous subunits: the guanylate cyclase activity is located in the carboxyterminus and an autoinhibitory, heme-binding domain exists in the aminoterminus. NO binds the iron in the heme and disrupts the autoinhibitory domain to stimulate the receptor [19]. Although biotin does not bind iron, it can react with proteins. Indeed, biotin is normally covalently attached to its companion enzyme via an amide bond between its carboxyl group and the ε-amino group of lysine in the enzyme; such a reaction is called biotinylation. Alternatively, biotin can be coupled to chromatin proteins, such as histones H2A, histone H3, and histone H4 [20]. Many of the lysines modified in these histones can also be acetylated; and because such lysines cannot be both biotinylated and acetylated, the two modifications are mutually exclusive. This reciprocal alteration is important in that acetylation is associated with transcription, and its prevention by biotinylation results in the repression of transcription. As such, it seems unlikely that histone biotinylation is involved with biotin action, because biotin induces genes involved with epidermal differentiation. However, it is possible that biotin might covalently modify the aminoterminus of the sGC and suppress its inhibitory activity. Regardless of the mechanism of sGC stimulation, the basis of transcription activation is probably a result of the phosphorylation of transcripiton factors by cGMP-activated PKG. For example, NF-κB is a transcription factor that mediates stress responses, and it is both modulated by biotin and phosphorylated by PKG [21], suggesting that the former may acting via the latter.

ULTRAVIOLET LIGHT STRESS MARKERS

Molecules elevated during stress can also be recruited as hormones. For example, ATP is the energy currency of cells and high mobility group proteins (HMG) are chromatin proteins that participate in DNA packaging and transcription. Neither would occur in the extracellular fluid unless they had leaked from damaged cells. That is, extracellular ATP or HMG is evidence of stress. Through evolution, these molecules were recruited to be stress hormones; now, in addition to their original function, both ATP and HMG are actively secreted during stress to signal other cells of danger [22]. Vitamins D and A are both light sensitive and would be in an ideal position to act as sensors of ultraviolet (UV) damage.

Vitamin D

Vitamin D is actually a precursor of the active hormone, DHCC; this conversion requires several steps in three different tissues (Figure 2). First, 7-dehydrocholesterol is transported to the skin where UVB light nonenzymatically breaks a ring to yield previtamin D_3, which then isomerizes to vitamin D_3. Vitamin D_3 next goes to the liver where it is hydroxylated on the 25 position. The final step is the hydroxylation of the 1 position in the kidney to form DHCC. Classically, DHCC is considered a hormone whose receptor is a ligand-regulated transcription factor, the vitamin D receptor (VDR), which mediates many of the effects of DHCC on calcium absorption in the gastrointestinal tract and, with parathyroid hormone, on bone resorption. However, DHCC can also trigger damage responses, especially in the skin: for example, it can stimulate the proliferation and differentiation of keratinocytes to replace damaged cells and it can promote the synthesis and secretion of antimicrobial peptides to defend compromised tissue until repairs are made [23]. The fact that its synthesis is sensitive to UV light allows DHCC levels to reflect, in part, UV light exposure.

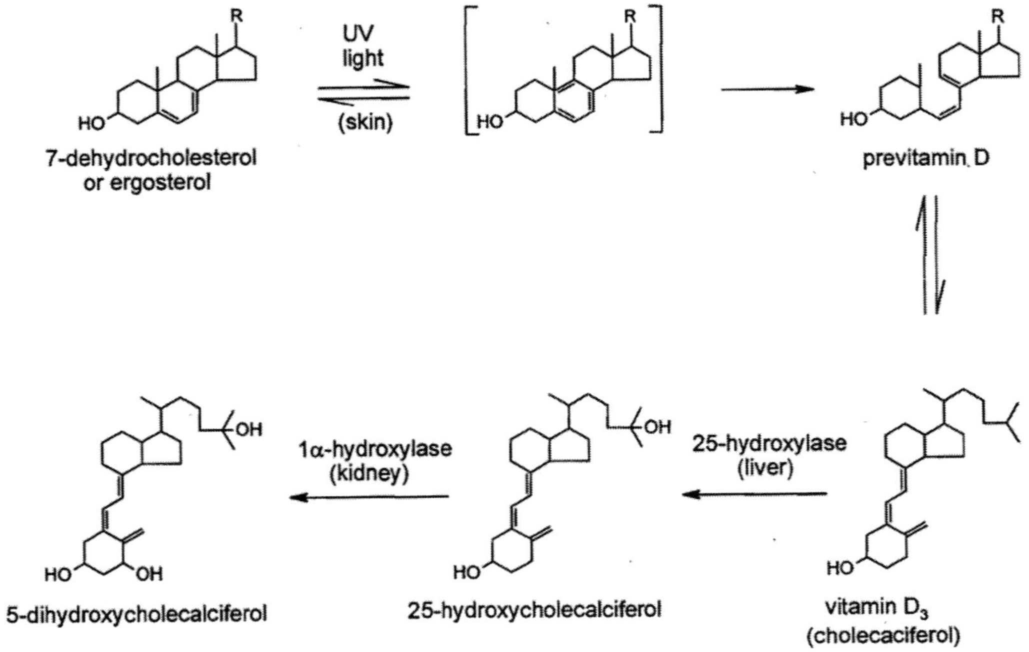

Figure 2. Synthesis of 1,25-dihydroxycholecalciferol (DHCC).

The acquisition of this nonclassical activity has been accompanied by an equally nonclassical mechanism [24]: the DHCC-VDR complex can directly activate several enzymes involved with cell signaling [25,26]. In essence, this is the reverse of what is seen with many vitamins which began as coenzymes and later acquired the ability to bind and activate receptors. This regulatory expansion of NR function is an ongoing process and, as such, is hardly surprising. Initially, NRs appeared to be regulated by post-translational modifications. In vertebrates, NRs acquired allosteric sites for hydrophobic metabolites, whose metabolism the NR regulated (Table 1); and, eventually, the switch was made to hydrophobic hormones. This evolution is continuing as the NRs are now developing the means to affect cell functions by nongenomic means.

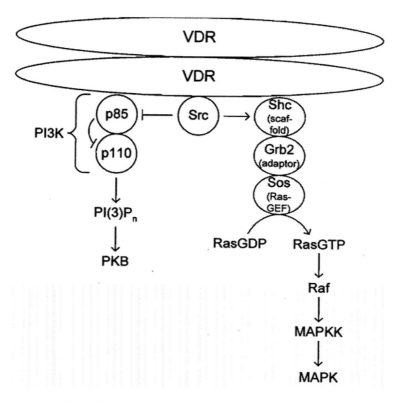

Figure 3. Schematic depiction of the nongenomic effects of the vitamin D receptor (VDR). Grb2, an adaptor; p85, regulatory subunit of PI3K; p110, catalytic subunit of PI3K; PI3K, phosphoinositide 3-kinase; PI(3)P$_n$, phosphoinositide phosphorylated on position 3; PKB, protein kinase B; RasGEF, Ras GNP exchange facilitator; Shc, a scaffold; Src, a soluble tyrosine kinase.

The VDR can activate several enzymes that can propagate its defense response (Figure 3). First, it can recruit Src, a soluble tyrosine kinase, to phosphorylate a number of substrates involved with cell signaling. For example, the phosphoinositide 3-kinase (PI3K) consists of an inhibitory subunit (p85) and a catalytic subunit (p110); VDR binds PI3K which leads to the phosphorylation and inhibition of p85. The catalytic subunit can then synthesize a special phospholipid that activates protein kinase B (PKB), also called Akt. PKB is strongly antiapoptotic by virtue of its ability to phosphorylate many molecules involved in apoptosis and block their activities. In addition, Src can phosphorylate Shc, a molecular scaffold that can initiate a protein kinase cascade leading to the stimulation of the MAPK. As the name implies, MAP kinase is critically involved in cell proliferation. As a result, both the antiapoptotic effects of PKB and the proliferative effects of MAP kinase augment the transcriptional function of VDR in the damage response.

Vitamin A

Vitamin A is also light sensitive: retinal is a photopigment in the retina. Although there is no evidence that it acts as a UV sensor in the skin, it is deposited in the skin in hypervitaminosis A and gives the skin a yellow-orange coloration. Furthermore, β-carotene, the precursor to vitamin A, is used to treat sun sensitivity in erythropoietic protoporphyria via its ability to absorb, and therefore screen out, light. As a hormone, it binds to either the retinoic acid receptor (RAR) or the RXR: RAR mediates the proliferation of normal epidermis, although it inhibits hyperproliferative disorders; and RXR promotes differentiation [23]. Retinoic acid also promotes wound healing by inducing collagen synthesis, inhibiting collagenases, and stimulating fibroblast proliferation. Therefore, like vitamin D, vitamin A is light sensitive and triggers defense responses. Also like the VDR, RAR has developed a nongenomic output to augment its defense response: RAR can directly bind and activate protein kinase Cδ (PKCδ) [27]. Although the exact mechanism for this activation is not known, PKCδ can be stimulated by tyrosine phosphorylation; therefore, a reasonable hypothesis would be for RAR to recruit a soluble tyrosine kinase, like Src, to phosphorylate PKCδ, just as it is recruited by VDR to phosphorylate PI3K and Shc. PKC, like MAP kinase, has been associated with cell proliferation.

OXIDATIVE STRESS MARKERS

Another form of stress is represented by the production of reactive oxygen species. In the case of oxidative stress, what could be a better sensor than coenzymes that possess antioxidant activity.

Lipoic Acid

In addition to it role in lipogenesis, lipoic acid possesses both antioxidant and antiapoptotic activities. The former is a result of its disulfide loop; in this respect, it resembles the antioxidant mechanism of glutathione. However, the basis for its antiapoptotic activity had remained obscure until it was discovered that lipoic acid could bind and activate the insulin receptor. Insulin is also antiapoptotic and is frequently added to culture media to maintain cell viability. This activity is primarily a result of its activation of PKB via the stimulation of PI3K, which generates a phospholipid essential for PKB activation. As noted above, PKB phosphorylates many mediators of apoptosis and inhibits their activities. Essentially, because lipoic acid can be oxidized, it can act as a redox sensor; and its recruitment as an insulin-like hormone further enables it to trigger a survival response to complement its antioxidant properties.

Vitamin E

The vitamins E, or the tocopherols, belong to the chromanol family of quinones, which also include vitamin K and coenzyme Q (chapter 15 in reference [3]). Although tocopherols are a dietary requirement in humans, no specific coenzyme role has been identified with this vitamin. Because of their structural similarities, some authorities have suggested that tocopherols may substitute for coenzyme Q in the electron transport system, but this hypothesis has never been proven. Rather, vitamin E appears to be a major antioxidant, especially important in protecting membrane lipids from free radicals and organic peroxides. For this reason, tocopherols have been tested as chemopreventative agents in prostate cancer; indeed, clinical trials have shown that men taking vitamin E had a one-third reduction in the incidence of prostate cancer. Further examination of the mechanisms of action of this vitamin reveals a second anticancer pathway: tocopherols are very potent antiandrogens [28]. They bind the androgen receptor with high affinity and block the action of endogeneous androgens. This effect appears to be physiological, since the IC_{50} is within normal serum levels of this vitamin. Therefore, both the antioxidant activity and the antiandrogen activity complement each other in the chemoprevention of cancer in male reproduction tissues.

Vitamin K_3

As noted above, vitamin K also belongs to the quinone superfamily and is sensitive to the redox potential of cells. This effect resides in the ability of vitamin K_3 to react with the catalytic cysteine in protein tyrosine phosphatases (PTP) to inhibit the phosphatases. Since PTPs reverse the activation of receptor and soluble tyrosine kinases, PTP inhibition will prolong the activation of these tyrosine kinases and their downstream signaling molecules. One such transducer is the MAPK, which triggers stress responses.

MISCELLANEOUS VITAMINS WITH DUAL ACTIONS

The vitamins discussed so far have multiple activities that tend to complement each other. Such a relationship allows one to propose a simple evolutionary scheme of diversification to explain these several functions. However, there is at least one vitamin that has multiple activities that are not so easily integrated into a single scheme.

Vitamin B_6

Pyridoxal phosphate (PLP) is the active form of vitamin B_6; it can be synthesized from either the aldehyde (pyridoxal), hydroxyl (pyridoxine), or the amine (pyridoxamine) forms (chapter 14 in reference [3]). The core mechanism for all the reactions catalyzed by PLP is the formation of a Schiff base between its aldehyde and the amino group in the substrate. From this basic structure, the Schiff base can be reversed in a nonstereospecific manner (racemization), nearby bonds can become labile (decarboxylation, β and γ elimination, side chain cleavage), or the amino group can be removed and added to another molecule (transamination). PLP can also participate in many other types of enzymatic reactions. However, in addition to its coenzymatic functions, PLP also possesses anticancer activity: vitamin B_6 deficiency is characterized by an increased incidence of cancers, low PLP plasma levels have been documented in patients having a variety of cancers, and the growth of several different cancer cell lines in culture can be reduced by PLP [29-31].

There are several mechanisms by which PLP might inhibit growth. First, PLP can antagonize several growth promoting hormones. For example, both estrogens and androgens promote the proliferation of certain reproductive tissues, and PLP can bind to and block the transcriptional activity of their steroid receptors [32]. PLP can also affect the secretion of certain growth factors: PLP can inhibit the release of growth hormone (GH) from pituitary cells in vitro [33]. Finally, PLP can directly attack the DNA replication machinery: PLP can suppress the activity of the DNA polymerase by competing with nucleotides for their binding site on this enzyme [34]. Unfortunately, PLP is involved with over 100 enzymes so that it is impossible to correlate its anticancer activity with any particular reaction or group of reactions. In the absence of such a correlation, one cannot speculate on why or how the noncoenzymatic activity of PLP arose.

Table 2. A summary of vitamins having nongenomic (vitamins A and D) or noncoenzymatic activities and their possible mechanisms

Vitamin	Classic function	Novel functions	Possible mechanisms for novel functions
A	RAR and/or RXR activation	Activate PKCδ (nongenomic)	Direct binding to PKCδ
B_6	Coenzyme in multiple reactions	Inhibition of proliferation	Inhibition of DNA polymerase, steroid receptors, and/or GH secretion
D	VDR activation	Activate MAPK, PI3K, and PLCγ (nongenomic)	Direct binding of Src with phosphorylation of Shc, PI3K, and PLCγ
E	Antioxidant	Inhibit prostate carcinoma	Androgen receptor antagonist
K	Coenzyme in γ-carboxylation of glutamate	Bone gene induction; MAP kinase stimulation	SXR activation; cysteine modification
Biotin	Coenzyme in carboxylation	Epidermal gene induction; insulin-like activity	cGMP elevation; lysine modification
Lipoic acid[a]	Coenzyme for oxidative decarboxylation of α-oxoacids	Antiapoptotic	PKB stimulation via insulin receptor activation
Nicotinic acid	Coenzyme precursor in redox reactions (H⁺/e⁻ carrier)	Vasodilation; antilipolytic	Decrease cAMP; activation of μ-crystallin; mono-/poly(ADP-ribosyl)ation

[a]Required in the diet of some organisms but not humans.

CONCLUSION

Coenzymes occupy pivotal positions in metabolic pathways and can, therefore, provide important information to the cell about its metabolic status. Recruitment as signaling molecules would be a natural development of their functional role. In addition, it would allow the coenzymes to regulate related processes via their hormone-like activities in order to improve coordination (Table 2). Vitamins A and D were already hormones that may have been originally recruited by virtue of their photoabsorptive properties. However, their receptors are ligand-regulated transcription factors and gene induction is a relatively slow process. Therefore, in this case, the development of nongenomic mechanisms of action would provide for complementary pathways that were faster. Essentially, two different vitamin groups have converged toward similar regulatory mechanisms.

ACKNOWLEDGEMENT

Work in the author's laboratory was supported, in part, by a grant from the South Carolina Research Foundation at the University of South Carolina.

REFERENCES

[1]   Bolander, FF. Vitamins: Not just for enzymes. *Curr Opin Invest Drugs* (2006) 7, 912-915.

[2]   Bolander, FF. Molecular Endocrinology. 3rd ed. San Diego: Elsevier; 2004.

[3]   Metzler, DE. Biochemistry: The Chemical Reactions of Living Cells, vol 1. 2nd ed. San Diego: Harcourt Academic Press; 2001.

[4]   Butcher, RW; Baird, CE; Sutherland, EW. Effect of lipolytic and antilipolytic substances on adenosine 3',5'-monophosphate levels in isolated fat cells. *J Biol Chem* (1968) 243, 1705-1712.

[5]   Armbruster, BN; Li, X; Pausch, MH; Heritze, S; Roth, BL. Evolving the lock to fit the key to create a family of G protein-coupled receptors potently activated by an inert ligand. *Proc Natl Acad Sci USA* (2007) 104, 5163-5168.

[6]   Wang, J; Wu, X; Simonavicius, N; Tian, H; Ling, L. Medium-chain fatty acids as ligands for orphan G protein-coupled receptor GPR84. *J Biol Chem* (2006) 281, 34457-34464.

[7]   Suzuki, S; Suzuki, N; Mori, J; Oshima, A; Usami, S; Hashizume, K. μ-Crystallin as an intracellular 3,5,3'-triiodothyronine holder *in vivo*. *Mol Endocrinol* (2007) 21, 885-894.

[8]   Ichikawa, T; Horie-Inoue, K; Ikeda, K; Blumberg, B; Inoue, S. Steroid and xenobiotic receptor SXR mediates vitamin K_2-activated transcription of extracellular matrix-related genes and collagen accumulation in osteoblastic cells. *J Biol Chem* (2006) 281, 16927-16934.

[9]   Owen, GI; Zelent, A. Origins and evolutionary diversification of the nuclear receptor superfamily. *Cell Mol Life Sci* (2000) 57, 809-827.

[10] Scott, GK; Atsriku, C; Kaminker, P; Held, J; Gibson, B; Baldwin, MA; Benz, CC. Vitamin K3 (menadione)-induced oncosis associated with keratin 8 phosphorylation and histone H3 arylation. *Mol Pharmacol* (2005) 68, 606-615.

[11] Diesel, B; Kulhanek-Heinze, S; Höltje, M; Brandt, B; Höltje, HD; Vollmar, AM; Kiemer, AK. α-Lipoic acid as a direct binding activator of the insulin receptor: Protection from hepatocyte apoptosis. *Biochemistry* (2007) 46, 2146-2155.

[12] Zempleni, J. Uptake, localization, and noncarboxylase roles of biotin. *Annu Rev Nutr* (2005) 25, 175-196.

[13] Fritsche, A. Biotin verändert das Zytokeratinmuster von kultivierten Keratinozyten. DVM thesis, Faculty of Veterinary Medicine, University of Zurich, Switzerland.

[14] Bonomi, A; Quarantelli, A; Sabbioni, A; Sperchi, P. L'integrazione delle razioni per le bovine le latte con Biotina in forma rumino-protetta. Effetti sull'efficienza produttiva e riproduttiva (contributo sperimentale). *La rivista de Scienza dell'Alimentazione* 25 (Suppl 1, 1996), 49-68.

[15] Zimmerly, CA; Weiss, WP. Effects of supplemental dietary biotin on performance of Holstein cows during early lactation. *J Dairy Sci* (2001) 84, 498-506.

[16] Fernandez-Mejia, C. Pharmacological effects of biotin. *J Nutr Biochem* (2005) 16, 424-427.

[17] De La Vega, L; Stockert, RJ. Regulation of the insulin and asialoglycoprotein receptors via cGMP-dependent protein kinase. *Am J Physiol* (2000) 279, C2037-C2042.

[18] Solórzano-Vargas, RS; Pacheco-Alvarez, D; León-Del-Rio, A. Holocarboxylase synthetase is an obligate participant in biotin-mediated regulation of its own expression and of biotin-dependent carboxylases mRNA levels in human cells. *Proc Natl Acad Sci USA* (2002) 99, 5325-5330.

[19] Pyriochou, A; Papapetropoulos, A. Soluble guanylyl cyclase: more secrets revealed. *Cell Signal* (2005) 17, 407-413.

[20] Kothapalli, N; Camporeale, G; Kueh, A; Chew, YC; Oommen, AM; Griffin, JB; Zempleni, J. Biological functions of biotinylated histones. *J Nutr Biochem* (2005) 16, 446-448.

[21] He, B; Weber, GF. Phosphorylation of NF-κB proteins by cyclic GMP-dependent kinase: A noncanonical pathway to NF-κB activation. *Eur J Biochem* (2003) 270, 2174-2185.

[22] Degryse, B; de Virgilio, M. The nuclear protein HMGB1, a new kind of chemokine? *FEBS Lett* (2003) 553, 11-17.

[23] Reichrath, J; Lehmann, B; Carlberg, C; Varani, J; Zouboulis, CC. Vitamins as hormones. *Horm Metab Res* (2007) 39, 71-84.

[24] Dixon, KM; Deo, SS; Norman, AW; Bishop, JE; Halliday, GM; Reeve, VE; Mason, RS. *In vivo* relevance for photoprotection by the vitamin D rapid response pathway. *J Steroid Biochem Mol Biol* (2007) 103, 451-456.

[25] Gniadecki, R. Activation of Raf-mitogen-activated protein kinase signaling pathway by 1,25-dihydroxyvitamin D-3 in normal human keratinocytes. *J Invest Dermatol* (1996) 106, 1212-1217.

[26] Buitrago, C; Pardo, VG; De Boland, AR. Nongenomic action of $1\alpha,25(OH)_2$-vitamin D_3: Activation of muscle cell PLCγ through the tyrosine kinase c-Src and PtdIns 3-kinase. *Eur J Biochem* (2002) 269, 2506-2515.

[27] Kambhampati, S; Li, Y; Verma, A; Sassano, A; Majchrzak, B; Deb, DK; Parmar, S; Giafis, N; Kalvakolanu, DV; Rahman, A; Uddin, S; Minucci, S; Tallman, MS; Fish, EN; Platanias, LC. Activation of protein kinase δ by all-*trans*-retinoic acid. J Biol Chem (2003) 278, 32544-32551.

[28] Thompson, TA; Wilding, G. Androgen antagonist activity by the antioxidant moiety of vitamin E, 2,2,5,7,8-pentamethyl-6-chromanol in human prostate carcinoma cells. *Mol Cancer Ther* (2003) 2, 797-803.

[29] Molina, A; Oka, T; Munoz, SM; Chikamori-Aoyama, M; Kuwahata, M; Natori, Y. Vitamin B_6 suppress growth and expression of albumin gene in a human hepatoma cell line HepG2. *Nutr Cancer* (1997) 28, 206-211.

[30] DiSorbo, DM; Wagner, R; Nathanson, L. In vitro and in vivo inhibition of B16 melanoma growth by vitamin B_6. *Nutr Cancer* (1985) 7, 43-52.

[31] Shultz, TD; Santamaria, AG; Gridley, DS; Stickney, DR; Slater, JM. Effect of pyridoxine and pyridoxal on the in vitro growth of human malignant melanoma. *Anticancer Res* (1988) 8, 1313-1318.

[32] Tully, DB; Allgood, VE; Cidlowski, JA. Modulation of steroid receptor-mediated gene expression by vitamin B6. *FASEB J* (1994) 8, 343-349.

[33] Ren, SG; Melmed, S. Pyridoxal phosphate inhibits pituitary cell proliferation and hormone secretion. *Endocrinology* (2006) 147, 3936-3942.

[34] Modak, MJ. Observations on the pyridoxal 5'-phosphate inhibition of DNA polymerases. *Biochemistry* (1976) 15, 3620-3626.

In: Micronutrients and Health Research
Editor: Takumi Yoshida, pp. 279-291

ISBN: 978-1-60456-056-5
© 2008 Nova Science Publishers, Inc.

Chapter X

PROTECTIVE EFFECT OF VITAMINS IN INDUCED MUTAGENESIS

E.S. Voronina, A.D. Durnev, A.K. Zhanataev, V.A. Nikitina and N.P. Bochkov

Research Center for Medical Genetics RAMS, Moscow, Russia;
State Zakusov Institute of Pharmacology RAMS, Moscow, Russia.

ABSTRACT

The *in vitro* cytomutagenetic study was carried out in intact and mutagen-treated (cadmium chloride, dioxidine, bleomycin) peripheral lymphocytes obtained in G_2 phase of the cell cycle from healthy donors within and after 14- and/or 30-day period of supplementation with vitamin and vitamin and mineral complexes.

It was established that the supplementation with complexes containing vitamins at total doses exceeding the daily allowances, does not increase the spontaneous mutagenesis and reduces the sensitivity of human cells to the chemical mutagens. Besides, the vitamin complexes of different quantity and quality contents were found able to induce *in vitro* the comutagenic modification of cell susceptibility to the effect of certain mutagens used in certain concentrations.

The revealed antimutagenic and comutagenic modifying effects were shown to depend upon the duration of consumption, amount and quality content of vitamin complexes used, the nature of mutagen and the level of induced cytogenetic damages.

INTRODUCTION

Supplementation with vitamins and other micronutrients as various complexes and nutritional supplements is valid not only in the prevention of vitamin deficiency and related pathological manifestations, but also as a preventive measure of cardiovascular and oncologic diseases which pathogenesis is associated with DNA oxidative damage and mutagenesis [1–

5]. Along with that, the experimental data provided by genotoxic studies of vitamins showed them to have both positive antimutagenic and negative comutagenic and even mutagenic effects [6]. For instance, depending on experimental design, vitamin C demonstrated the antimutagenic, comutagenic and mutagenic effects [7]. So, on the one hand it is not possible to make an *a priory* conclusion about unconditionally safe vitamin consumption, on the other hand, a direct extrapolation of data obtained experimentally to the human condition appears obviously inaccurate due to the interspecies differences in vitamin metabolism.

Studies aimed to evaluate the influence of alimentary factors, including vitamins, upon human sensitivity towards the mutagenic exposures are under very early development [8]. Single results showed that the susceptibility of human peripheral lymphocytes to chemical mutagens and/or genotoxicants exposures may depend on vitamin content in blood plasma, and it changes depending on individual dietary profile [9,10]. However, it remains unclear what influence the regular supplementation with vitamins at cumulative doses over the daily allowances may exert on the spontaneous mutagenesis and cell sensitivity to the cytogenetic effect of chemical mutagens exposure in humans. These effects were not evaluated in view of their dependence upon the duration of vitamin consumption, qualitative and quantitative contents of supplemented vitamin complexes, the nature of mutagens and concentrations in which they lead to cytogenetic damages of different severity.

The present work deals with a comparative cytogenetic investigation of spontaneous and chemical mutagens-induced *in vitro* mutagenesis in peripheral lymphocytes of healthy volunteers prior, after and throughout the period of supplementation with different vitamin and mineral complexes.

MATERIALS AND METHODS

The following mutagens have been used.

Dioxidine (Pharmacon, Russia) – 1,4-di-N-oxide-2,3-bis-(oximethyl)xinoxaline, an antibacterial agent with a wide spectrum of action. The mutagenic properties of dioxidine are well known [6]. In cytogenetic experiments the mutagen was used at doses of 0.01, 0.03 and 0.1 mg/ml.

Bleomycin (Sigma, Germany) – a polypeptide, *Str. Verticillus* vital activity product, an antitumor antibiotic. The mutagenic properties are well known [6]. In cytogenetic experiments the mutagen was used in concentration of 0.1 and 1.0 U/ml.

Cadmium chloride – a commonly encountered ecotoxicant, the cytogenetic activity is well evaluated, including studies in peripheral lymphocytes cultures [6]. The mutagen was used at a dose of 0.02 mg/ml.

Table 1 outlines the quantitative and qualitative contents of used vitamins and vitamin and mineral complexes which were registered and approved for use in Russian Federation as biologically active food supplements. Complexes 1 and 2 were given as one tablet twice daily regimen (morning and evening) after meal. Complex 3 was given as water solution twice a day, morning and evening after meal. To determine the real assimilation rate the dynamics of changes in plasma vitamin levels were measured, the obtained results were reported earlier [11].

Table 1. Quantity and quality contents of vitamin and vitamin + mineral complexes

Vitamins and vitamin-like compounds and minerals	Daily consumption			Daily allowances
	Complex 1[*]	Complex 2[**]	Complex 3	
Vitamin A (beta-carotene)	3200 IU	6700 IU	6500 IU	3333 IU
Vitamin C	90 mg	500 mg	60 mg	70-100 mg
Vitamin E	98,2 IU	100 IU	7 IU	10-12 IU
Vitamin B_1	20 mg	25	1,2 mg	1,1-2,1 mg
Vitamin B_2	20 mg	25	1,2 mg	1,3-2,4 mg
Vitamin B_5 (Pantothenic acid)	30 mg	50 mg	6 mg	10-12 mg
Vitamin B_6	12 mg	25 mg	1,2 mg	1,8-2,0 mg
Vitamin B_{12}	100 µg	125 µg	2 µg	3,0 µg
Vitamin D	600 IU	200 IU	300 IU	100 IU
Vitamin K	20 µg	-	-	65-80 µg
Niacinnamide	50 mg	25 mg	13 mg	14-28 mg
Biotin	60 µg	25 mg	14 µg	30-100 µg
Folic acid	800 µg	200 mg	400 µg	200 µg
Paraaminobenzoic acid	-	25 mg	-	-
Inositol	-	25 mg	-	-
Choline	-	25 mg	-	-
Chromium	13 µg	30 µg		50-200 µg
Calcium	300 mg	125 mg		80-800 mg
Copper	2 mg	-		1,5-2,0 mg
Iodine	300 µg	-		150 µg
Iron	8 mg	9 mg		10-18 mg
Magnesium	100 mg	62,5 mg		400 mg
Molybdenum	50 µg	-		75-250 µg
Nickel	2,5 µg	-		-
Potassium	60 mg	49,6		-
Selene	40 µg	30 µg		20-100 µg
Silicon	20 µg	-		-
Vanadium	20 µg	-		-
Manganese	3 mg	7,5 mg		2,0-5,0 mg
Phosphorus	230 mg	25 mg		1200 mg
Zink	15 mg	15 mg		15 mg

* Complex 1 also contained: *Panax radix* (100 mg), guarane (350 mg), echinacea , spiruline, chlorella, royal jelly, Alphalf's powder , 50 mg of each, the daily dose is indicated in parenthesis.

** Complex 2 also contained: octacosanole (15 mg), lecithin (16,6 mg), rutin (5 mg), hesperidine (25 mg), RNA (16,6 mg), DNA (2,67 mg), bacillus acidophilus (8,33 mg); the aminoacids: lysin (8,33 mg), arginine (4,17 mg), glutamic acid (10 mg), methionine (8,33 mg); the extracts of: wild cherry, *Taraxacum officinale* folia, echinacea, fennel, Foti herb, ginger, gotu cola, parsley, papaya folia, red raspberry leaf, rice, sarparilla, slippery elm (*Ulmus fulva*), yellow dock (*Rumex crispus*) - 30 mg of each; as well as spiruline (75 mg), aloe vera (50 mg), bilberry (1 mg), proantacyanide (2 mg), peppermint folia (1 mg), *ChimaphilaUmbellata* folia (1 mg), *Ginkgo Biloba* (0,1 mg), the daily dose is indicated in parenthesis.

For the trials healthy volunteers were invited who had neither occupational exposure to chemicals or other harmful substances nor ionizing radiation exposure, neither subjected to X-ray examination nor suffered from virus infectious diseases over the period of one year prior investigation, as well as not addicted to tobacco smoking (Table 2). Throughout the whole period of investigation they followed habitual individual diet, working schedule and life-style. All subjects gave written informed consent to the trial procedure.

Table 2. Characteristics of donors included in the study

Parameters	Complex 1	Complex 2		Complex 3		
	Experiments with dioxidine and cadmium chloride	Experiments with dioxidine	Experiments with bleomycin	Experiments with dioxidine	Experiments with bleomycin 0.1 U/ml	Experiments with bleomycin 1.0 U/ml
Number of donors per group	15 8 female, 7 male	15 8 female, 7 male	11 5 female, 6 male	11 5 female, 6 male	13 7 female, 6 male	15 8 female, 7 male
Age	24 – 48 years	21 – 48 years	23 – 53 years	21 – 48 years	21 – 43 years	22 – 43 years
Mean age	32.5 ± 2.3	32.5 ± 2.3	32.1 ± 2.2	25.5 ± 1.9	25.4 ± 2.5	30.3 ± 2.1
Intake duration	14 and 30 days	14 days	14 days	14 days	14 days	14 days

The blood samples were collected fasting by the venipunction, twice – prior and 24 hrs after ending of course of complexes 2 and 3 intake, or three times – prior, after 14 days and 24 hrs after ending of course of complex 1 intake. Heparin was used as an anticoagulant agent.

The standard D.A. Hungerford's techniques with modifications by N.P. Bochkov [12] were employed to prepare the whole blood culture. The cultured mixture contained the following components: medium RPMI-1640 with glutamine (Sigma, Germany) in tests with complex 1 or Eagle's medium with glutamate (PanEco, Russia) in tests with complex 2 and 3 – 75% (7.5 ml); fetal calf serum (BioClot, Germany) – 15% (1.5 ml); whole blood – 10% (1 ml). To stimulate the lymphocyte division the culture was added with phytohemagglutinin P (Difco, USA) in the amount of 0.02 ml. Culturing was performed in sterile polypropylene vials 15 ml of volume.

The mutagens were added to cultures on hour 50 of culturing (G_2 phase of the cell cycle), culturing duration made in total 54 hrs.

For cell hypotonization 0.55% potassium chloride was used, glacial acetic acid + ethanol (or methanol with complex 1) mixed at a ratio of 1:3 were used for cell fixing. Air-dried cytogenetic slides were coded and microscopically examined using the double blind method.

The chromosome aberrations were analyzed following the International Guidelines without metaphase karyotyping [12,13]. The single and paired fragments, chromosome and chromatid exchanges, and cells bearing multiple aberrations (more than 5 per cell) were accounted.

The results were considered significantly different at $p < 0.05$ and less, Fisher's (φ) test was used in this statistical analysis.

RESULTS

The results obtained from the cytogenetic study are summarized in Table 3 and 4.

Table 3. Main results from cytogenetic studies in healthy donors

Experiment version	Number of donors	Follow-up period					
		COMPLEX 1					
		Prior supplementation		After 14 days		After 30 days	
		Number of cells	Aberrant metaphases (%)	Number of cells	Aberrant metaphases (%)	Number of cells	Aberrant metaphases (%)
Spontaneous level	15	4800	$2,8 \pm 0,2$	4500	$3,0 \pm 0,2$	4800	$2,7 \pm 0,2$
Cadmium chloride	15	4800	$5,5 \pm 0,3^a$	4800	$5,2 \pm 0,4^a$	4600	$4,3 \pm 0,3$ [a,b] ($\downarrow$22%)
Dioxidine 0,03 mg/ml	15	4800	$10,0 \pm 0,6^a$	4600	$8,1 \pm 0,4^{a,6}$ ($\downarrow$19 %)	4600	$7,2 \pm 0,5$ [a,b,c] ($\downarrow$28%)
Dioxidine 0,1 mg/ml	15	5100	$17,1 \pm 0,8^a$	4500	$16,3 \pm 0,6^a$	5100	$14,8 \pm 0,6$ [a,b] ($\downarrow$15%)
		COMPLEX 2					
		Prior supplementation		After 14 days			
		Number of cells	Aberrant metaphases (%)	Number of cells	Aberrant metaphases (%)		
Spontaneous level	15	4081	$3,2 \pm 0,3$	4049	$3,4 \pm 0,3$		
Dioxidine 0,01 mg/ml	15	7266	$5,8 \pm 0,3^a$	7888	$4,6 \pm 0,2$ [a, b,d] ($\downarrow$21%)		
Bleomycin 0,1 U/ml [d]	11	2769	$7,3 \pm 0,5^a$	3090	$7,5 \pm 0,5$ [a,d]		
Bleomycin 1,0 U/ml	11	2512	$16,6 \pm 0,7^a$	2785	$15,1 \pm 0,7^a$		
		COMPLEX 3					
		Prior supplementation		After 14 days			
		Number of cells	Aberrant metaphases (%)	Number of cells	Aberrant metaphases (%)		
Spontaneous level	11	3168	$2,4 \pm 0,3$	2807	$2,8 \pm 0,3$		
Dioxidine 0,01 mg/ml	11	5877	$5,5 \pm 0,3^a$	5601	$4,8 \pm 0,3$ [a,d]		
Bleomycin 0,1 U/ml	13	3792	$7,8 \pm 0,4^a$	3376	$8,5 \pm 0,5$ [a,d]		
Bleomycin 1,0 U/ml	15	4378	$14,5 \pm 0,5^a$	3968	$16,8 \pm 0,6$ [a,b,d] ($\uparrow$16%)		

Percentage of statistically significant decrease ($\downarrow$) or increase ($\uparrow$) in mutagen cytogenetic effect.

[a] – significant differences vs. corresponding values for spontaneous mutations;

[b] – significant differences vs. mutagen effect prior supplementation;

[c] – significant differences vs. mutagen effect 14 days after supplementation;

[d] – significant differences in some individuals indicating the antimutagenic or comutagenic; modification (see text and Table 5 for details).

Effect of Vitamin Complexes on the Spontaneous Mutation

The incidence of the aberrant cells in complex 1 treated donors varied from 1.3% to 4.3% before, from 1.7% to 4.3% 14 days after, and from 2.0% to 4.7% 30 days after administration. The mean incidence of cells bearing chromosome aberrations in group made $2.8 \pm 0.2\%$ prior vitamin complex intake, $3.0 \pm 0.2\%$ 14 days after intake, and $2.7\% \pm 0.2\%$ 30 days after intake (Table 3).

In donors received complex 2 during 14 days, the level of aberrant cells amounted to $3.2 \pm 0.3\%$ before, and $3.4 \pm 0.3\%$ after administration ($p > 0.05$). The incidence of aberrant cells varied from 1.3% to 5.2% before, and from 1.6 to 4.7% 14 days after the last dose.

In donors given complex 3 the level of aberrant metaphases made $2.4 \pm 0.3\%$ before, and $2.8 \pm 0.3\%$ after 2-week intake ($p > 0.05$). The incidence of aberrant cells varied from 1.0 to 3.3% before, and from 1.3 to 4.0% 14 days after administration.

Thus neither of tested mutagens was found to produce the mutagenic activity.

Cytogenetic Effects of Cadmium Chloride

The results derived from cytogenetic examination of cells obtained at different stages of complex 1 administration and treated with cadmium chloride *in vitro* are presented in Table 3 and 4.

Table 4. Chromosome aberration types in healthy donors blood prior and after supplementation with vitamins

COMPLEX 1

Experiment version	Number of donors	Prior supplementation Cells/Aberrations	Single fragments	Paired fragments	Ex-changes	After 14 days Cells/Aberrations	Single fragments	Paired fragments	Ex-changes	After 30 days Cells/Aberrations	Single fragments	Paired fragments	Ex-changes
Spontaneous level	15	4800/143	24	5	2	4500/142	25	3	3	4800/133	24	3	1^{a,c}*
Cadmium chloride	15	4800/282	49	7	4	4800/266	47	5	3	4600/203	39*,c	3	2*
Dioxidine 0,03 mg/ml	15	4800/508	94	10	4	4600/397	77*	7	2*	4600/348	70**	4^{a,c}	2*
Dioxidine 0,1 mg/ml	15	5100/971	175	10	4	4500/827	166	11	6	5100/841	155**	6**,c	3**,c*

COMPLEX 2

Experiment version	Number of donors	Prior supplementation Cells/Aberrations	Single fragments	Paired fragments	Ex-changes	MD	After 14 days Cells/Aberrations	Single fragments	Paired fragments	Ex-changes	MD
Spontaneous level	15	4081/134	31	2	0.4	0	4049/142	34	1	0.2	0
Dioxidine 0,01 mg/ml	15	7266/432	57	2	0.1	0.1	7888/369	45***	1*	0.1	0
Bleomycin 0,1 U/ml	11	2769/210	74	14	0	6	3090/234	72	4	0.3	6
Bleomycin 1,0 U/ml	11	2512/498	183	14	1	19	2785/487	165*	9*	1	18

COMPLEX 3

Experiment version	Number of donors	Prior supplementation Cells/Aberrations	Single fragments	Paired fragments	Ex-changes	MD	After 14 days Cells/Aberrations	Single fragments	Paired fragments	Ex-changes	MD
Spontaneous level	11	3168/80	24	2	0.1	0	2807/78	27	1	0	0
Dioxidine 0,01 mg/ml	11	5877/328	53	5	0.3	0.5	5601/272	47	1	0.2	0
Bleomycin 0,1 U/ml	13	3792/307	75	13	0.2	8	3376/308	85	6	0.3	8
Bleomycin 1,0 U/ml	15	4378/739	155	13			3968/714	167	12	0.7	25***

Significant differences vs. pre-vitamin recordings (*p < 0.05; **p < 0.01; ***p < 0.001). For complex 1 – «a» - compared to baseline recordings, «c» - compared to recordings on Day 14 of experiment.

MD – cells bearing multiple chromosome damages (more than 5 chromosome aberrations per cell).

The mean incidence of cells with chromosome aberrations made $5.5 \pm 0.3\%$ before the first dose of complex 1, $5.2 \pm 0.4\%$ 14 days after, and $4.3 \pm 0.3\%$ 30 days after the last dose. All results obtained are significantly higher than values typical to the spontaneous mutagenesis, and thus confirm the data of studies on the cytogenetic activity of cadmium chloride [14].

The comparison of results evidencing the cytogenetic activity of cadmium chloride showed that the rate of chromosome damages in blood samples taken on Day 30 are significantly higher than those collected prior administration. Aberrant cell frequency ranged $4.0 - 7.0\%$ before, $2.3 - 7.3\%$ and $2.0 - 6.3\%$ 14 and 30 days after complex intake respectively. Scoring of aberration types before and after administration of complex 1 revealed a significant decline in the number of single fragments and exchanges (Table 4).

The reduction of cytogenetic damages while on complex 1 administration was observed not only when average intergroup scores were compared, but it was also found in two (No 4 and No 5) out of 15 donors at the end of the supplementation with complex tested (Table 5).

Thus, the 30-day administration of complex 1 increased the peripheral lymphocytes resistance towards the cytogenetic effect of cadmium chloride.

Table 5. Significant differences in cytogenetic mutagen effects on individual donors prior and after supplementation with different vitamins

Donor No, Sex (age)	Prior supplementation					After 14 days					At the end of supplementation				
	Cells	Single fragments	Paired fragments	Exchanges	Aberrant metaphases M±m%	Cells	Single fragments	Paired fragments	Exchanges	Aberrant metaphases M±m%	Cells	Single fragments	Paired fragments	Exchanges	Aberrant metaphases M±m%
		per 100 cells					per 100 cells					per 100 cells			
Complex 1 (cadmium chloride)															
4M(48)	300	5.3	1.3	1.0	7.0±1.5	300	5.7	-	-	5.0±1.3	300	1.7	-	0.3	2.3±0.9***a
5F(25)	300	5.3	2.0	1.0	6.0±1.4	300	5.0	1.7	0.3	7.0±1.5	300	1.7	0.7	-	2.0±0.7***a
Complex 1 (dioxidine 0.03 mg/ml)															
2M(24)	400	12.8	1.5	0.8	13.8±1.7	400	7.0	1.3	0.8	7.5±1.3**a	300	10.7	0.7	0	11.0±1.8
7M(31)	300	9.7	1.0	1.0	11.7±3.4	300	9.7	1.7	-	11.3±1.8	300	7.0	0.3	-	7.0±1.5*a
10M(47)	300	12.3	0.3	0	11.7±3.4	300	6.3	0.7	0	6.3±1.4**a	300	5.7	0	0	6.7±1.4**a,c
12F(42)	300	11.7	0.3	0.3	11.0±1.8	300	6.0	0.3	0	6.3±1.4**a	300	6.3	0	0.3	6.0±1.4*a,c
13M(25)	300	13.0	0	0.6	13.0±1.9	300	7.7	0.3	0	7.3±1.5**a	300	5.3	0	0	5.0±1.3***a,c

Donor No, Sex (age)	Prior supplementation						At the end of supplementation					
	Cells	Single fragments	Paired fragments	Exchanges	MD	Aberrant metaphases M±m%	Cells	Single fragments	Paired fragments	Exchanges	MD	Aberrant metaphases M±m%
		per 100 cells						per 100 cells				
Complex 2 (dioxidine 0.01 mg/ml)												
6F(25)	277	7.6	0.4	0	0.4	7.9±1.6	600	4.3	0.2	0	0	4.5±0.9*
12M(23)	600	7.5	0.7	0	0	8.0±1.1	600	3.8	0.2	0	0	3.8±0.8**
Complex 3 (dioxidine 0.01 mg/ml)												
1M(22)	600	9.7	0	0	0.2	9.8±1.2	600	5.5	0.3	0	0	5.3±0.9**
8F(22)	600	6.3	0.3	0	0	6.7±1.0	600	3.5	0.2	0.2	0	3.8±0.6*
Complex 2 (bleomycin 0.1 U/ml)												
2M(43)	300	5.9	0	0	0.7	5.0±1.3	300	11.0	0.7	0	1.0	11.6±1.8**
5F(25)	221	11.8	0	0	0.5	10.9±2.1	236	4.2	0.4	0.4	0.8	5.5±1.5*
Complex 3 (bleomycin 0.1 U/ml)												
12F(24)	300	8.3	0.3	0	0	7.7±1.5	226	18.1	1.8	0	3.1	18.6±2.9*
13F(25)	300	9.0	0.3	0	0	7.3±1.5	300	14.7	0.3	0	0.7	13.0±1.9*
Complex 3 (bleomycin 1 U/ml)												
7F(35)	300	22.0	1.3	0	2.0	20.0±2.3	300	11.7	1.0	0	0.3	12.0±2.0**
1M(26)	250	15.6	0.8	0.4	0	14.4±2.0	300	29	2.7	0	3.7	28.3±2.6***
12F(27)	228	16.2	1.8	0	0	15.8±2.4	300	26.3	2.3	0	2.0	27.7±2.6***
13F(28)	300	11.3	1.0	0.3	0.6	11.7±2.0	300	17.0	1.7	0	2.0	18.3±1.5*
5M(24)	300	16.3	2.7	0	1.7	16.7±2.1	300	10.3	1.3	0	0.7	9.3±1.7**

* - $p < 0.05$; ** - $p < 0.01$; *** - $p < 0.001$. For complex 1 – «a» - compared to baseline recordings, «c» - compared to recordings on Day 14 of experiment.

MD – cells bearing multiple chromosome damages (more than 5 chromosome aberrations per cell).

Cytogenetic Effects of Dioxidine while on Supplementation with Different Complexes

The results derived from cytogenetic examination of cells obtained before and after administration of different complexes treated with dioxidine *in vitro*, are presented in Table 3 and 4. Under any experimental conditions the results obtained with dioxidine were significantly higher comparing to those from control cultures of the same donors, further supporting the available data on the cytogenetic activity of dioxidine studied *in vitro* [6].

A) Complex 1

In cell cultures examined prior complex 1 administration, dioxidine at a dose of 0.03 mg/ml caused damages in $10.0 \pm 0.6\%$ of studied cells.

After 14 days of complex 1 intake the rate of mutagen-induced aberrant metaphases made $8.1 \pm 0.4\%$, and 30 days after administration it was $7.2 \pm 0.5\%$. The rate of aberrant metaphases varied at all three experimental stages ranging as $6.0 - 13.8\%$, $6.3 - 11.3\%$ and $4.7 - 11.0\%$, accordingly. Comparison of data obtained revealed that the number of cells bearing damages induced by 0.03 mg/ml of dioxidine diminished significantly as early as 14 days after the beginning of complex 1 administration ($p < 0.01$), 30 days after supplementation these changes became more significant ($p < 0.001$).

A significant reduction in the amount of cytogenetic damages was observed in donors No 2, 7, 10, 12 and 13 after 14 days and/or the last dose of complex 1 (Table 5).

The comparison of aberration types frequency at all experimental stages demonstrated that after administration of complex 1 the number of single fragments and chromosome exchanges significantly decreased 14 days after administration, and the number of aberrations of all types reduced 30 days after administration.

With dioxidine used as 0.1 mg/ml the intergroup rate of aberrant metaphases made prior complex 1 intake $17.1 \pm 0.8\%$. 14 days after administration it made $16.3 \pm 0.6\%$, and 30 days after the last dose this value was significantly lower than the baseline level and it made $14.8 \pm 0.6\%$ (Table 3).

Aberration types comparison showed a significant lower proportion of single and paired fragments and chromosome exchanges after 30-day treatment as compared to baseline values (Table 4).

B) Complex 2

The intergroup level of 0.01 mg/ml dioxidine-induced aberrant metaphases amounted prior intake of complex 2 to $5.8 \pm 0.3\%$, whereas 14 days after administration it was found significantly lower that the baseline values and made $4.6 \pm 0.2\%$ (Table 3).

A significant decrease in the number of single and paired fragments was found (Table 4). Besides, the comparison of individual data revealed a significant reduction of mutagen-damaged cells yield following complex administration in two (No 6 and No 12) out of 15 donors studied (Table 5).

C) Complex 3

In experiments carried out before administration of complex 3 the mutagen at a dose of 0.01 mg/ml caused damages in 5.5 ± 0.3%, and at the end of 14-day intake it made 4.8 ± 0.3% of cells (p > 0.05). The scores variations ranged 4.3 – 9.8% and 3.2 – 6.3% respectively. Interestingly, while no differences in average values between the groups were observed, they were found in 2 of 11 donors studied (No 1 and No 8) whose amount of dioxidine-damaged cells was significantly lower after vitamin intake period as compared to the beginning of the study (Table 5).

Cytogenetic Effects of Bleomycin while on Supplement with Different Complexes

Under any experimental conditions the results obtained with bleomycin were significantly higher when compared with those from control cultures of the same donors, thus further supporting the data earlier obtained from *in vitro* studies on the cytogenetic activity of bleomycin [15].

A) Complex 2

After the whole blood cells cultures were treated with 0.1 U/ml of bleomycin, the aberrant metaphases were detected in 7.3 ± 0.5% before and 7.5 ± 0.5% after administration of complex 2. The individual variations ranged from 4.0% to 12.8% of aberrant metaphases before, and from 5.5% to 11.6% after treatment. The comparison of these results showed no significant differences. However, while no difference in the average group scores was observed it was found between the results obtained "before" and "after" in two (No 2 and No 5) out of 11 donors studied (Table 5). The first donor demonstrated significantly increased yield of damaged cells, whereas the second showed a significant decline therein.

The proportions of chromosome aberrations of various types remained unchanged before and after complex 2 intake (Table 4).

With bleomycin at a dose of 0.1 U/ml prior complex 2 intake there was observed 16.6 ± 0.7% of aberrant metaphases, 14 days after administration aberrant metaphases amount made 15.1 ± 0.7% (p > 0.05). The incidence of aberrant cells varied from 11.0% to 28% prior complex 2 intake, and ranged from 8.0% to 23.6% after the end of administration.

It is remarkable that scoring of "aberrant metaphases percent" showed no significant differences, they emerged, however, after the numbers of single and paired fragments were compared (Table 4). We believe that this finding reflects the elevation of cell resistance towards the mutagenic exposure.

B) Complex 3

The comparison of results obtained from bleomycin-treated (0.1 U/ml) blood cultures of complex 3 given donors, revealed no significant differences between the average group scores; before complex 3 administration the percent of aberrant cells made 7.8 ± 0.4%, and after administration it was 8.5 ± 0.5%. After comparing the rate of chromosome damages of different types these differences were neither observed. The individual variability ranged 4.7

– 16.7% before, and 4.3 – 18.1% after administration. A significant increase in damaged cells yield after complex 3 intake was observed in two (No 12 and No 13) out of 13 donors studied (Table 5).

In the following experimental series bleomycin was used as 1 U/ml. Under this dosage 14.5 ± 0.5% of aberrant metaphases was found after administration of complex 3, the individual variations ranged from 11.3% to 20.0%. After complex 3 intake the average group rate made 16.8 ± 0.6%, the individual variations range was 9.5% to 28.3%.

The comparison of results showed that along with significantly increased amount of damaged metaphases (Table 3), after complex 3 administration a significant increase in the number of cells bearing multiple chromosome damages was observed (Table 4). Worthy is to note that in 5 donors significant differences between the results obtained before and after administration were revealed. In 4 donors (No 7, 11, 12 and 13) the post-treatment recordings were significantly higher, whereas in one subject (No 15) significantly lower compared to those obtained at the end of experiment (Table 5).

Thus, the administration of complex 3 elevated the sensitivity of donor cells to the cytogenetic action of bleomycin used at a dose of 1.0 U/ml.

CONCLUSION

The obtained data (Table 3 and 4) provide evidence that tested vitamin and vitamin and mineral complexes of different quality and quantity contents, including those containing vitamins at doses significantly exceeding the daily allowances (Table 1), caused no damages to chromosome structures in peripheral lymphocytes from healthy donors. The results obtained from all experimental series are consistent with currently available data on the incidence of peripheral lymphocytes bearing chromosome aberrations among population in Russia. Ratios of aberration types agree with values which characterize the spontaneous mutagenesis within a population. The single fragments (24 – 34 per 1000 cells) constitute the largest proportion. The ratios of aberrations of different types are almost similar as compared between groups studied, thus being in agreement with those observed in cytogenetic population studies [16].

Supplementation with complex 1 and 2 containing excessive vitamin amounts, either elevated the resistance of peripheral blood cells towards the action of mutagens *in vitro*, or exerted no significant effects. Besides, with an evidently regularity the antimutagenic modification was substantially better expressed under long-term vitamin supplementation. Along with that, its expression was dependent not only upon the duration of vitamin consumption, but the concentration of mutagen used *in vitro*, and consequently, the level of cytogenetic damage. In particular, with dioxidine used in comparable as to the cytogenetic effect doses of 0.01 and 0.03 mg/ml, the decline of its cytogenetic activity was observed after one and two weeks following complex 1 and 2 supplementation, whereas a more pronounced cytogenetic effect of dioxidine at 0.1 mg/ml was corrected only over a 4-week period of supplementation with complex 1.

The 14-day administration of complex 3 containing low doses of vitamins did not modify the effect of dioxidine and increased the sensitivity of cells to the cytogenetic action of bleomycin at a dose of 1.0 but not 0.1 U/ml.

In most of experiments with bleomycin an interesting trend was observed, and namely there were seen significant and differently oriented individual variations of sensitivity to its cytogenetic action. Even in this single experiment variant which provided average group values evidencing the comutagenic modification of sensitivity to mutagen effect, the individual variations were found within the group (donor No 7 and No 14) that indicate the reduction of sensitivity to the action of mutagen tested. Similar, although less evident, results were obtained from comparison of individual variations of sensitivity to dioxidine action. These findings when viewed in general context are in agreement with classical fundamentals of pharmacological genetics, however as to methodology, the investigations performed suggest to use those cell samples allowing reliable recordings of both the average group and individual differences.

However, it remains unclear to what extent the modification effects observed with mutagen treatment *in vitro* could be extrapolated to *in vivo* conditions. Nevertheless, the reported studies we referred above [6] demonstrate the protective effects of certain vitamin complexes evaluated in cytogenetic studies *in vivo*, thus allowing to believe that the used complex 1 and 2 would produce a real antimutagenic action *in vivo*. Additionally, in all experimental variants with complex 1 supplementation ("with" and "without" mutagen treatment) a significant decline in exchanges level was observed 30 days after the end of complex intake As it is classically acknowledged, the exchange-type aberrations do not occur in G_2 phase of the cell cycle and so, the obtained result may be regarded as an evidence benefiting donor chromosome structures protection *in vivo*.

The comparison of the effects exerted by all three supplemented complexes makes it obvious that not only the amounts and contents of a complex, but the duration of its administration may play a crucial role in determining the direction of its modification effect in human. So, it is apparent that the antimutagenic efficacy of complex 1 rises along with the duration of supplementation therewith. This finding is of a great interest because in the experiments we conducted in parallel it was shown that while on supplementation with studied complexes, the level of main antioxidant vitamins and group B vitamins was stabilized by the end of the second week of supplementation [11].

The experiments designing mutagens addition during G_2 phase of the cell cycle assume the occurrence of single and paired fragments mediated through the action of reactive oxygen species. Such prooxidant mechanism underlying the cytogenetic effect is well known [6], and described earlier for cadmium chloride [6,17], dioxidine [18] and bleomycin [6,19]. The cytogenetic effect of these compounds was shown to decrease *in vitro* under the action of antioxidant enzymes SOD and catalase and chemical antioxidants [6]. These data allow the relationship between the increase in cell resistance towards the mutagenic exposure and the protective effect of vitamins-antioxidants as well as non-organic nutrients as co-factors of antioxidant protection enzymes.

Thus, the obtained data taken together allow to assume that the supplementation with complexes containing vitamins at total doses over the daily allowances does not increase the spontaneous mutation and diminishes the human cell sensitivity to the cytogenetic effect of chemical mutagens. Along with that, vitamin complexes at certain amounts and of certain contents (complex 3) are obviously capable of inducing *in vitro* a comutagenic modification of cell sensitivity to the action of certain mutagens used in certain concentrations.

The observed modifying effects depend upon the duration of supplementation, quantity and quality contents of used vitamin complexes, mutagen nature and the rate of induced cytogenetic damages.

REFERENCES

[1] Yuen B., Furrer L., Ballmer P.E. Antioxidant vitamin supplementation in the prevention of cardiovascular disease. *Ther. Umsch.*, 2005, V. 62, P. 615-618.

[2] Vitaglione P., Morisco F., Caporaso N., Fogliano V. Dietary antioxidant compounds and liver health. *Crit. Rev. Food Sci. Nutr.*, 2004, V. 44, P. 575-586.

[3] Thomas D.R. Vitamins in health and aging. *Clin. Geriatr. Med.*, 2004, V. 20, P. 259-274.

[4] Gerber M., Boutron-Ruault M.C., Hercberg S., Riboli E., Scalbert A., Siess M.H. Food and cancer: state of the art about the protective effect of fruits and vegetables. *Bull. Cancer*, 2002, V. 89, P. 293-312.

[5] Luft F.C. Somatic DNA oxidative damage and coronary disease. *J. Mol. Med.*, 2005, V. 83, P. 241-243.

[6] Durnev, A.D. Seredenin, S.B. *Mutagenes: Screening and pharmacological prevention of exposure.* Moscow: Meditsina Publishers, 1998.

[7] Shamberger R.J. Genetic toxicology of ascorbic acid. *Mutat. Res.*, 1984, V. 133, P. 135-159.

[8] Fenech M., Ferguson L.R. Vitamin/minerals and genomic stability in humans. *Mutat.Res.*, 2001, V. 475, P. 1-6.

[9] Fenech M. Chromosomal damage rate, aging, and diet. *Ann. NY Acad. Sci.*, 1998, V. 854, P. 23-36.

[10] Dusinska M., Kazimirova A., Barancokova M., Beno M., Smolkova B., Horska A., Raslova K., Wsolova L., Collins A.R. Nutritional supplementation with antioxidants decreases chromosomal damage in humans. *Mutagenesis*, 2003, V. 18, P. 371-376.

[11] Vrzhesinskaia O.A., Beketova N.A., Nikitina V.A., Pereverzeva O.G., Kharitonchik L.A., Isaeva V.A., et al. Effects of biologically active food additives with different contents of vitamins on the vitamin status in humans. *Voprosy pitaniia*, 2000, V. 69, P. 27-31.

[12] Bochkov N.P. *Method of registration of chromosome damage as a biological indicator of environmental factors influence on humans.* Moscow, 1974.

[13] Ishidate M. Data book of chromosomal aberration test in vitro. Elservier, Amsterdam-NY-Oxford, 1988.

[14] Fahmy M.A., Aly F.A. In vivo and in vitro studies on the genotoxity of cadmium chloride in mice. *J. Appl. Toxicol.*, 2000, V. 20, P. 231-238.

[15] Povirk L.F., Austin M.J. Genotoxicity of bleomycin. *Mutat. Res.*, 1991, V. 257, P. 127-143.

[16] Bochkov N.P., Chebotarev A.N., Katosova L.D., Platonova V.I. The database for analysis of quantitative characteristics of chromosome aberration frequencies in the culture of human peripheral blood lymphocytes. *Genetika*, 2001, V. 37, P. 549-557.

[17] Fotakis G., Cemeli E., Anderson D., Timbrell J.A. Cadmium chloride-induced DNA and lysosomal damage in a hepatoma cell line. *Toxicol In Vitro,* 2005, V. 4, P. 481-489.

[18] Durnev A.D., Dubovskaya O.Yu., Nigarova E.A., Seredenin S.B. Role of free radicals in mechanism of mutagenic action of photrinum and dioxidine. *Pharmaceutical Chemical Journal,* 1989, V. 23, P. 1289-1291.

[19] Korkina L.G., Cheremisina Z.P., Suslova T.B., Durnev A.D., Seredenin S.B., Velichkovskiy B.T. Bleomycin and oxygen free radicals. *Pharmaceutical Chemical Journal,* 1989, V. 23, P. 901-904.

In: Micronutrients and Health Research
Editor: Takumi Yoshida, pp. 293-307

ISBN: 978-1-60456-056-5
© 2008 Nova Science Publishers, Inc.

Chapter XI

SRTXRF ANALYSIS OF TRACE ELEMENT ON INFLAMMATORY IMMUNE RESPONSE

O.L.A.D. Zucchi[1,*], L.H. Faccioli[2], A. Nomizo[2],
S. Moreira[3], A. Sá-Nunes[2], R.M.F. Bolzoni[2],
L.L. Santos[1] and M.J. Salvador[1,4,*]

[1]Faculdade de Ciências Farmacêuticas de Ribeirão Preto, Universidade de São Paulo
(USP), Depto. Física e Química, Ribeirão Preto (SP), Brasil;
[2]Faculdade de Ciências Farmacêuticas de Ribeirão Preto, Universidade de São Paulo,
Depto. Análises Clínicas, Toxicológicas e Bromatológicas, Ribeirão Preto (SP), Brasil;
[3]Faculdade de Engenharia Civil, Universidade Estadual de Campinas (UNICAMP),
Depto. de Recursos Hídricos, Caixa Postal 6021, CEP 13083-970, Campinas (SP), Brasil;
[4]Instituto de Pesquisa e Desenvolvimento, Universidade do Vale do Paraíba (UNIVAP),
Av. Shishima Hifumi, 2911, CEP 12244-000, São José dos Campos (SP), Brasil and
Instituto de Biologia, Universidade Estadual de Campinas (UNICAMP), Curso de
Farmácia, Caixa Postal 6109, CEP 13083-971, Campinas (SP), Brasil

ABSTRACT

Using synchrotron radiation total-reflection X-ray fluorescence spectrometry
(SRTXRF), it was possible to determine the concentration of several elements in lung,
spleen, thymus, lymph nodes and liver samples of BALB/c mice infected with *Toxocara
canis* nematode and in healthy group, as a control. The elements P, S, Cl, K, Ca, Ti, Cr,
Mn, Fe, Ni, Cu, Zn, As, Rb, Ba and Pb were detected with concentration between 0.16
(Ni-liver) and 5091 (P-thymus) $\mu g.g^{-1}$. The measuring time was 100 seconds and
detection limits varied from 0.20 $\mu g.g^{-1}$ for Ni to 25.88 $\mu g.g^{-1}$ for P. Moreover,
inflammatory immune response was evaluated, by chemometric techniques, such as

---

* Correspondence concerning this article should be addressed to: olzucchi@fcfrp.usp.br or
mjsalvador1531@yahoo.com.br.

principal component and cluster analyses using the elemental concentrations data. Lung, spleen and thymus showed a characteristic pattern between 12 and 24 days post infection, whereas lymph nodes, between 24 and 48 days post infection; liver did not show remarkable features. Since spleen, thymus and lymph nodes have a significant role in immune response, these days could point out a peak of leukocytes activation for each organ.

Keywords: Trace elements; Immune response; Inflammation; X-ray Fluorescence; SRTXRF; Synchrotron radiation total-reflection X-ray fluorescence spectrometry.

INTRODUCTION

Several elements are responsible for many biochemical, imunological and physiological activities in the body [1]. Furthermore, there is an association between levels of some trace elements in body fluids or tissues and the presence of various diseases [2].

Some trace elements are of significant importance on immune system and depending on the particular metal, concentration and several other factors, it may lead to either immunostimulatory or immunosuppressive mechanisms [3]. For example, chromium increases the humoral immune response at lower concentrations, whereas higher doses depress the phagocytic activity of alveolar macrophages [4].

Copper deficiency alters the responses of several effector cells involved in the circulatory component of inflammation, affects the ability of the leukocytes to destroy bacteria and also causes the release of immature leukocytes [5,6].

Iron deficiency and iron overload can exert subtle effects on immune status by altering the proliferation of T and B cells [7]. In addition, the local concentration of iron and iron-binding proteins vary not only between serum and different tissues but also during disease states [8].

Zinc deficiency causes thymic atrophy and a high frequency of infections. It also induces cytokines, as IL-1, IL-6 and TNF-α, showing an immense immunoregulative capacity, and these effects are highly specific for this metal [9].

Moreover, quantitative changes in the level of a particular element in body are known to cause changes with respect to other elements [10]. Therefore, several elements should be analyzed in a single sample.

SRTXRF is a suitable technique for evaluation of trace element alterations of tissues in pathological states, due to its simultaneous, multielemental character, high sensitivity, and low sample consumption and short analysis time [11]. The X-ray fluorescence is based on the measure of the intensities of characteristic X-rays emitted by the elements that constitute the sample, and can be done through the dispersion of wave length (WDXRF) or energy (EDXRF). Fundamentally this technique consists of three stages: excitement of the elements that constitute the sample, dispersion and detection of characteristic x-rays emitted and measuring of these X-rays. Other analytical techniques such as atomic absorption spectrometry (AAS), inductively coupled plasma atomic emission spectrometry (ICP-AES) and neutron activation analysis (NAA) also can be used for heavy metal determination;

however, need extensive sample preparation, which usually is troublesome, time consuming and prevents in situ analysis [12,13].

Thus, the aim of this work is the use of SRTXRF to determine element levels in tissues of BALB/c mice infected with *Toxocara canis* nematode, in order to assess the dynamic of immune response by host.

MATERIAL AND METHODS

Instrumentation

Measurements were performed in an X-ray fluorescence beamline at National Synchrotron Light Laboratory, in Campinas City, Brazil. For the X-ray detection a Si(Li) detector was employed, with 165 eV resolution at 5.9 keV (Mn K_α line). For the excitation, a polychromatic (E_{max} = 22 keV) beam from a storage ring (1.37 GeV and 100 mA) with 2.0 mm width and 1.0 mm height under total reflection conditions was used [14]. The spectra were analyzed and quantitative calculations performed with the AXIL 3.5 software, Analysis of X-rays Spectra by Iterative Least Squares Fitting [15]. The samples and the standards were irradiated during 100s.

Reagents

Multi-elemental standard solutions for calibration by TXRF were prepared by appropriate dilution, with purified water in a Milli-Q system, of Al, Si, K, Ca, Ti, Cr, Fe, Ni, Zn, Ga, Se, Sr, Mo, Cd, Ba, Pt, Tl, and Pb, covering the range of atomic numbers from 13 (Al) to 82 (Pb). In order to digest the samples, HNO_3 (65%) and H_2O_2 (30%) were used.

Samples

Female BALB/c mice weighing 12-15 g were infected with *Toxocara canis* eggs by gastric intubation. Infective doses were 500 embryonated eggs in 0.6 mL of saline. Control group animals received only 0.6 mL of saline. At 3, 12, 24 and 48 days post infection, mice were sacrificed and lung, liver, thymus, spleen and lymph nodes were the collected organs. Samples were stored at -20 °C until analysis.

Sampling and Sample Treatment

Pieces of analysed tissue (Table 1) were carefully prepared according the following procedure. A determined amount of tissue was digested in an open system, heated at temperature of 120-130 °C, with HNO_3 and H_2O_2 [16], until the solution became clear. After digestion, final volume for lung, spleen, thymus and lymph nodes samples was 1 mL and for liver samples, 5 mL. Afterwards, 1 mL of each solution was taken and 10 µL of Ga (stock solution 1000 µg mL^{-1}) were added as internal standard in sample. Then an aliquot of 5 µL was pipette onto a Perspex disk and dried under an infrared lamp. All samples were prepared in triplicate.

Table 1. Mean weight (g) of tissues used in sample preparation for control and treated samples

Organ	3 days	12 days	24 days	48 days
Lung	0.033 ± 0.010 (7)	0.059 ± 0.026 (6)	0.049 ± 0.007 (7)	0.061 ± 0.010 (10)
Spleen	0.050 ± 0.032 (8)	0.080 ± 0.033 (8)	0.089 ± 0.031 (8)	0.081 ± 0.019 (11)
Thymus	0.075 ± 0.020 (8)	0.022 ± 0.014 (7)	0.017 ± 0.017 (7)	0.017 ± 0.008 (12)
Lymph nodes	0.025 ± 0.010 (8)	0.023 ± 0.013 (8)	0.027 ± 0.017 (8)	0.018 ± 0.008 (12)
Liver	0.182 ± 0.037 (8)	0.224 ± 0.057 (8)	0.203 ± 0.093 (8)	0.245 ± 0.027 (12)

Note: mean weight ± standard deviation, in g of tissue; in parenthesis, number of samples.

TXRF Calibration Procedure

The samples and standards analyzed, deposited in the Perperx disk, were taken to the spectrometer in order to measure the characteristic X-ray of all elements present in the samples. TXRF calibration was performed using a fitted non-dimensional sensitivity curve, with Ga addition as the internal standard to eliminate errors caused by excitation/detection geometry. Five multi-elemental standard solutions, containing Al, Si, K, Ca, Ti, Cr, Fe, Ni, Zn, Se – K fluorescent lines and Sr, Mo, Cd, Ba, Pt, Tl, Pb – L fluorescent lines, were prepared at different and well-known concentrations. All sensitivity values in the atomic number range from 13 (Al) to 82 (Pb) were then obtained after fitting.

TXRF Quantitative Analysis

After pulse spectres were obtained, in a previous calibrated spectrometer (channel number *versus* energy), the peaks energy presented in theses spectres and theirs characteristics X-ray intensity were estimated. The quantitative, based on the relationship between the fluorescent intensity, analysis can be made by Eqn (1), since the sample can be considered as a thin film, whose absorption and enhancement effects are negligible [17].

$$R_i = S_i \cdot C_i \tag{1}$$

where R_i is the fluorescent intensity of element i (cps), S_i (cps µg^{-1} mL) is the sensitivity for this element and C_i the concentration (µg mL^{-1}).

In order to correct the geometric effect, was added gallium as internal standard in each sample and standard (Eqn 2):

$$\frac{R_i}{R_{Ga}} = \frac{S_i}{S_{Ga}} \cdot \frac{C_i}{C_{Ga}} \tag{2}$$

where R_{Ga}, S_{Ga} and C_{Ga} = fluorescent intensity (cps), elemental sensitivity (cps.μg^{-1}mL) and concentration of the element Ga (10 μg mL^{-1}), respectively.

Being defined S'_i and Q_i :

$$S'_i = \frac{S_i}{S_{Ga}} \tag{3}$$

and

$$Q_i = \frac{R_i}{R_{Ga}} \cdot C_{Ga} \tag{4}$$

S'_i = relative sensitivity of element i (adimensional); Q_i = product of the relative intensity by the concentration of Ga (μg mL^{-1}), therefore:

$$Q_i = S'_i \cdot C_i \tag{5}$$

In the multielementar standard samples the Q_i is directly proportional to C_i; thus, the angular coefficient represents the relative sensitivity for the element i. By S'_i values of each element in standard solution, it was obtained Eqn (6), where Z_i is the atomic number:

$$\ln S''_i = b_0 + b_1.Z_i + b_2.Z_i^2 + b_3.Z_i^3 \tag{6}$$

Figure 1 show the sensitivity curves obtained for elements of K and L lines emission, covering atomic numbers ranging from 13 (Al) to 82 (Pb). Statistical parameters for each element in sensitivity curve are showed in Table 2.

The limits of detection were calculated for tissue samples [18] (Eqn 7), for a counting time of 100 s.

$$LOD_i = 3 \cdot \sqrt{\frac{RB_i}{T}} \cdot \frac{C_{Ga}}{R_{Ga} \cdot S'_i} \tag{7}$$

where RB_i: the background area under the element i peak (cps); T: the time of detection (s).

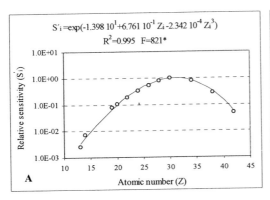
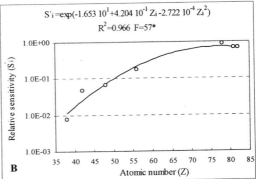

Figure 1. Sensitivity curves (experimental and calculate) for the K and L fluorescent lines (A and B, respectively).

Table 2. Statistical parameters of fitted sensitivity curve (K and L lines)

Elements	Mean	S.D.	Lower CI	Upper CI
Al	2.51E-03	6.15E-04	2.34E-03	2.68E-03
Si	7.02E-03	8.32E-03	4.74E-03	9.31E-03
K	7.83E-02	8.12E-02	5.59E-02	1.01E-01
Ca	1.06E-01	2.00E-02	1.00E-01	1.11E-01
Ti	1.80E-01	3.86E-02	1.70E-01	1.91E-01
Cr	3.22E-01	2.72E-02	3.14E-01	3.29E-01
Fé	5.30E-01	7.01E-02	5.10E-01	5.49E-01
Ni	7.71E-01	4.85E-02	7.57E-01	7.84E-01
Zn	1.02E+00	8.04E-02	9.93E-01	1.04E+00
Se	7.74E-01	1.49E-01	7.33E-01	8.15E-01
Sr (X-Kα)	2.71E-01	3.67E-02	2.61E-01	2.81E-01
Mo (X-Kα)	4.76E-02	1.08E-02	4.46E-02	5.06E-02
Sr (X-Lα)	7.58E-03	3.33E-03	6.59E-03	8.57E-03
Mo (X-Lα)	4.70E-02	8.03E-02	2.30E-02	7.09E-02
Cd	6.66E-02	9.26E-02	3.90E-02	9.42E-02
Ba	1.76E-01	6.14E-02	1.58E-01	1.95E-01
Pt	8.77E-01	3.37E-01	7.77E-01	9.77E-01
Tl	6.80E-01	2.93E-01	5.93E-01	7.68E-01
Pb	6.51E-01	2.59E-01	5.73E-01	7.28E-01

Note: SD, standard deviation; CI, confidence interval.

RESULTS AND DISCUSSION

Calibration curve for SRTXRF was obtained by X-ray intensities from standard samples. Figure 1A and Figure 1B show the sensitivity curve for K and L lines, respectively. The curves are described by Eqs. 8 and 9 for elements whose atomic number ranges $13 \leq Z \leq 42$ and $42 \leq Z \leq 82$, respectively.

$$S'_i = \exp\left(-1.398 \ 10^1 + 6.761 \ 10^{-1} \ Z_i - 2.342 \ 10^{-4} \ Z_i^3\right) \quad\quad (8)$$

$$S'_i = \exp\left(-1.653 \ 10^1 + 4.204 \ 10^{-1} \ Z_i - 2.722 \ 10^{-4} \ Z_i^2\right) \quad\quad (9)$$

In Eq. (8) (Figure 1A), it can be observed an absolute maximum for Z=31, namely, the function is increasing for Z<31 and is decreasing for Z>31. This fact is explained because Ga (Z=31) was used as internal standard (S_{Ga} = 1.0, theoretical). When Z=31 is substituted in Eq. (7), a relative sensitivity of 1.000013 was obtained, showing a error of 0.0013 %.

In analyses of samples by AXIL software, we employed a criterion described by this way: the count rate for an element i must be, at least, three-fold the count rate obtained in standard deviation for the same element. Furthermore we also used Chi-Square value (X^2), that is decreased when it detects element i and residual value, that shows the dispersal of values. These procedures were used to say if there was an element or not.

Concentration of free metal ions and metalloenzymes in living organisms are very sensitive characteristics. The relationship between the structure of compounds and the metal ions included in their structure is so tight that the diseases associated with the functioning of metal-containing agents may be manifested either increasing or decreasing of trace levels with respect to normal values [19].

However, trace element concentrations in tissues show a great variability, depending on age, sex, diet, genetic factors, healthy/disease states and specific organ [20]. Table 3 shows maximum and minimum concentrations of each element, for lung, spleen, thymus, lymph nodes and liver samples, and it is possible to remark a large range of concentrations.

Table 3. Range of minimum and maximum concentration (µg g^{-1}) measured in control and treated samples, respective relative standard deviation (RSD %) for each element (between triplicates) and mean limit of detection (LOD - µg g^{-1})

Element	Lung	Spleen	Thymus	Lymph nodes	Liver	RSD (%)	LOD (µg g^{-1})
P	881.9 – 1395	1985 – 5091	158.9 – 4628	1201 – 2296	1106 – 3337	1.87	25.88
S	624.1 – 1136	1067 – 2414	652.9 – 1285	656.3 – 1142	1310 – 3096	1.90	15.85
Cl	20.43 – 84.87	21.45 – 296.9	30.94 – 153.1	50.61 – 220.6	12.30 – 153.8	14.75	10.67
K	1318 – 2361	2542 – 5982	2148 – 3521	1664 – 2616	1695 – 4225	0.89	3.21
Ca	148.2 – 300.9	91.98 – 285.1	73.78 – 2096	136.4 – 349.8	136.0 – 316.0	1.86	1.86
Ti	nd	nd	1.60 – 28.28	2.57 – 10.21	1.31 – 22.95	16.90	0.88
Cr	4.67 – 9.73	4.17 – 10.44	4.67 – 27.21	6.26 – 19.78	1.32 – 2.71	5.01	0.42
Mn	0.34 – 0.76	Nd	nd	0.58 – 1.81	1.40 – 2.31	14.36	0.23
Fe	92.18 – 175.7	124.1 – 285.6	30.69 – 198.2	55.59 – 181.9	88.16 – 196.5	1.10	0.23
Ni	0.30 – 0.79	0.21 – 1.78	0.33 – 2.75	1.20 – 6.19	0.16 – 0.66	13.62	0.20
Cu	2.97 – 5.78	1.39 – 3.63	1.50 – 9.95	1.39 – 5.35	4.41 – 8.69	4.70	0.25
Zn	16.97 – 37.08	16.06 – 36.88	11.27 – 40.60	14.22 – 27.92	25.15 – 43.34	1.27	0.35
As	1.75 – 4.70	2.48 – 4.24	1.64 – 16.29	4.10 – 9.34	2.33 – 8.10	5.56	0.42
Rb	2.43 – 3.86	2.97 – 9.36	2.89 – 16.27	2.23 – 5.20	4.33 – 8.41	10.13	2.00
Ba	7.44 – 15.45	5.93 – 10.36	5.96 – 34.13	9.14 – 30.28	5.37 – 12.06	5.17	0.72
Pb	0.44 – 0.52	1.46 – 3.03	1.53 – 10.21	0.70 – 6.91	0.46 – 3.70	13.04	1.08

Note: nd, non-detected element.

Elements as copper, zinc, iron and chromium, that play a significant role in immune response, were detected in low concentrations. Moreover, other elements, in high or trace levels, could exert unknown effects in immune system. Hence, a very sensitive and multielemental technique, such as SRTXRF, is suitable [11 and mean limits of detection (LOD) obtained for samples are presented in Table 3. Minimum LOD obtained was 60.06 ng g^{-1} for Ni and maximum, 76.66 µg g^{-1} for P. The experimental detection limits were obtained each kind of sample by Eq. (7). A typical spectrum (lymph node sample) with all the detected elements is shown in Figure 2.

The precision was evaluated between replicas, as relative standard deviation (% RSD) values, for all the analyzed elements (Table 3). As expected, these values depended on the concentration of the element of interest and its LOD [1]. For example, in the case of Mn and Ni, whose levels in tissues were close to the limit of detection of the method, the mean precision ranged from 9.72 to 21.66%, depending on the concentration of the elements. On the other hand, for K, Fe and Zn, the precision ranged from 0.44 to 2.28%. The levels of these elements were more than 10 times higher than their corresponding detection limits.

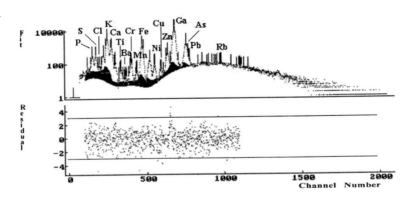

Figure 2. Experimental X-ray spectrum of lymph nodes measured for 100 s with SRTXRF.

In order to assess the potential relationships between the element content in each group of samples and immune response, pattern recognition methods (principal component analysis – PCA and cluster analysis – CA) were used. The data pre-treatment used was the half range (hr) – central value (cv) transformation:

$$hr = \frac{x_{max} - x_{min}}{2} \qquad cv = \frac{x_{max} + x_{min}}{2} \qquad z_i = \frac{x_i - cv}{hr}$$

where x_{max} and x_{min} are the maximum and the minimum concentration for each variable, respectively. All the variables (x_i), were transformed into values of a standardized variables, z_i [21].

From each organ samples, PCA and CA were carried out. For PCA, the three first principal components used to plot graphics (data not showed) are described in Table 4. In the statistical analyses the principal component analysis (PCA) validate the cluster analysis [22-

23]. In these chemometric analysis, Euclidean Distance was used as similarity measurement for each organ (Figure 3), and similar results were obtained when comparing CA to PCA.

Table 4. PCA parameters used for each analyzed organ

Organ	Axis X	Axis Y	Axis Z
Lung	Ni ($\lambda_1 = 6.16$) – 34.23%	Pb ($\lambda_2 = 5.54$) – 30.76%	Ba ($\lambda_3 = 2.28$) – 12.67%
Spleen	Cu ($\lambda_1 = 6.06$) – 40.38%	As ($\lambda_2 = 5.02$) – 33.46%	Cl ($\lambda_3 = 1.57$) – 10.47%
Thymus	Fe ($\lambda_1 = 10.23$) – 63.97%	Rb ($\lambda_2 = 2.51$) – 15.70%	Ca ($\lambda_3 = 1.75$) – 10.90%
Lymph nodes	Cu ($\lambda_1 = 9.01$) – 56.34%	Ni ($\lambda_2 = 2.47$) – 15.43%	Ni ($\lambda_3 = 1.78$) – 11.14%
Liver	Cu ($\lambda_1 = 8.48$) – 52.,99%	Pb ($\lambda_2 = 2.75$) – 17.17%	Ba ($\lambda_3 = 2.16$) – 13.52%

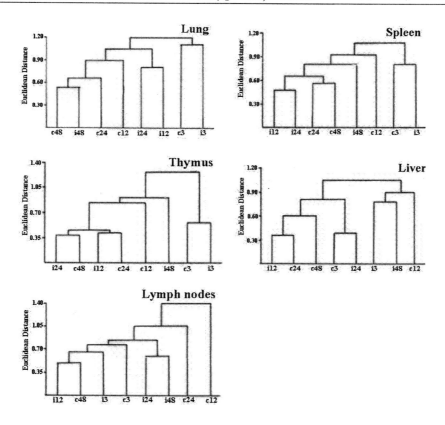

Figure 3. Cluster analysis for each analyzed organ (time: 3, 12, 24, and 48 days; i: infected; c: control).

Data obtained in CA displayed similarities for lung and spleen, that is: i12 and i24 samples (12 and 24 days post infection) clustering them and CA similarity may reflect the immunological cells stimulation in these organs. In fact, it is known that in 18th day post infection with *T. canis* there is a peak of IL-5 (interleukin-5) cytokine production by leukocytes [24], an important marker for infection that is correlated with Th2 pattern of immune response [25]. Furthermore, IL-5 synthesis was verified in spleen and lungs of *T. canis*-infected mice [26]. Thus, tissues with a characteristic cluster between i12 and i24 samples show the strong correlation with studies related with immune response in lungs and spleen during *Toxocara canis* infection [27-28], opening the possibility to use trace element analysis to assess the manifestation of immune response *in vivo* in secondary lymphoid organs as spleen and tissues, as lung. We also showed a slight cluster between i12 and i24 samples (i24, c48, i12 and c24 formed a cluster) in thymus, a typical primary lymphoid organ, but it was not as clear as lung and spleen dendrograms.

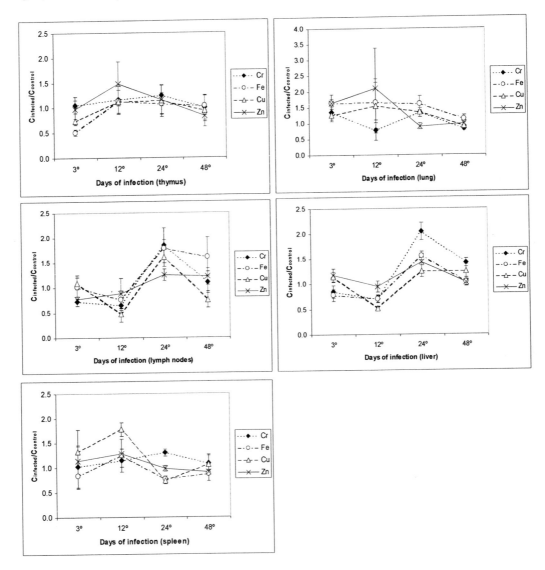

Figure 4. Relative concentration of Cr, Fe, Cu and Zn in analyzed organs.

Thymus has a significant role in the T cell differentiation, and its function is also related with zinc. This metal is essential for thymus by a zinc-dependent thymic hormone called thymulin [29]. As observed in Figure 4, there was an increase of zinc levels in 12th post infection (about 50%), maybe meaning an increase of thymus activity during *T. canis* infection. This observation is very interesting because in the typical immune response to infection occurs the mobilization and activation of differentiated T-cells present in peripheral secondary lymphoid tissues as spleen and lymph nodes. Zinc levels increased suggest that thymus is functionally in the infected mice and that T cell differentiation in the thymus is required to mount full immune response to *T. canis* in the periphery.

In lung samples there was an increase of iron levels, as expected in an infection [8] (Figure 4). *T. canis* infection induces a strong inflammatory response with predominant eosinophils leukocytes in the lung. These findings suggest that a high level of iron is correlated with presence of the inflammatory response in the lung. This organ also has a central role during *T. canis* mice infection, due to the migratory route of this nematode, constituted by two phases: visceral, in first week of infection, when *T. canis* larvae migrate to liver and lung tissues, and afterwards, miotropic/neurotropic phase, when larvae migrate to several organs and standing in muscular and cerebral tissues [30].

Lymph nodes are important lymphoid tissues because within them the adaptative immune response coming up with strong activation of T and B-lymphocytes. Our results show that the lymph nodes displayed a cluster between i24 and i48 samples. This could mean a peak and persistence of immune response, respectively. Also it is observed a peak of concentration for Cr, Fe, Cu and Zn in 24th day post infection in lymph nodes (Figure 4). All together, these observations suggest that the formed cluster could be related with lymphocyte activation.

In liver was not possible to observe a characteristic pattern, maybe owing to complex biochemical reactions carried out by this organ. Though, liver showed a similar behavior with respect to lymph nodes, that is, an increase of Cr, Fe, Cu and Zn levels in 24th day post infection (Figure 4). Furthermore, zinc-bound metallothioneins (enzymes involved in zinc homeostasis and related with immune system and ageing) are mainly produced into liver, and the maximum concentration of zinc was measured in this organ (43.34 μg g^{-1}) and in thymus (40.60 μg g^{-1}), that produces thymulin (zinc-dependent hormone) [31], thus indicating that extrathymic lymphocytes differentiated in the liver may also participate during the immune response to *T. canis*.

Copper has an involvement in immune function and its levels increase in infection and neoplasia, due to to increased synthesis of ceruloplasmin [6]. It was observed that in lung, spleen and thymus samples, copper levels tend to increase around 12th day post infection, whilst in lymph nodes and liver, around 24th day (Figure 4). Furthermore, copper deficiency causes attenuated intravascular adhesion of leukocytes to the vascular endothelium, a main step in response to inflammatory stimuli [5]. Copper probably has an important role in the leukocyte migration from blood to lymphoid tissues, since in three organs (spleen, lymph nodes and liver) this element was the first principal component of PCA (Table 4).

In Table 5, Pearson correlation coefficients are displayed for Fe, Cr, Cu and Zn. These elements showed good correlations among them, meaning some relationship with immune response. High correlation between Fe and Cr was observed in all organs, showing that these elements could play important functions, especially to during the activation of immune cells in inflammatory/immune response *in vivo*. Zinc is an essential trace element for the immune system and the zinc homeostasis is involved in the regulation of the immune system. Zinc deficiency compromises the function of primarily T cells but also of several other immune cells. However, zinc homeostasis can have relationship with immunity [32]. On the other hand, Iron-containing compounds stimulates TNF-α production, antigen presenting cell activity and cellular immune response in normal mice [33].

Table 5. Pearson correlation coefficients for Fe, Cr, Cu and Zn

Correlation	Lung	Spleen	Thymus	Lymph nodes	Liver
Fe-Cr	0.716	0.696	0.791	0.706	0.940
Fe-Cu	0.823	0.558	0.622	0.368	0.671
Fe-Zn	0.768	0.555	0.635	0.544	0.598
Zn-Cu	0.882	0.822	0.571	0.472	0.517
Zn-Cr	0.425	0.707	0.609	0.610	0.497
Cu-Cr	0.628	0.522	0.524	0.714	0.623

The life of an organism is critically dependent on the proper regulation of uptake, assimilation, intracellular compartmentation and intercellular translocation of trace metals. The message which is the key to the understanding of the specific biological function of an element in nature is carried out by the species: oxidation state, metalloorganic moiety, or complex with a bio-ligand. The identification of the elemental species involved is a critical step toward a complete understanding of the nutritional aspects and toxicity of these elements and a key to the understanding of many metal-involving biochemical and immunochemical process in the cell. Understanding the functional connections between genes, proteins, metabolites and mineral ions was referred to as one of biology's greatest challenges in the post-genomic era [34]. The biochemistry of a cell needs to be characterized not only by its characteristic genome and proteome, but also by the distribution of metals and metalloids among the different species and cell compartments, the metallome. Metallogenomics, metalloproteomics and metallomics are among the emerging disciplines which are critically dependent on spatially resolved concentration maps of trace elements in the cell, on information on chemical speciation and on metal-binding coordination sites. Advances in analytical techniques capable of providing this type of information are therefore required to study metal-dependent biochemical processes. Therefore, mineral elements, often at the trace levels, play a considerable role in physiology and pathology of biological systems.

It is noticeable that few elements have been studied with respect to immune response, and it is recognized that there are potential connections among several elements owing to maintain homeostasis in organisms. The method used and SRTXRF seems to be a suitable analytical technique for the simultaneous determination of trace element alterations in some tissues, leading to informations about the course of immune response during *T. canis* infection.

CONCLUSION

Synchrotron radiation total-reflection X-ray fluorescence spectrometry is shown to be a useful technique for trace element determination in biological samples. *Toxocara canis*-mice infection is a suitable model to study immune response and to establish relationships with changes in element levels. After cluster analysis, it was observed for lung, spleen, thymus and lymph nodes a peak of immune response during infection period, while liver displayed none characteristic pattern. This work shows for the first time that different element levels changes in primary and secondary lymphoid organs during the parasite infection and argue for the possibility to use this methodology to study the different patterns of immune response.

ACKNOWLEDGEMENTS

Research was partially performed at the National Synchrotron Light Laboratory (proj. D09B-XRF-1146). To Fundação de Amparo à Pesquisa do Estado de São Paulo (FAPESP) for the financial support and fellowship given to the L.L.Santos (proj. FAPESP 03/00336-7).

REFERENCES

[1]   Marcó P LM; Jiménez E; Hernández C EA; Rojas A; Greaves ED. Determination of Zn/Cu ratio and oligoelements in serum samples by total reflection X-ray fluorescence spectrometry for cancer diagnosis. *Spectroch. Acta (part B)*. 2001; 56:2195-2201.

[2]   Geraki K; Farquharson MJ. Radiat. An X-ray fluorescence system for measuring trace element concentrations in breast tissue. *Phys. Chem.* 2001; 61:603-605.

[3]   Lawrence DA; McCabe Jr MJ. Immunomodulation by metals. *Int. Immunopharmacol.* 2002; 2:293-302.

[4]   Shrivastava R; Upreti RK; Seth PK; Chaturvedi UC. Effects of chromium on the immune system. *FEMS Immunol. Méd. Microbiol.* 2002; 34:1-7.

[5]   Schuschke DA; Saari JT; Miller FN. Leukocyte-endothelial adhesion is impaired in the cremaster muscle microcirculation of the copper-deficient rat. *Immunl. Lett.* 2001; 76:139-144.

[6]   Moreno T; Artacho R; Navarro M; Pérez A; Ruiz-López MD. Serum copper concentrations in HIV-infection patients and relationships with other biochemical indices. *Sci. Total Environ.* 1998; 217:21-26.

[7]   Weiss G; Wachter H; Fuchs D. Linkage of cell-mediated immunity to iron metabolism. *Immunol. Today.* 1995; 16:495-500.

[8]   Wilson ME; Britigan BE. Iron acquisition by parasitic protozoa. *Parasitol. Today.* 1998; 14:348-353.

[9]   Wellinghausen N; Kirchner H; Rink L. The immunobiology of zinc. *Immunol. Today.* 1997; 18:519-521.

[10]   El-Khatib AM; Bahnassy AA; Denton M. Radiat. Trace elements in the human scalp hair and finger nails as affected by infection with *Schistosoma mansoni*. *Phys. Chem.* 1995; 45:141-145.

[11]   Bellisola G; Pasti F; Valdes M; Torboli A. The use of total-reflection X-ray fluorescence to track the metabolism and excretion of selenium in humans. *Spectroch. Acta (part B)*. 1999; 54:1481-1485.

[12] Tölg, G; Klockenkämper, R. The role of total reflection X-ray fluorescence in atomic spectroscopy. *Spectrochim. Acta Part B*.1993; 48:111-127.

[13] Holynska, B; De Koster, CG; Ostachowicz, J; Samek, L; Wegrzynek, D. Determination of metals in polycarbonate foils by energy dispersive X-ray fluorescence methods. *X-ray Spectrom.* 2000; 29:291-296.

[14] Pérez CA; Radtke M; Sánchez HJ; Tolentino H; Neuenshwander RT; Barg W; Rubio M; Bueno MIS; Raimundo IM; Rohwedder JJR. Synchrotron radiation X-ray fluorescence at the LNLS: beamline instrumentation and experiments. *X-Ray Spectrom.* 1999; 28:320-326.

[15] Van Espen P; Nullens H; Adams FA. A computer analysis of X-ray fluorescence spectra. *Nucl. Instrum. Meth.* 1977; 142:243-250.

[16] Ward AF; Marciello LF; Carrara L; Luciano VJ. Simultaneous determination of major, minor and trace elements in agricultural and biological samples by inductively coupled argon plasma spectrometry. *Spectrosc. Lett.* 1980; 13:803-831.

[17] Klockenkämper R; Von Bohlen A. Total reflection X-ray fluorescence moving towards nanoanalysis: a survey. *Spectrochim. Acta (part B)*. 1989; 44:461-469.

[18] Ladisich W; Rieder R; Wobrauscheck P; Aiginger H. Total reflection X-ray fluorescence spectrometric determination of elements in nanogram amounts. *Nucl. Instrum. Meth.* 1993; 330:501-506.

[19] Kolmogorov Y; Kovaleva V; Gonchar A. Analysis of trace elements in scalp hair of healthy people, hyperplasia and breast cancer patients with XRF method. *Nucl. Instrum. Meth. (part A)*. 2000; 448:457-460.

[20] Kubala-Kukus A; Braziewicz J; Bana D; Majewska U; Gozdz S; Urbaniak A. Trace element load in cancer and normal lung tissue. *Nucl. Instrum. Meth. (part B)*.1999; 150:193-199.

[21] Moreda-Piñeiro A; Fischer A; Hill SJ. The classification of tea according to region of origin using pattern recognition techniques and trace metal data. *J. Food Compos. Analysis*. 2003; 16:195-211.

[22] Geladi P. Chemometrics in spectroscopy. Part 1. Classical chemometrics, Spectrochim. *Acta Part B*. 2003, 58:767-782.

[23] Zucchi OLAD; Moreira S; Salvador, MJ; Santos LL. Multi-element analysis of soft drinks by X-ray fluorescence spectrometry, *J. Agr. Food. Chem.* 2005, 53:7863-7865.

[24] Rogério AP; Sá-Nunes A; Albuquerque DA; Aníbal FF; Medeiros AI; Machado ER; Souza AO; Prado Jr. JC; Faccioli LH. *Lafoensia pacari* extract inhibits IL-5 production in toxocariasis *Parasite Immunol.* 2003; 25:393-400.

[25] Higa A; Maruyama H; Abe T; Owhashi M; Nawa Y. Effects of *Toxocara canis* infection on hemopoietic stem cells and hemopoietic factors in mice. *Int Arch Allergy Appl Immunol.* 1990; 91:239-243.

[26] Hiratochi M; Takamoto M; Tatemichi S; Sugane K. Inhibition of interleukin 5 production with no influence on interleukin 4 production by an anti-allergic drug, tranilast, in *Toxocara canis*-infected mice. *Int. J. Immunopharmacol.* 2000; 22:463-471.

[27] Takamoto M; Sugane K. Mechanisms of eosinophilia in *Toxocara canis* infected mice: in vitro production of interleukin 5 by lung cells of both normal and congenitally athymic nude mice. *Parasite Immunol.* 1993; 15:493-500.

[28] Reiterová K; Tomasovicová O; Dubinsky P. Influence of maternal infection on offspring immune response in murine larval toxocariasis. *Parasite Immunol.* 2003; 25:361-368.

[29] Mocchegiani E; Muzzioli M; Cipriano C; Giacconi R. Zinc, T-cells pathways, aging: role of metallothioneins. *Mech. Ageing Dev.* 1998; 106:183-204.

[30] Abo-Shehada MN; Herbert IV. The migration of larval *Toxocara canis* in mice II. Post-intestinal migration in primary infections. *Vet. Parasitol.* 1984; 17:75-83.

[31] Mocchegiani E; Giacconi R; Cipriano C; Muzzioli M; Fattoretti P; Bertoni-Freddari C; Isani G; Zambenedetti P; Zatta P. Zinc-bound metallothioneins as potential biological markers of ageing *Brain Res. Bull.* 2001; 55:147-153.

[32] Rink L; Haase, H. Zinc homeostasis and immunity. *TRENDS in Immunology* 2007, 28:1-4.

[33] Blazi MP; Hrvacic B; Zupanovic Z; Hadzija M; Stanic B; Polancec D. Differing effects on experimental arthritis, TNF-α levels and immune response in mice. *Int. Immunopharmacol.* 2003; 3:1743-1749.

[34] Lahner B; Gong J; Mahmoudian M; Smith EL; Abid KB; Rogers EE; Guerinot ML; Harper JF; Ward JM; McIntyre L; Schroeder JI; Salt DE. Genomic scale profiling of nutrient and trace elements in *Arabidopsis thaliana. Nat. Biotechnol.* 2003; 21:1215-1221.

INDEX

B

D

E

F

H

N

O

P

S

T

U

V